Physics and Measurement for Anesthesia

Craig Birch • Stacey Byers
Julian Dimech • Nicholas Lightfoot
Nic Randall • Amanda Siu
Matthew Taylor • Michael Webb
Andrew Wong
Editors

Physics and Measurement for Anesthesia

Basic Science Essentials for Anesthesia and Critical Care Exams

Springer

Editors
Craig Birch
Anaesthesia & Pain Medicine
Middlemore Hospital
Auckland, Auckland, New Zealand

Stacey Byers
Anaesthesia & Pain Medicine
Middlemore Hospital
Auckland, Auckland, New Zealand

Julian Dimech
Anaesthesia & Pain Medicine
Middlemore Hospital
Auckland, New Zealand

Nicholas Lightfoot
Medical and Health Sciences,
Anaesthesiology
University of Auckland
Auckland, Auckland, New Zealand

Nic Randall
Intensive Care Medicine
Middlemore Hospital
Otahuhu, Auckland, New Zealand

Amanda Siu
Anaesthesia & Pain Medicine
Middlemore Hospital
Auckland, Auckland, New Zealand

Matthew Taylor
Anaesthesia & Pain Medicine
Middlemore Hospital
Auckland, Auckland, New Zealand

Michael Webb
Faculty of Anaesthesia
University of Auckland
Auckland, Auckland, New Zealand

Andrew Wong
Epsom Anaesthesia Group
Auckland, Auckland, New Zealand

ISBN 978-3-031-65059-8 ISBN 978-3-031-65060-4 (eBook)
https://doi.org/10.1007/978-3-031-65060-4

This Springer imprint is published by the registered company Springer Nature Switzerland AG
The registered company address is: Gewerbestrasse 11, 6330 Cham, Switzerland

Preface

Anaesthesia is a practical, clinically based medical science. Its conduct requires anaesthetists/anaesthesiologists and intensivists to learn and understand the principles of applied physics (as well as a range of other basic and applied sciences), related to equipment responsible for the clinical care of patients.

This book has been written primarily for anaesthetic registrars/residents and their teachers to assist with preparation for the postgraduate, basic science examinations in anaesthesia and critical care medicine.

Each topic is systematically covered using first principles, contextual examples and illustrations to explain and demonstrate complex concepts. The book arose from the work of Dr. Alan McLintic, a highly respected clinician, anaesthetist and teacher. For over 25 years, he gave weekly tutorials on physics, clinical measurement and statistics for postgraduate students of anaesthesia and critical care who were preparing for their examinations. He compiled and constantly updated a set of teaching notes, and this became a valuable resource. Prior to his sudden and untimely death in September of 2020, he decided to turn the notes into a textbook. We have taken his work, extended his notes and edited the material to make it as accessible and relevant as possible.

The uniqueness of this book has been recognised by the Australian and New Zealand College of Anaesthetists (ANZCA), which has identified the importance of these topics and endorsed the book which covers the examinable content for the primary examination of ANZCA.

No other text offers such a comprehensive and up-to-date compilation of these topics, and it will be hugely beneficial for residents or registrars and teachers in Australasia. ANZCA has recognised this and will add it to its recommended reading list for postgraduate students of anaesthesia and intensive care medicine. The UK postgraduate anaesthesia and intensive care exam syllabus is similar to that of ANZCA, and we expect that it will also be useful for anaesthetists there and internationally, since these scientific principles can easily be applied to any operating theatre or intensive care unit around the world.

Auckland, New Zealand
Craig Birch

Obituary: Dr. Alan John McLintic

Alan John (AJ) McLintic (1958–2020) died suddenly and unexpectedly of heart disease at age 62. He was a specialist anaesthetist at Middlemore Hospital, Auckland, and an Honorary Senior Lecturer at the University of Auckland, New Zealand.

An old friend and colleague, Leyla Sanai, summed AJ up as "a consultant anaesthetist, academic teacher, medical ethicist, philosopher, talented artist, musician, bon viveur, iron man, marathon runner, swimmer, mountaineer, skier, rugby player, proud Scot, dry wit, sparkling friend, the cleverest person I knew."

Alan was born of Scottish parents in Dar es Salam, Tanzania. His family moved back to Scotland when he was a young boy, and he was raised in Dollar, a small town where he and his sister, Anne, attended the excellent local school, the Dollar Academy. He was a very good scholar and went on to Glasgow University where he studied medicine. He was an all-rounder who lived a full student life, enjoying the academic, sporting and social activities on offer. He was an active member of the rugby club and played the guitar in a rock band.

After university, Alan remained in Glasgow where he worked as a junior doctor and a cardiology registrar and then joined the West of Scotland training scheme. During this time, he was a member of the "Shock Team," a medical retrieval team.

AJ was extraordinarily talented in many spheres of his life. He embraced whatever he was doing with incredible energy and dedication. He was not driven by the need to impress others or any particular reward. Rather, the pleasure for him was in the journey that included learning and persisting until the job was done. And the standard was rarely short of excellent.

He started public speaking at university, and this continued through his career. His talks were keenly anticipated and did not disappoint. He would research the subject extensively and then deliver a talk, which was as memorable for the delivery as it was for the content. His dry wit, self-deprecating nature and ability to hold a broad audience meant that the listeners left feeling enriched and entertained. Alan was particularly good at exposing long-held beliefs as myths and explaining how these misconceptions are perpetuated. At the NZSA ASM meeting in 2018, an Australian visiting speaker described AJ's talk on "The motivations behind science denial" as the best and the most interesting he had attended at any conference on any subject, anywhere in the world. Alan's talk at the ANZCA ASM in 2012 titled "The real and perceived genetics of race in medicine" was widely regarded as the talk of the conference. Many of his talks would go on to become journal publications

(McLintic 2019a, b). He loved science and philosophy, and he managed to marry these interests in his talks and his writing. One of the joys of his life included attending scientific conferences and sceptics meetings. He would return home fizzing with ideas which he would enthusiastically share.

Alan was a superb and respected clinician, but his most impressive legacy at work will be as a teacher. He would have had an influence on almost all the anaesthetic registrars training in the Auckland area over the past 25 years, having tutored the part 1 registrars at Middlemore every Thursday morning. He taught the "gnarliest" subjects: physics, measurement and statistics. Even after 25 years, he continued to tweak these tutorials, keeping them relevant and interesting. Prior to his death, he dedicated himself to writing a textbook which covered this syllabus.

Alan started painting in the early 2000s and, in more recent years, cut down on his time at Middlemore Hospital in order to develop his career as an artist. He painted, among other styles, beautiful oil landscapes, which many of his colleagues and friends have on their walls. In recent years, demand for his work increased, and it was exhibited and sold in local galleries. No doubt he could have gone on to make this his sole profession, such was his skill.

He started playing the guitar at school and played in a band in his high school and university years. The band stuck together in spite of living on different continents, and the most recent gig was at one of the members' 60th birthday. AJ would fly back to the UK for these reunions. At home in Auckland, he loved playing music with friends. He organised many memorable musical evenings, which involved printing songbooks and encouraging everyone to join in, including those of us with lesser musical ability.

Alan was an accomplished endurance multisport athlete, competing in events for many years (including the iconic Coast to Coast twice!) and until just months before he died.

His most recent sporting passion was for golf. His unbridled enthusiasm for playing and practicing was infectious and inspired a group of friends to play regularly. The golf epitomised his pursuit of excellence, but he played primarily for the fun of it and for the joy of forging a deeper connection with friends.

Despite his myriad talents, Alan was understated and modest. He could bring humour to the most mundane of topics. He loved relaxing with friends and discussing issues over a beer. He listened intently, and after due consideration, he would respond with a worthy and insightful reply.

Alan was an extraordinarily talented man in so many ways. He was also a kind, generous and thoughtful human being. We are so fortunate to have known him as a friend and a colleague. He enriched our lives and made the world we live in a better place.

References

McLintic A. The motivations behind science denial. N Z Med J. 2019a;132(1504):88–94.

McLintic A. Reifying race in medicine. Australas Anaesth. 2019b:299–308.

Department of Anaesthesia and
Pain Medicine, Counties Manukau Health,
Auckland, New Zealand

Craig Birch

Contents

Force, Pressure and Tension

1

Alan McLintic and Andrew Wong

Force

Definition

A force is that which, when unopposed, changes the state of rest or motion of an object. If there is no force acting on an object, it is either stationary or moving at constant velocity. A force acts upon a mass to change its velocity:

$$\text{Force} = \text{Mass} \times \text{Acceleration}$$

A force can be described both in magnitude and direction, giving it a vector quantity.

Units of Force

- The SI unit of force is newton (N). This 1 N is the force required to give a 1 kg mass an acceleration of 1 $m.s^{-2}$.
- One newton can also be expressed in base units = 1 $kg.m.s^{-2}$.
- Dyne is the force required to give 1 g an acceleration of 1 $cm.s^{-2}$. It is 1/100,000 the force of a newton.
- Gravity gives objects an acceleration of 9.81 $m.s^{-2}$.
- The gravitational force experienced by 1 kg is 9.81 N or 9.81 $kg.m.s^{-2}$. This is referred to as a 1 kg weight.

A. McLintic · A. Wong (✉)
Epsom Anaesthesia, Auckland, New Zealand

C. Birch et al. (eds.), *Physics and Measurement for Anesthesia*,
https://doi.org/10.1007/978-3-031-65060-4_1

Pressure

What Is Pressure?

Pressure is the perpendicular force applied to the surface of an object per unit area:

$$\text{Pressure} = {}^{\text{Force}}\!/_{\text{Area}}$$

A system under pressure also has the potential to do work on its surroundings, and thus pressure can be expressed in terms of energy stored per unit volume, joules per unit volume.

Pressure can also be measured by its ability to displace a vertical column of liquid such as water or mercury.

SI Units of Pressure

- SI unit of pressure is pascal (Pa).
- 1 pascal (Pa) = 1 N/m^2.
- 1 kPa = 1000 Pa.

Pressure Conversion Table

What Is 1 Bar?

- 1 bar is a metric unit of pressure developed for meteorology that is exactly 100 kPa (Table 1.1). Sometimes, it is called technical atmospheric pressure. 1 atmosphere is 101.325 kPa and is the average at sea level.

Table 1.1 Pressure unit conversion

Conversion factor table		
1 atmosphere (average at sea level)		101.325 kPa
1 bar ('technical atmosphere')		100 kPa
Unit 1	**Unit 2**	**Conversion (some units rounded up)**
1 bar	kPa	100 kPa
1 bar	hPa (hectopascal)	1000 hPa
1 bar	Pa	100,000 Pa
1 bar	mbar (millibar)	1000 mbar
1 bar	cmH_2O	1020 cmH_2O
1 bar	mmHg	750 mmHg
1 bar	Torr	750 torr
1 bar	Psi (lb/in^2)	14.5 psi
1 bar	$Dyne.cm^{-2}$	9.8×10^5 $dyne.cm^{-2}$
1 hectopascal	Pascals	100 Pa
1 hectopascal	cmH_2O	1.02 cmH_2O

Gauge Pressure and Absolute Pressure

Absolute Pressure

This is pressure relative to a complete vacuum, a pressure of 0 Pa.

Gauge Pressure

Gauge pressure is the pressure above or below atmospheric pressure. It makes sense that, for example, when a cylinder is 'empty', we want the gauge to read zero, not 1 bar or 100 kPa. Most of the pressures we use in clinical practice, including blood pressure, are gauge pressures:

- Absolute pressure in a full cylinder oxygen = 138 bar.
- Gauge pressure in full cylinder oxygen = 137 bar (Table 1.2).

When working with gas and other physical laws, you must use absolute pressures, or the calculations will be wrong.

How Much Oxygen Is Available from a Full Cylinder If It Is Released at Atmospheric Pressure and Temperature Is Constant?

- Boyle's law: PV = constant.
- Absolute pressure full cylinder oxygen = 13,800 kPa.
- Atmospheric pressure (1 bar) = 100 kPa.
- Volume cylinder = 10 L.
- Total volume oxygen = 13,800/100 × 10 L = 1380 L.
- Subtract 10 L for the volume of oxygen remaining in cylinder = 1370 L.

Table 1.2 Useful pressures

	Some useful pressures	
Pipeline pressure		420 kPa
Full cylinder oxygen	Gas	13,700 kPa or 15,000 kPa
Full cylinder nitrous oxide	Liquid + vapour (20 °C)	~5000 kPa
Full cylinder CO_2	Liquid + vapour (20 °C)	~5500 kPa

Different manufacturing standards cite filling pressures at 15 °C, in which case the CO_2 and N_2O pressures will be lower

Surface Tension

What Is Meant by the Term Tension?

Tension can be described as a pulling force transmitted axially. This can be seen as the opposite of compression.

Cohesive Versus Adhesive Forces

There are mutual attractive forces between similar molecules of a liquid (cohesion). In a liquid, these forces act on neighbouring molecules such that all are pulled equally, with net effect being zero. At the surface, the molecules are also attracted to different molecules such as surface or air (adhesion). If cohesive forces are greater, then they will tend to form droplets rather than spread out and wet the surface. The balance of these forces determines the contrasting shape of the meniscus of water and mercury.

Meniscus Shape and Capillarity

Meniscus

In a mercury manometer, the cohesive forces are stronger than the adhesive forces, causing accumulation in the middle of the glass tube and a convex meniscus. In a water manometer, the adhesive forces of water are stronger than the cohesive forces. Water thus tends to spread outwards over the surface and then up a glass tube. This causes a concave meniscus and a tendency to draw the fluid column up the tube (Fig. 1.1).

In both situations, the reading should be taken from the midpoint of the meniscus.

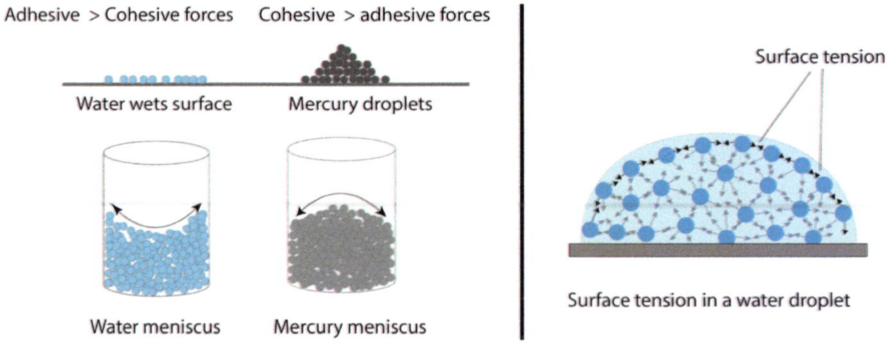

Fig. 1.1 Meniscus

Capillarity

Capillarity is seen in a very thin tube dipped into a reservoir of the liquid. The adhesive forces draw a column of liquid up the tube until the gravitational force of the increasing mass of liquid in the column overcomes the adhesive force:

- Water manometer over-reads by 4.5 mm in a 6 mm diameter tube.
- Mercury under-reads by 1.5 mm.

What Is Surface Tension?

Molecules at the surface of a liquid/air interface have no neighbouring liquid molecules above. The molecules are therefore pulled together and down, and the surface contracts to its minimal size per unit volume. This is why bubbles are spheres and a water meniscus is curved. It also explains how some objects which have densities greater than water can remain at the surface. The enhancement of the cohesive forces between surface neighbouring molecules is called surface tension.

Units of Surface Tension

The surface tension of a simple flat surface is expressed as the force required to break surface tension over a certain distance (Fig. 1.2):

$$\text{Surface tension} = {}^{\text{Force}}\!/_{\text{Unit length}}$$

- SI units: $N.m^{-1}$.

Measuring Surface Tension

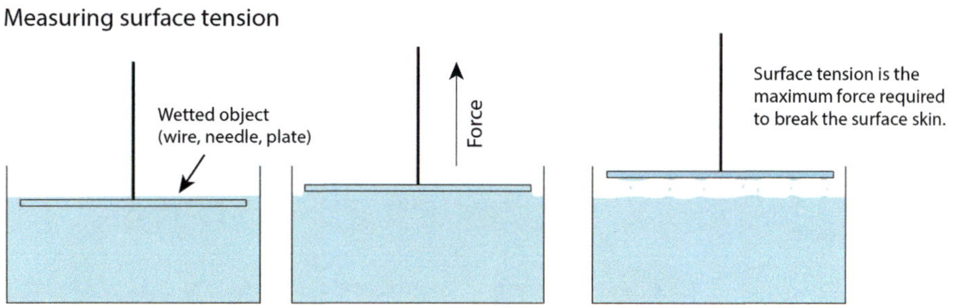

Fig. 1.2 Surface tension measurement

Laplace's Law (Young-Laplace Equation)

This states the relationship between wall tension, internal pressure and radius of a distensible vessel in a static situation.

It is not clear what part Laplace had to play in the set of equations that have been given his name, nor why his name became attached to them. There were several nineteenth-century contributors to this work.

Laplace Equations

What Sort of Vessels Does it Apply to?

This can be applied to curved surfaces under tension between two different fluids, such as water and air. There must be an interface. Therefore, bubbles and other liquid/air interfaces can be applied. It also applies to distensible objects if the vessel walls are very thin (Fig. 1.3).

Why Does Wall Tension Vary with Radius?

Wall tension is a lateral force on a curved surface that produces a net inward force. The wall contracts down until the net inward force balances the net outward force of air and equilibrium is reached. The outward force of the internal pressure is now balanced by the inward force of wall tension plus the surrounding pressure. The internal pressure therefore exceeds the external pressure.

At larger radii, the lateral force of wall tension is more tangential to the internal pressure and requires to be greater to produce an adequate balancing inward force (Fig. 1.4). In an infinite-sized balloon, there would be no inward force so the internal pressure would be atmospheric.

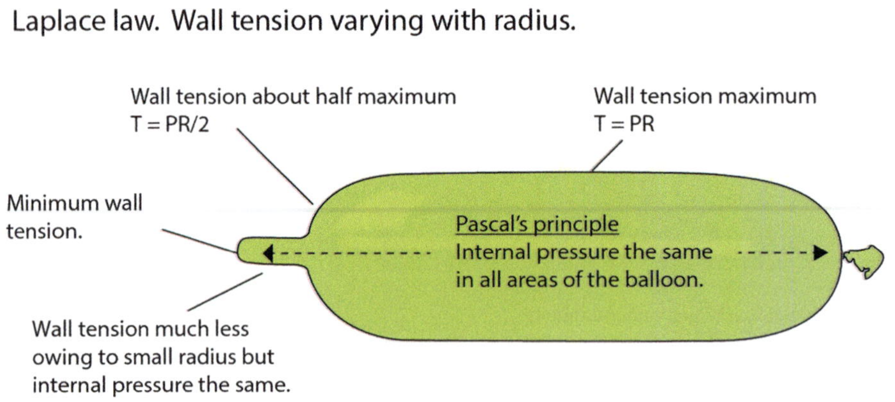

Fig. 1.3 Laplace law and radius

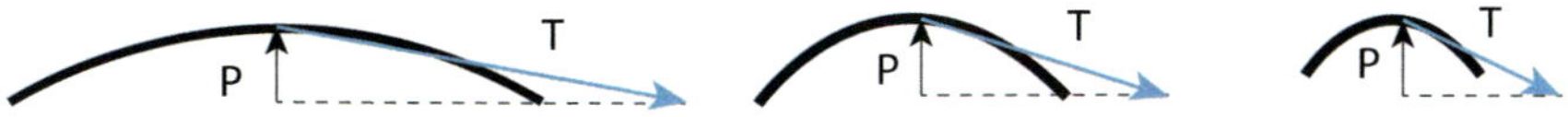

The wall tension opposing the internal pressure is applied more indirectly as radius increases. This means that the required tension must be greater to balance the internal pressure. The length of line T represents the magnitude of surface tension.

Fig. 1.4 Wall tension and radius

Table 1.3 Surface tension calculation of different shapes

Object	Notes	Equation
Sphere	One internal surface. Two perpendicular circumferences in a sphere, each with a radius. Pressure (P) is the difference between internal and external pressure but can be thought of as internal gauge pressure	$P = \frac{T}{R_1} + \frac{T}{R_2} = \frac{2T}{R}$
Bubble	Inner and outer surfaces both contribute to the total tension	$P = \frac{4T}{R}$
Cylinder	Only one radius	$P = \frac{T}{R}$

Laplace's Law and Anaesthesia Significance

Laplace's law refers to an idealised vessel with a very thin wall and may not explain real-life situations where walls may be thick and muscular or where elastic properties change with stretch. The following are common examples where Laplace's laws might be discussed in exams.

Two-Bubbles/Two-Alveoli Analogy

YouTube demonstrations show two soap bubbles being inflated to different sizes and then connected together. The smaller one empties into the larger one and collapses, while the larger one expands further. Why?

There is an assumption that the surface tension is the same or nearly the same in each bubble (Table 1.3). In this case, the internal pressure must be higher in the smaller bubble ($P = 4\ T/R$). Thus, air flows from smaller to larger bubble until the small one collapses (Fig. 1.5).

This analogy is used to remind us of the property of surfactant in reducing surface tension as the radius decreases. The internal pressure is stabilised despite changes in radii.

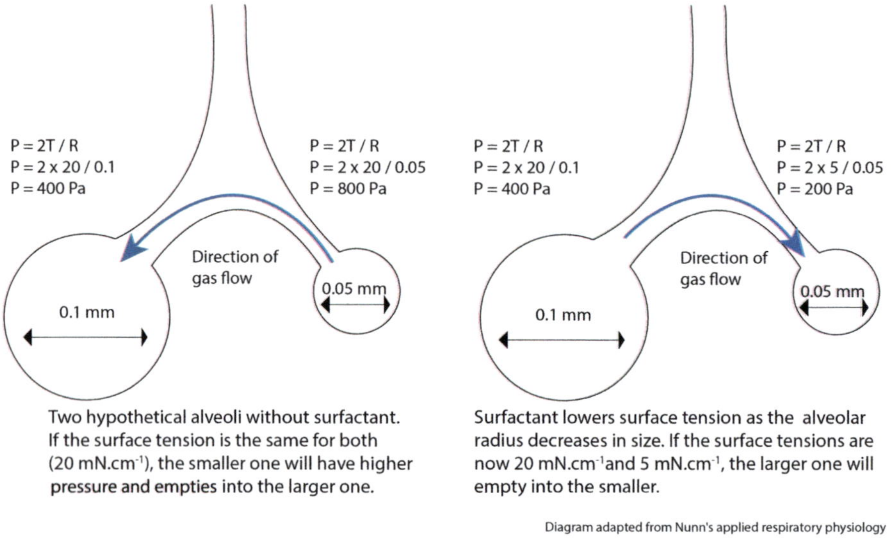

Fig. 1.5 Laplace and alveoli

Dispute

The Laplace 'bubble model' of surfactant reducing lung recoil and stabilising alveoli as lung volume decreases is disputed because:

- Alveoli are not spheres. Describing them as such is a gross oversimplification. It is more a polygonal structure, with additional parenchymal structures resulting in additional forces acting on the alveoli.
- Differing surface tensions should not occur if there is a continuous fluid lining between alveoli.

Alternative Explanation

Alternative explanations include surfactant 'rafts' on the alveolar lining fluid, which cause dry areas that break up the surface tension.

Distensible Vessels and Wall Tension

In contrast to the liquid surface tension in the bubbles example, the wall tension of distensible vessels increases as the radius increases:

- A dilated LV requires to be at higher tension if pressure is to be maintained. This increases metabolic demand. One response is to make more muscle. This spreads the load to oppose the internal pressure. Wall stress is an indication of the net force acting on an area of myocytes and is equal to wall tension/wall thickness.
- A dilated aneurysm requires higher wall tension to withstand internal pressure. If that tension cannot be achieved, it will dilate further. A vicious cycle develops that will eventually lead to rupture.

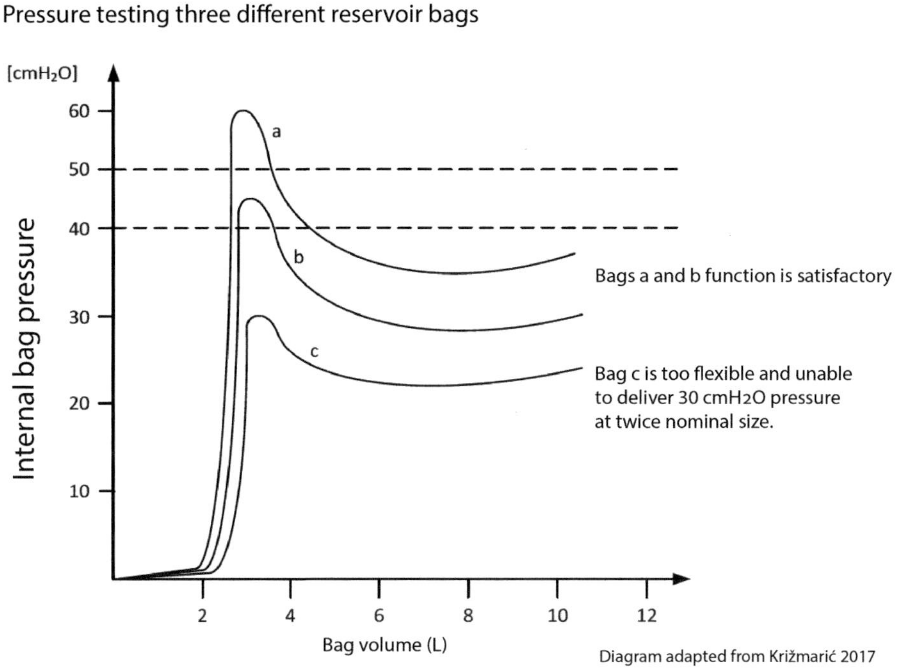

Fig. 1.6 Reservoir bag volume and pressure

Laplace Law and Reservoir Bag Safety

If the APL valve is closed and the bag inflated, what happens to the internal pressure in an ideal Laplace context? The flexibility of the reservoir bag means that as the radius rises the wall tension rises, but as tension acts increasingly tangentially (Table 1.3), the internal pressure remains constant ($P = 2\ T/R$). This provides patient protection.

The reality is that the elastic properties of the bag change as it is stretched, so the relationship is not predictable purely by Laplace. Usually, there is an early peak followed by a plateau.

ISO Safety Standards for Reservoir Bags

If you fill the bag to twice its nominal volume, the minimum pressure must be 30 cmH_2O and not exceed 60 cmH_2O (Fig. 1.6).

Fig. 1.7 Bourdon gauge

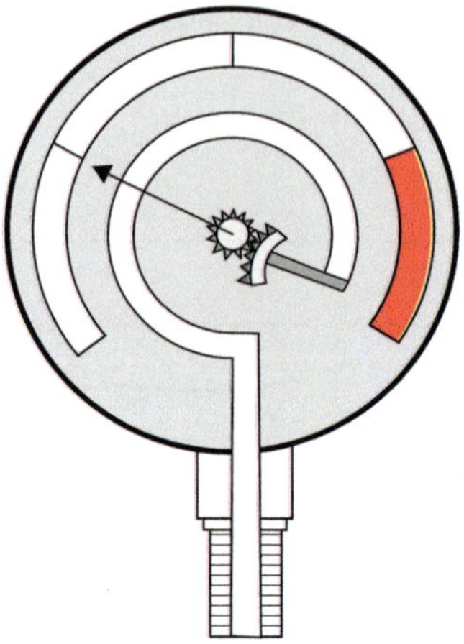

Pressure Gauges

Mercury Manometers

This type of gauge has advantages in terms of simplicity and reliability with no moving or mechanical parts. It does not require calibration. The pressure supporting 7.5 mm mercury will support 10.2 cmH_2O. The gauge must be open at the top so as to equilibrate with surrounding atmospheric pressure. The fluid column must not be tilted.

The diameter of the tubing is not critical. The gravitational force increases with the mass of the column, but the pressure remains the same. It is the height of the column that is important. This holds true until capillarity plays a part when the column becomes very narrow.

Bourdon Gauges

This is a type of aneroid gauge, meaning that there is no liquid (Fig. 1.7). It is the most common type used to measure gas pressure in cylinders and is a direct application of Boyle's law where the product of pressure and volume is constant for a given quantity of gas at specified temperature:

$PV = k$ where k is constant

Increasing gas pressure causes a steel tube to uncoil and drive a pointer across a scale.

Bellows Gauges

This is another type of aneroid gauge where expansion or contraction of bellows drives a pointer.

Diaphragm Strain Gauge

In this type of gauge, the fluid pressure acts directly to deform a diaphragm. The movement of the diaphragm is then sensed by either:

- Changing resistance of a wire or foil strip adhered to surface: Resistance is measured in Wheatstone bridge (see Electricity section). This is referred to as a piezoresistive transducer.
- Optically: Reflection of light off bulging diaphragm changes the amount detected by photoelectric cell. Used in fibre-optic intracerebral pressure monitors.
- Capacitance: The diaphragm is one plate of a capacitor. Distance from the other plate varies with the movement of diaphragm.
- Inductance: Diaphragm attached to a magnet which is moving between coils as the diaphragm bulges. An electrical potential is induced.

Piezoelectric Transducers

A solid-state alternative to the diaphragm uses a thin piezoelectric element that flexes in response to pressure changes and generates a voltage.

Further Reading

Middleton B, Phillips J, Stacey S. Physics in anaesthesia, 2nd ed. Scion Publishing; 2021.

Fluids

2

Alan McLintic and Andrew Wong

Fluid Flow Defined

What Is a Fluid?

Fluids are substances that continually deform (or show lack of resistance to deformation) and have the ability to flow under an applied shear stress. They are unable to resist any shear force applied to them. They include liquids, gases and plasmas.

What Is Shear Stress?

Shear stress is a force applied parallel to a material in cross section that causes layers to slide over each other. This is in contrast to normal stress that is applied perpendicular to the material cross section.

Laminar Flow

Characteristics

This type of flow is characterised by smooth movement of fluid in axial layers with very little or no mixing of the layers in the fluid column. The fluid motion is in one direction without eddies. Friction between layers results in a velocity gradient with

A. McLintic · A. Wong (✉)
Epsom Anaesthesia, Auckland, New Zealand

C. Birch et al. (eds.), *Physics and Measurement for Anesthesia*,
https://doi.org/10.1007/978-3-031-65060-4_2

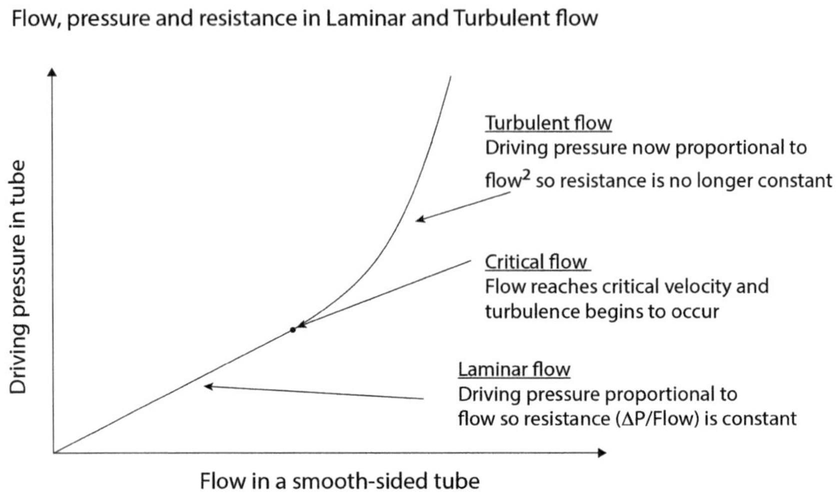

Fig. 2.1 Flow/pressure in laminar vs. turbulent flow

the velocity being greatest in the centre of the fluid column and least (sometimes zero) at the walls:

- Flow rate is proportional to the driving pressure along the tube (Fig. 2.1).
- Flow rate is inversely proportional to resistance.
- Resistance is constant no matter the flow rate. Flow = Δ Pressure / Resistance.

Hagen-Poiseuille Relationship

This gives the relationship of flow and the pressure drop in laminar flow of a non-compressible liquid in a constant cross-sectional area of a cylindrical tube. This can be applied to airflow in the very small airways of the lungs:

- Flow α Δ pressure
- Flow α r^4
- Flow α 1/length
- Flow α 1/viscosity (η)
  - Increasing temperature may increase flow by decreasing viscosity:

$$\text{Flow} = \pi.\Delta P.r^4 \big/ 8l.\eta \quad \text{or Flow} = \pi.\Delta P.d^4 \big/ 128l.\eta$$

Viscosity

Viscosity is the property of a fluid that causes it to resist flow through internal frictional forces. It is an expression of the frictional forces acting between layers as a fluid flows along a tube.

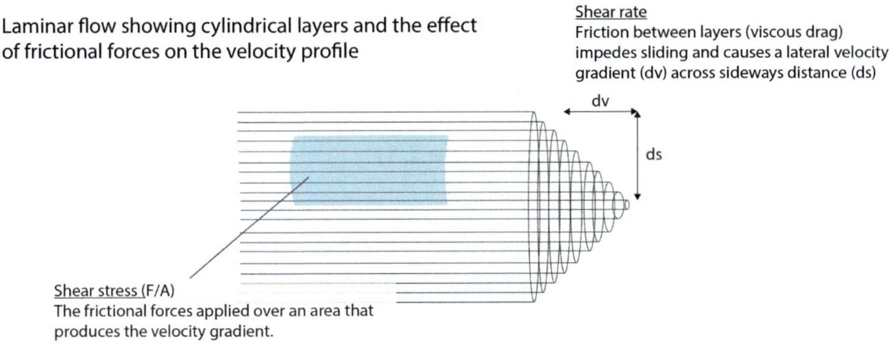

Fig. 2.2 Laminar flow and shear stress/rate

Dynamic Viscosity (η)

Random lateral movement of particles causes friction between the sliding layers (viscous drag). This impedes sliding and causes the velocity of layers to fall (dv) across the tube over a 'sideways' distance (ds). This results in a lateral velocity gradient (dv/ds) called the shear rate (Fig. 2.2).

The frictional force applied over an area on the surface of a layer (F/A) that produces this gradient is called the shear stress. This force is proportional to the viscosity of the fluid and the velocity gradient.

Thus, a substance with high viscosity has large frictional forces per given velocity gradient:

$$\eta = \text{Shear stress} / \text{Shear rate} = \frac{F}{A} \bigg/ \frac{dv}{ds}$$

Units of Dynamic Viscosity

- SI units: Pascal.second or N.s.m^{-2}
- CGS units: Dyn.s.cm^{-2} or poise

Newtonian Fluids

Newtonian fluid is a fluid in which the dynamic viscosity is not affected by the flow rate itself. To get one layer to slide over another twice as fast, you have to double the force required to overcome resistance. The shear stress is proportional to the relative motion of the layers, and thus dynamic viscosity is constant. Hagen-Poiseuille only applies to Newtonian fluids. A non-Newtonian fluid is one in which the shear stress and shear rate relationships are more complex and non-constant.

Is Blood Newtonian or Non-Newtonian?

Strictly speaking, it is non-Newtonian. This is particularly seen at low flow rates where RBC aggregation occurs. At higher flow rates, this factor loses importance and it can be regarded as near Newtonian.

Table 2.1 Temperature and viscosity

Fluid	Viscosity	Density
Liquid	Decreases	Decreases
Gas	Increases	Decreases

Effect of Warming on Viscosity (Table 2.1)

Kinematic Viscosity

Kinematic viscosity (ν) is dynamic viscosity divided by density. It can be used to combine viscosity and density in a single value in Reynold's number.

Measuring Viscosity

Viscometer

The viscometer is used for fluids where the viscosity does not vary with flow conditions. There are numerous designs, but all produce relative motion between the fluid and a surface. Either an object moves through a stationary fluid or the fluid flows past a stationary object.

In the rotational version, a cone-shaped bobbin sits in spinning sample of fluid and is rotated by viscous drag from the fluid. The bobbin's movement is displayed on a scale.

Turbulent Flow

Characteristics

This type of flow is characterised by random and chaotic changes in pressure and velocity when measured at a specific point in the fluid. It occurs when the kinetic energy in the fluid exceeds the dampening effects of the fluid viscosity. It occurs in situations of high flow, especially if there exist irregularities in the tube. It is characterised by swirls and eddies. Velocity profile becomes flat and is no longer maximal in the centre of the tube. The driving pressure becomes more dependent on density rather than viscosity. Resistance is no longer constant and may change with flow velocity.

Relationship Between Flow, Pressure and Resistance

Various algebraic relationships exist for particular fluids, tubes and orifices. Most are approximations fitted to empirical data.

As with laminar flow, an increase in driving pressure will increase flow, but the relationship is non-linear and may be complex depending on the tube shape. At its simplest, for a tube without branches, the driving pressure is proportional to the square of the flow (Table 2.2).

Table 2.2 Laminar vs. turbulent flow

	Laminar flow	Turbulent flow
ΔP ∝	Flow	$Flow^2$
ΔP ∝	Length	Length
ΔP ∝	Viscosity	Density
ΔP ∝	$1/r^4$	$*1/r^?$

* ΔP needs to be higher for a given radius if flow is turbulent but is not expressible as a simple power

Orificial Flow

This is the flow through a tube that has length less than the radius. The flow through an orifice is always partially turbulent.

Reynold's Number

This can be used to predict whether flow is likely to be laminar or turbulent. It is a ratio of inertial forces (velocity and density) to frictional forces (viscosity). The greater the inertial forces relative to the frictional, the more likely is turbulence. The predictive thresholds are based on empirical data and vary between texts. Thresholds are smaller with irregular tubes:

$$\text{Reynold's number} = \frac{v.\rho.d}{\eta}$$

v is the linear velocity in the tube. ρ is the density. d is the diameter of the tube. η is the viscosity.

Reynold's thresholds for a cylindrical smooth tube:

- Laminar <~2000.
- Turbulent >~2000.
- For an irregular tube, turbulence may occur with Reynold's of 300.

Role of Viscosity and Density in Turbulence

A highly viscous fluid tends to reduce turbulence by dampening down inertial disturbances, while low viscosity promotes turbulence. The inertial forces (v ρ) of swirls and eddies tend to persist when density increases as more energy is retained within the eddies. Thus, high density promotes turbulence.

Areas of Relevance in Anaesthesia

Variation in Flow Characteristics within Respiratory Tree

Airflow through small airways is at lower velocity than in large airways, and laminar flow dominates compared to that in the large and upper airways.

Table 2.3 Viscosity and density of gas mixtures

	Viscosity	Density
Oxygen	1.11	1.11
70% N_2O/30% O_2	0.89	1.41
80% He/20% O_2	1.08	0.33

Table 2.4 Critical flow and turbulence

Tube diameter	Critical flow at which turbulence begins
9 mm	9 L min^{-1}
15 mm	15 L min^{-1}
22 mm	22 L min^{-1}

Helium/Oxygen Mixture

Helium/oxygen mixture has significantly lower density than oxygen or air (Table 2.3). Its use reduces the likelihood of turbulence in large airways, thereby reducing resistance and work of breathing in upper airway obstruction.

Oxygen/N_2O

O_2/N_2O is less viscous than O_2/air and reduces driving pressure in laminar flow. The density of O_2/N_2O is greater, though, so turbulence is theoretically more likely.

Temperature

Warm gases have reduced density and increased critical velocity, and therefore turbulence is less likely.

Pneumotachograph

Pneumotachograph relies on laminar flow between the pressure sensors.

ETT and Equipment

The narrower the ETT, the greater the velocity for a given flow rate and the more likely there will be turbulence (Table 2.4). Irregularities in breathing equipment also promote turbulence.

Bernoulli Principle and the Venturi

The Bernoulli Principle

An increase in the velocity of a fluid occurs simultaneously with a decrease in potential energy and static pressure of the fluid. This conforms to the conservation of energy principle in that, during steady fluid flow, the sum of all forms of energy along the streamline is the same at all points along the flow line.

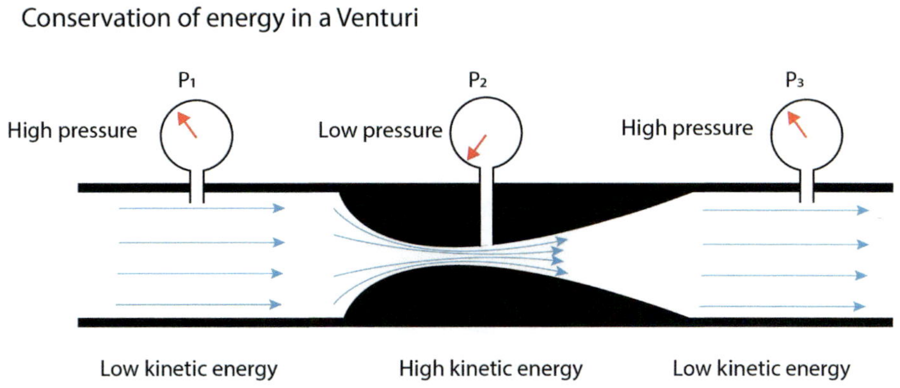

Fig. 2.3 Venturi

Thus, an increase in velocity (kinetic energy) occurs with simultaneous decrease in potential energy including static pressure.

There are multiple applications of Bernoulli's principle including explanation of pressure differences across an aircraft wing. This principle is applied in medicine in the use of the Venturi.

Venturi

A Venturi is a tube with a smooth constriction in which the cross section gradually decreases and then increases. If flow is kept constant, the pressure will be lowest at the narrowest point where velocity and kinetic energy are the greatest (Fig. 2.3).

Applications in Anaesthesia

- Injectors such as oxygen in mainstream, with air entrained at P_2
- Suction devices
- Nebulisers where liquid is entrained into the oxygen mainstream at P_2
- Also involves 'jet entrainment' caused by friction of oxygen at high velocity pulling air along with it

The Coanda Effect

The Coanda effect is the phenomenon of wall attachment of a stream of fluid due to a region of low pressure. If a high-velocity stream flows along a wall surface, there is no room for air to be entrained when the stream attaches to the wall surface (Fig. 2.4).

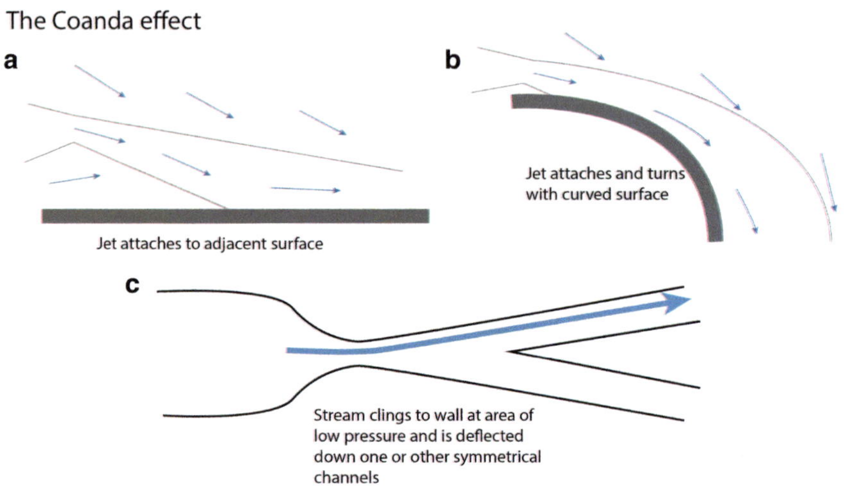

Fig. 2.4 The Coanda effect

Suggested Relevance in Anaesthesia

- This effect has applications in medical fluidics where the Coanda effect may be used for switching or amplification purposes. These are found in fluid logic ventilators. In diagram (c) (Fig. 2.4), a puff of air introduced at the narrowest point can cause stream to move from one limb to the other, thus switching from inspiratory to expiratory phases.
- It may also explain the cause of myocardial infarct in the distribution of a normal coronary artery and similarly uneven distribution of airflow in bronchi.

Gas Laws

3

Alan McLintic and Andrew Wong

What Is a Gas?

What Is the Elemental Composition of Gases?

Gases may be made up of either single atoms (argon), elemental molecules (oxygen) or compound molecules (CO_2).

What Distinguishes a Gas from a Solid or Liquid?

Unlike solids or liquids, gases possess higher kinetic energy. There is *vast separation* of gas particles and negligible interaction between them (Fig. 3.1).

Gaseous States Are Described Through Which Physical Properties?

Gases can be described by physical properties of pressure, volume, amount (number of particles) and temperature.

Relationship Between Temperature and Pressure

The pressure exerted by a gas is the result of collisions of the particles with the walls of the vessel. Pressure varies with the rate of these collisions, while the rates of collision are determined by the kinetic energy of the molecules. Gas temperature is a

A. McLintic · A. Wong (✉)
Epsom Anaesthesia, Auckland, New Zealand

C. Birch et al. (eds.), *Physics and Measurement for Anesthesia*,
https://doi.org/10.1007/978-3-031-65060-4_3

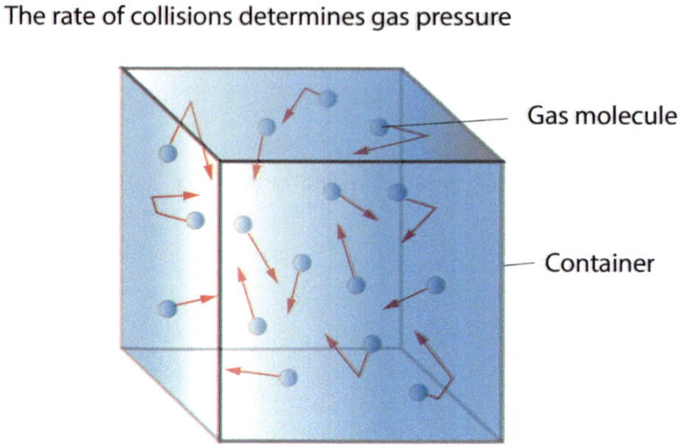

Fig. 3.1 Gas molecules and motion

direct measure of the kinetic energy of the gas. It therefore stands that the higher the temperature, the higher the pressure of a gas.

Ideal Versus Real Gases

The gas laws include 3 of at least 23 equations of state, with descriptions of state of matter under a given set of physical conditions.

Ideal Gas

The gas laws are concerned with *ideal gas*. This is a hypothetical situation in which gas particles are assumed to have zero volume and there are no intermolecular forces acting between molecules. Furthermore, collisions are described as elastic, in that the total energy of the molecules remains unchanged due to these collisions.

The terms ideal gas and perfect gas are often used synonymously. Others distinguish a perfect gas as one whose heat capacity is constant under all circumstances.

Real Gas

Gas laws in real-life situations involve real gases which vary from ideal in the above and other ways. There are, for example, weak van der Waals forces caused by momentary polarization of particles. For most practical purposes, they can be ignored.

The Gas Laws

The mass of a gas cannot be easily measured as with a solid or liquid. However, we can easily measure the volume of a gas, its pressure and temperature to determine its mass using the gas laws. It is important to note that these laws apply to closed systems only.

Boyle's Law

At constant temperature, the volume of a given mass of a gas is inversely proportional to its absolute pressure(Fig. 3.2):

$$V \propto {}^{1}\!/_{P} \text{ and } PV = k$$

Relevance in Anaesthesia

- Allows the volume available from an oxygen cylinder to be calculated from the measured cylinder pressure
- Lung volume calculations from a body plethysmograph

Charles' Law

At constant pressure, the volume of a given mass of gas varies directly with the absolute temperature (Fig. 3.3):

$$V \propto T \text{ and } V = kT$$

Relevance

- Mole of gas occupies more space at BTPS than ATPS or STP.

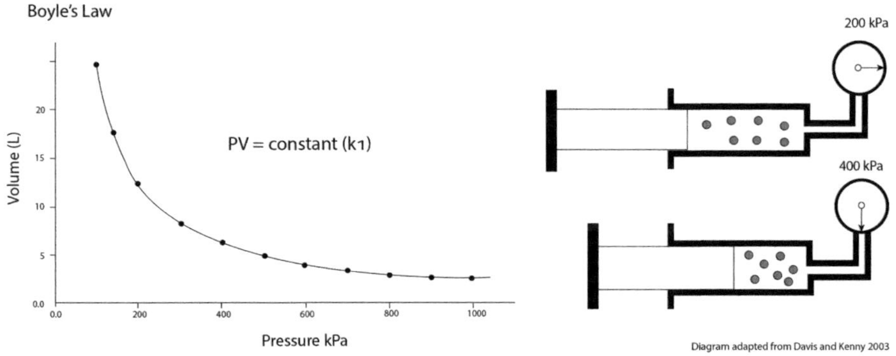

Fig. 3.2 Boyle's law

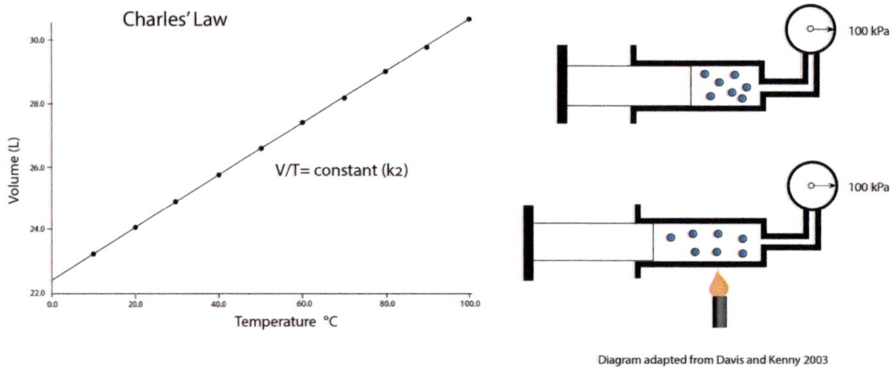

Fig. 3.3 Charles' law

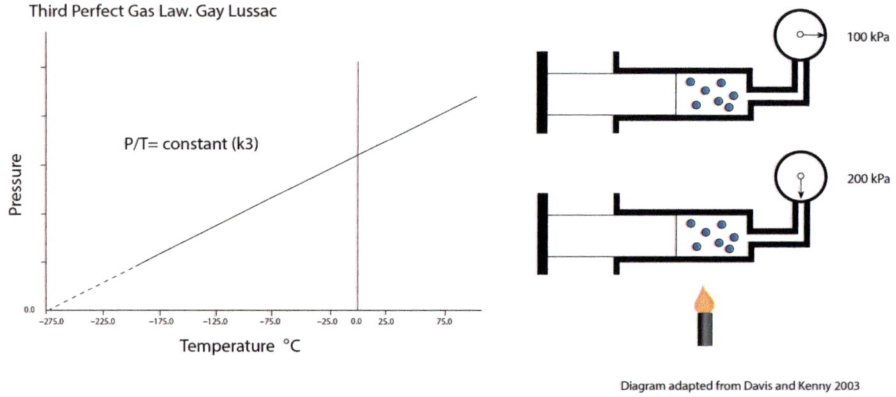

Fig. 3.4 Gay-Lussac's law

Third Gas Law (Gay-Lussac)

At constant volume, the absolute pressure of a given mass of gas varies directly with the absolute temperature of the gas, when the volume is kept constant (Fig. 3.4):

$$P \propto T \text{ and } P = kT$$

Relevance

- Bourdon gauge temperature sensor
- Explosion potential of heated cylinders

Ideal Gas Law

The three gas laws can be combined such that

$$PV = nRT$$

n is the number of moles. R is the universal gas constant.

Universal Gas Constant (R)

The universal gas constant (also known as the molar gas constant and the ideal gas constant) is the kinetic energy change per unit temperature per mole gas. The value is approximately the same for any mole of gas:

- $R = 8.314\ J.K^{-1}.mol^{-1}$.
- For 1 mole of any gas, PV/T is constant (R).

The Boltzmann Constant

The average change in kinetic energy of a particle in a gas per Kelvin:

- $k_B = 1.381 \times 10^{-23}\ J.K^{-1}$.

Ideal Gas Applied to Real Gases

The above formula applies to ideal gases. For real factors, there are correction factors for forces between molecules and the volume occupied by molecules:

$$RT = \left(P + \frac{a}{V^2}\right)(V - b)$$

where (a) corrects for intermolecular forces and (b) corrects for volume of molecules.

Dalton's Law of Partial Pressures

In a mixture of gases, the pressure exerted by each gas is the same as it would exert if it was alone in the container. A gas is a mixture of molecules, like beads in a jar. From the ideal gas laws perspective, they are acting completely independently.

Add a cylinder of O_2 at 21 kPa to a cylinder of N_2 at 79 kPa. Final cylinder pressure will be 100 kPa and will contain 21% O_2 and 79% N_2 (Fig. 3.5).

Dalton's Law of Partial pressures

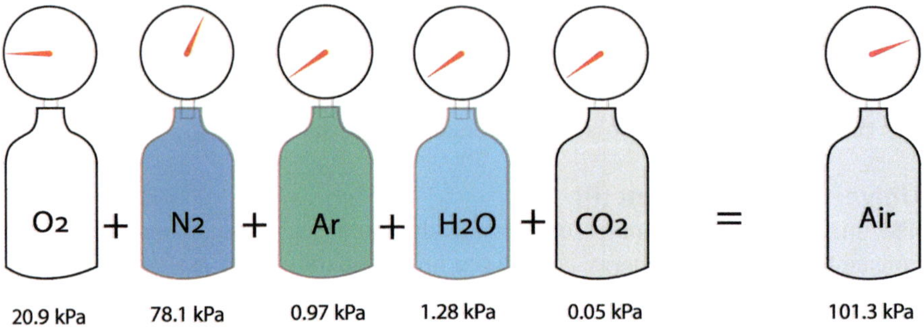

Fig. 3.5 Dalton's partial pressures

Standard Temperatures and Pressures

Table 3.1 Standard pressures and temperatures

Standards of temperature and pressure for describing gas states			
Conditions	Temperature	Pressure	Volume one mole
Standard temperature pressure (STP). * Traditional	0 °C	* 1 atmosphere (101.325 kPa)	22.4 L
Standard temperature pressure (STP). † Since 1982	0 °C	† 100 kPa (1 bar)	22.7 L
Standard laboratory conditions (Australasia)	25 °C	100 kPa (1 bar)	24.8 L
Ambient temperature pressure saturated	Ambient	Ambient	
Body temperature pressure saturated	37 °C	Ambient	

Avogadro's Law

Equal volumes of gases at the same temperature and pressure contain the same number of molecules (Fig. 3.6).

Derive the Volume of 1 Mole Gas at STP from the Universal Gas Equation

$$PV = nRT$$

$$\text{Volume per mole}(\text{STP}): V/_n = \frac{RT}{P} = \frac{(8.314 \times 273.15)}{101.325} = 22.413$$

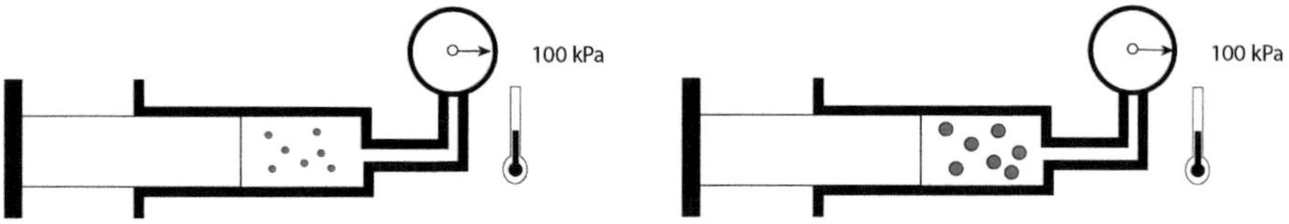

Gases at the same volume, pressure and temperature contain the same number of molecules.

Fig. 3.6 Relationship of volume/pressure and number of molecules

Hence, for gases of a given volume and at a given temperature, if the pressure of the gas is the same, they must contain the same number of molecules.

How Can this Be True?

The force exerted by an individual molecule of any ideal gas at a given temperature is the same despite differences in molecular mass. The force exerted by a molecule on a wall is equal to the rate of *change of momentum*. Thus, although a large molecule has greater momentum, it moves more slowly, and the time lapse between impacts is proportionately longer. The force and pressure of large molecules are, therefore, the same as those exerted by small molecules.

Calculate the Volume Remaining in a N_2O Cylinder at STP

- Mass of N_2O remaining = Mass cylinder − Mass empty cylinder (tare weight).
- Number of moles N_2O remaining = Mass N_2O/Molecular weight (44 g).
- Volume of N_2O remaining = Number of moles N_2O × 22.4 L (Table 3.1).

Although this has been a standard exam exercise, it must be remembered that:

(a) N_2O is a vapour at this temperature, and there will be inaccuracy from the ideal gas laws.
(b) At room temperature, the molar volume will be greater than 22.4 L.
(c) 22.4 L is measured at 1 atmosphere rather than 1 bar.

What Is a Mole?

In order to understand how the concept of a mole was developed, you must understand the basic atomic structure.

Basic Atomic Structure

Table 3.2 Relative charge and mass of atomic particles

Particle	Charge	Relative mass
Proton	Positive +1	1
Neutron	Neutral 0	1
Electron	Negative −1	0.0005

Note: Nucleon is a collective term for protons and neutrons

Atomic number (or proton number)	Number of protons in nucleus. Defines the element. No two elements have the same number of protons
Charge	In the usual neutral atom, the number of electrons equals the number of protons. Ions have different numbers of protons and electrons
Relevance of number of electrons	Determines the reactions and chemical behaviour. Thus, the proton number reveals a lot about an atom's chemical properties
Mass number	Number of protons and neutrons in an atomic nucleus
Atomic mass	Mass of protons, neutrons, electrons and nuclear binding energy (NBE) in the nucleus of a specific isotope. As electrons and the NBE have negligible mass for most applications, atomic mass ≅ mass number (Table 3.2)
Isotope	Atoms with the same number of protons but different numbers of neutrons. All have the same numbers of electrons, and so their chemical properties are the same
Importance of neutron number	The greater the number of neutrons, the more unstable the nucleus and the more likely to radioactively decay
Relative atomic mass	The average mass of all the isotopes. Not usually a whole number
Units of atomic mass	SI unit is the kg but is usually expressed as the Dalton, which is 1/12 of the mass of one carbon-12 atom. Thus, 1 Dalton is effectively the mass of one proton (or neutron). The masses of all atoms are whole-number multiples of this building block

Definition of the Mole

SI Definition Since November 2018

The mole (mol) is the SI unit of 'amount of substance'. One mole contains exactly 6.022×10^{23} elementary entities, which is Avogadro's constant. An elementary entity may be an atom, a molecule, an ion, an electron, any other particle or specified group of particles.

Thus, the new SI definition does not relate it to the method of arriving at the Avogadro's constant, unlike the previous definition.

Previous Definition and Explanation

The number of atoms in 12 g of carbon-12 (^{12}C): This has been measured at 6.022×10^{23}.

The mass of ^{12}C is the result of its 12 nucleons. By choosing 12 g of ^{12}C, we develop a simple relationship whereby the mass of a mole (the mass of 6×10^{23} molecules) is simply the mass number expressed in grams:

- Mass of one mole of ^{12}C atoms = 12 g
- Mass of one mole of ^{1}H atoms = 1 g
- Mass of one mole of ^{16}O atoms = 16 g
- Mass of one mole of ^{16}O molecules = 32 g

Thus, the mole was defined to provide a convenient comparative measure and then the number of particles determined. From 2018, the definition has been reduced to a unit of 'amount' that represents a specific number of particles.

Henry's Law

At a given temperature, the number of molecules of a gas dissolving in a liquid is proportional to the partial pressure of the gas above the liquid.

What Is Meant by Solubility?

The ability of a substance to dissolve in a solvent is known as its solubility. Dissolving implies a mixture between solute and solvent as distinct from a chemical reaction between the two. Solubility is gauged by the amount that will dissolve before a saturated solution occurs.

Factors Affecting Solubility

Generally, decreasing temperature increases the solubility of gases but decreases the solubility of solids and liquids. The solubility of gas increases with decreasing temperature and increasing partial pressure of the gas. Solubility is also dependent on the solute (N_2O more soluble than N_2) and the solvent (N_2O more soluble in blood than saline).

Table 3.3 Some commonly used proportionality constants

Variations		Notes
Partition coefficient	Ratio of amount in one phase: amount in other phase	Two phases to be of equal volume and temperature
Bunsen coefficient	Volume gas/unit volume solvent	Volume gas/unit volume solvent when gas is at 1 bar and 0 °C (STP)
Ostwald coefficient	Volume gas/unit volume solvent	Volume gas dissolved at ambient temperature and pressure. The Ostwald and Bunsen coefficients are identical (if temperature is the same [0 °C])
Oxygen solubility in blood	Vols%/mmHg	Oxygen in blood at 37 °C is 0.003 mL/dL/mmHg
CO_2 solubility in blood	mmol.L^{-1}/mmHg	CO_2 in blood at 37 °C is 0.03 mmol.L^{-1}/mmHg

Proportionality Constants

The ratio of dissolved phase to gaseous phase is called the proportionality constant and is specific for a certain gas and a certain liquid, at a given temperature. There are several ways to express the proportionality constant (Table 3.3).

Heat

4

Alan McLintic and Nic Randall

What Is the Difference Between Heat and Temperature?

Temperature is the measure of the thermal energy of a substance. It is an indication of the kinetic energy possessed by the molecules. Molecules with higher temperature move faster; having a greater kinetic energy means that more of this can be transferred.

Heat is the energy that is transferred from a substance with higher thermal energy (greater temperature, hotter) to one with a lower thermal energy (lower temperature, cooler) and has an associated time component (see below).

Temperature describes the thermal state of something, while heat describes thermal energy movement. So, a hot element (high kinetic energy) burns quickly as it transfers a large amount of energy in a short period of time (large amount of heat).

Units of Temperature, Heat and Watt

Temperature is measured in Kelvin (K) or Celsius (°C).

Zero Kelvin (OK) occurs at absolute zero when all atomic (kinetic) movement of atoms has stopped. The temperature scale Celsius is commonly used as it provides the convenient reference point of 0 °C (freezing point of pure unionised water). Note that when using the Kelvin scale, the degree symbol (°) is not used.

The Joule (J) is the SI unit of energy, it is equal to the work (force × distance) occurring to move an object 1 meter when a force of 1 newton (N) is applied. Pressure × Volume is the a form of work more commonly referenced in anaesthesia especially when talking about respiratory or cardiovascular performance. The derivation of this requires some mental gymnastics – pressure is force

A. McLintic · N. Randall (✉)
Department of Intensive Care Medicine, Counties Manukau Health, Auckland, New Zealand
e-mail: nic.randall@middlemore.co.nz

C. Birch et al. (eds.), *Physics and Measurement for Anesthesia*,
https://doi.org/10.1007/978-3-031-65060-4_4

over unit area (F/m^2); volume (m^3) is distance (m) multiplied by unit area (m^2), cancelling the unit area leaves the more familar equation.

When used to describe heat, a joule is the amount of energy dissipated (as heat) when an electric current (1 amp) is passed through a resistance of 1 ohm, over the period of 1 s.

The watt (J/s) is the amount of heat (J) transferred in a unit time (s), also referred to as power.

The terms calorie and kilojoule can be confusing, they both describe the same thing, *heat energy*, but have different numerical values. A calorie, is the amount of heat energy required to raise the temperature of 1 g of water by 1 °C, for a kilocalorie (kcal) the water volume would be 1 kg, the temperature rise remains 1 °C. Calorie comes from Latin *calor* (heat) and has its originates in work with steam and heat engines. It is equivalent to 4.184J. An electric kettle or jug is an energy transfer appliance, a kettle of approximately 4200 W would heat a litre of water (1 kg), 1 °C every second. Now that you understand the principal, you can predict the boiling time for your study break cup of tea, remember you will need to measure the starting water temperature first though! Different substances require different amounts of energy to change their temperature, this is know as the *specific heat capacity (see below).*

Heat Transfer: Definitions

Conduction

Heat transfer via exchange or transfer of kinetic energy through direct contact.

'Heat diffusion' without exchange of matter.

Radiation

Transfer of energy between bodies separated in space by electromagnetic radiation; this process does not require a medium. Energy is lost predominantly in the infrared spectrum and can be reflected, hence the use of metallic blankets, to retain heat.

Convection

Transfer of heat by the bulk movement of molecules within fluid; this is the dominant form of heat transfer in liquids and gases. When a gas or liquid is heated, the particles move faster and the space between them increases, this makes the heated fluid less dense, and it rises above cooler regions. Convection currents can be established if a constant source of heat is provided to the system.

Evaporation

Evaporation occurs when molecules at the surface of a liquid have enough energy to overcome their intermolecular bonds and enter the vapour phase. Evaporation can occur even at low temperatures, because some molecules at the surface will have enough kinetic energy to escape. Molecules acquire the escape energy from collisions within the liquid (latent energy); the consequence is that energy (heat) is lost from the liquid and cooling occurs. The more evaporation that occurs, the greater the cooling effect, as per the first law of thermodynamics (conservation of energy).

Heat Loss Under Anaesthesia

The majority of heat loss occurs through the skin; strategies to reduce this include pre-warming of patients, blankets and operating theatre. Pre-warming increases the thermal mass and is a form of heat banking; this is intended to help reduce heat loss due to redistribution to cooler surfaces (radiation, convection). Using tucked blankets (cocoons) and forced air warmers helps to reduce conduction and convection losses. Minimising skin and surgical wound exposure (especially abdominal) combined with keeping the patient dry reduces evaporative heat loss. The various contributions to heat loss are displayed in Table 4.1.

Table 4.1 Different contributions to heat loss under anaesthesia

Heat loss mechanisms under anaesthesia		
Radiation	40%	Pre-warming
Convection	30%	Blankets, coverings, forced air warmers
Conduction	5%	Pre-warmed fluids
Evaporative cooling	15%	Minimise skin exposure and wounds
Other factors	10%	

Pattern of temperature drop in anaesthesia

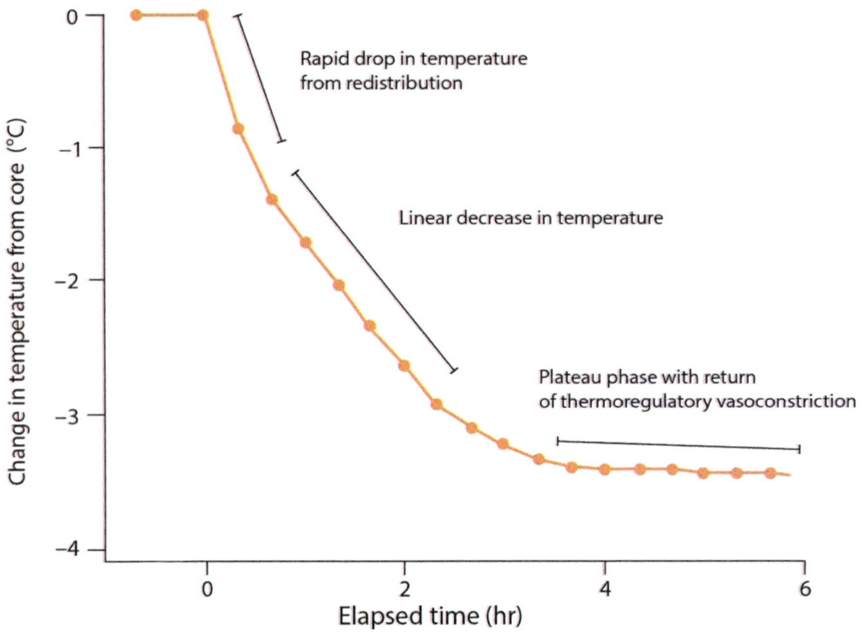

Fig. 4.1 Model of heat loss occurring during anaesthesia showing a triphasic pattern

Heat Loss Phases

Patients under anaesthesia demonstrate a typical temperature loss pattern, which can be described using the triphasic model (Fig. 4.1).

- Rapid decrease by 0.5–1.5 °C over 30 min:
  - Due to peripheral vasodilatation and redistribution.
  - The majority of temperature drop is due to heat redistribution, not heat loss.
- Linear decrease of approximately 0.3 $°Ch^{-1}$
  - Impaired vasoconstriction
  - Absent behavioural response
  - Decreased metabolic heat production
- Plateau phase of stabilisation:
  - Thermoregulatory vasoconstriction finally occurs.
- Heat loss during regional (epidural/spinal):
  - This demonstrates a similar pattern; however, the rate of loss is reduced, and temperature nadir is 0.5–1 °C higher than seen in with a general anaesthetic.
  - If general anaesthesia is combined with regional anaesthesia, the potential for heat loss is higher and an accelerated graph is seen.

Heat Capacity

Heat capacity is a physical property of a substance. It is defined as the amount of heat that is required to raise the temperature of an object.

Units are $J.K^{-1}$ or $J.°C^{-1}$.

Some objects get hotter than others, despite being supplied the same amount of 'heat'. The ability of a substance to absorb heat (energy) is related to the available quantum states, and whether it is homogeneous or a mixture. Because the heat capacity of a substance varies with temperature, pressure and state of the matter (liquid, solid or gas), the term 'specific heat capacity' is used. This relates to the 'specific' conditions for the measured value. For example, the table below shows the difference in the amount of energy required to change the temperature of H_2O in its different states.

	2093	J/K.kg	0 °C	101.325 kPa
Water	4185	J/K.kg	15 °C	101.325 kPa

Heat capacity is relevant to anaesthesia because it relates to the thermal mass of an object, determining the rate of heating or cooling that occurs.

What Determines the Temperature Rise of an Object?

ΔT = (Energy added/Mass) × Specific heat capacity

- Specific heat capacity of the material (a property of the atoms)
- The amount of heat/energy added
- The mass of the system

An object may have a high thermal mass because it either is of large mass or has high specific heat capacity or both. Practically, this is seen with the rapid cooling (and risk of overheating) of children during anaesthesia (confounded by their relatively larger surface area for this loss to occur) and temperature stability that can be achieved with equipment that use a 'heat sink'.

What Is a 'Heat Sink'?

A heat sink is a thermally stable reservoir that can absorb or release heat without a significant change in temperature. Heat sinks are used to stabilise temperature of the reference junction of thermocouples and to stabilise the temperature of vaporisers (see vaporisers).

What Physical Properties Must a Heat Sink Have?

High Thermal Mass

This is usually achieved through its large mass rather than the material having a high specific heat capacity.

An exception was the Boyle's bottle water bath, due to water having a very high specific heat capacity.

High Thermal Conductivity

Thermal conductivity is the ability of a material to transfer heat. In metals, this is predominantly through the flow of free electrons (an intrinsic property), and in gases, it is due to collisions between molecules. Thermal conductivity varies between gases and is also dependent on gas concentration.

Copper (and its alloys) are commonly used as heat sinks due to a high thermal conductivity. This allows an effective and efficient transfer heat; however, due to a low specific heat capacity, this means that they rely on their mass (kg) to provide the temperature stability required and therefore are often very heavy.

Vaporisers

5

Alan McLintic and Michael Webb

Vaporisers

Refer to the Previous Chapter and Be Able to Explain the Following Concepts

- Latent heat and evaporative cooling
- Heat capacity and the heat sink
- Evaporation, vapour pressure and determinants of SVP
- Anaesthetic vaporisers are devices designed to variably saturate inhaled gases with volatile anaesthetic agents, for the continuous induction and maintenance of anaesthesia. Many such devices exist, and with time, more complex technology has superseded what was initially a very simple design (Table 5.1). The advances in technology have come with the purpose of increasing the safety, accuracy, and precision of the devices. Knowledge of the early devices, and their underlying physical principles, provides a solid base of important anaesthetic basic science, including saturated vapour pressures, flow, and effects of thermal energy.

A. McLintic · M. Webb (✉)
Department of Anaesthesia and Pain Medicine, Counties Manukau Health, Auckland, New Zealand

C. Birch et al. (eds.), *Physics and Measurement for Anesthesia*,
https://doi.org/10.1007/978-3-031-65060-4_5

Table 5.1 Types and examples and vaporisers (adapted from Boumphrey et al. 2011)

Type of vaporiser		Examples
Draw over vaporiser		Oxford miniature vaporiser (OMV)
		Goldman inhaler
		Boyle's bottle
Plenum vaporisers	Variable bypass vaporisers	Datex-Ohmeda Tec series
		Aladin cassette
	Injection/gas-vapour blender/ measured flow	Draeger Diva
		Tec 6 Desflurane vaporiser

Classification of Vaporisers

Draw Over Vaporisers

Draw over vaporisers are now resigned to historical models, with the notable exceptions of those being used in the field (OMV). In the model, the carrier gas is "drawn over" the volatile agent by negative pressure created by the patient's work of breathing. The gas is saturated within the vaporiser and pulled downstream in the patient. This type of vaporiser may be placed within the breathing circuit but, given the nature of the energy used to deliver the gas, must have a very low resistance. The draw over vaporiser can be used in a circle system, with the caveats that it is placed in the inspiratory limb and with the warnings that recirculation of the gas increases volatile anaesthetic concentration and that wicks must be avoided as they can become saturated with water vapour. Gas flow rates and temperature can dramatically impact the delivery of anaesthetic vapours in this design. This device provides an un-calibrated delivery of gas that relies heavily on the experience of the operator.

Plenum Vaporisers

Plenum vaporisers are self-contained units in which volatile agents are housed. Fresh gases flow through the plenum vaporiser, collecting vaporised anaesthetic agents as they pass. A patient cannot create sufficient negative pressure to draw gas through the device, and pressure must be applied. Plenum vaporisers offer significant advantages in accuracy over the draw over models. This accuracy comes from the features of the housing unit, namely controlling the flow of gas into and through the unit, and the ability to control and account for the effects of temperature in the unit. Here, we will discuss the variable bypass vaporiser as the model for this class.

Variable Bypass Vaporisers

Basic Principles

The basic principles of these devices revolve around the concepts of flow diversion or splitting, saturation of fresh gases, and control of temperature and flow.

Splitting of Fresh Gas Flow

Fresh gas is directed towards the vaporisers from the flow meters in the anaesthetic machine. A dial or gauge is manually turned to split the fresh gas flow into two distinct streams. One stream (the majority of the fresh gas) bypasses the vaporiser entirely. A smaller portion of the flow is directed into the vaporiser. The ratio of the gases bypassing and entering the chamber is called the splitting ratio and ultimately decides the final output concentration delivered to the patient.

The fresh gas that is directed to the vaporising chamber picks up fully saturated vapour. Owing to one of the properties of the anaesthetic agent, its saturated vapour pressure, the volatile concentration within the plenum housing is predictable. Saturated vapour pressure is a constant parameter at room temperature. The known vaporising chamber flow (as a proportion of total flow in the circuit) that contains a known concentration of the volatile agent is then added back to the bypass flow and delivered to the patient.

It is worthwhile to note that the location of the control valve for gas flow into the vaporising chamber may be located either at the entry or at the outlet of this housing. Most modern vaporisers place it on the outlet. This is because vapour has been added to the flow entering the vaporising chamber, and therefore the volume leaving the chamber is larger and may make up a larger than anticipated share of the total gas flow leading to an inadvertent overdose of volatile agent.

The following example and figure (Fig. 5.1) will provide some clarity:

If the outlet splitting ratio of a sevoflurane vaporiser is 20:1, what is the vaporiser output concentration?

- The outlet splitting ratio means that, for every 100 mL/min leaving the vaporising chamber, 2000 mL/min is flowing through the bypass channel.
- The total flow leaving the vaporiser must be 2100 mL.
- The 100 mL leaving the VC is fully saturated with sevoflurane.
- SVP sevoflurane at 20 °C is 21 kPa (rounded down).
- The concentration in the VC is 21% (21 kPa/100 kPa, assuming atmospheric pressure at 1 bar for simplicity).

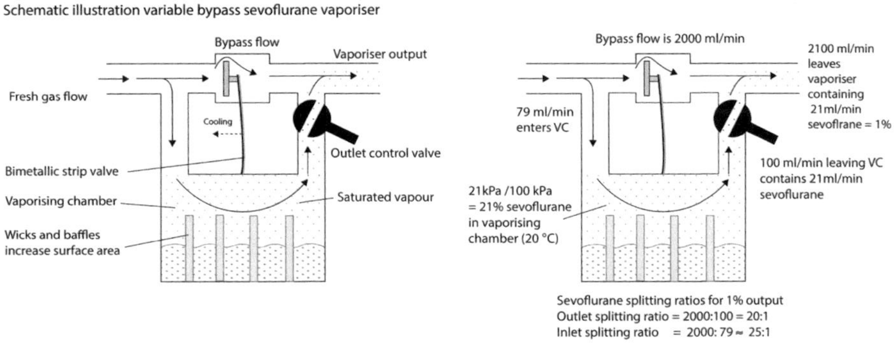

Fig. 5.1 Variable bypass sevoflurane vaporiser

- The 100 mL leaving the VC must contain 21 mL sevoflurane, and this is added back to the bypass flow so that the vaporiser output of 2100 mL now contains 21 mL of sevoflurane.
- The output is 21/2100 = 1% sevoflurane.

What was the inlet splitting ratio in this example?

- If 100 mL was exiting the VC, what volume was entering?
- If 21% of the volume in the VC was sevoflurane, that means that 79% must have been carrier gas.
- 79 mL of carrier gas must have entered the VC and picked up 21 mL of sevoflurane and left as 100 mL with a sevoflurane concentration of 21%.
- From before, the bypass flow was 2000 mL, and we now know that the VC inlet flow was 79 mL so the inlet splitting ratio was 2000/79 = 25:1 (rounded down).

Temperature Stability

Owing to the physical properties of the volatile anaesthetic agents, to accurately and safely administer them, temperature must be carefully controlled in the plenum vaporiser. These devices have inherent features that aim to keep a stable and predictable thermal environment. Fluctuations in ambient and vaporising chamber temperature will alter the saturated vapour pressure and therefore concentration of anaesthetic in the vaporiser chamber flow. This will lead to inaccuracies in calibration. Thermostabilisation is aided by a large mass of copper alloy casing.

The copper casing is a heat sink in that it has high thermal conductivity and high heat capacity. The latter is achieved mainly through its large mass rather than its specific heat capacity, which is relatively low for copper. Thus, changes in environmental and vaporising chamber temperature are somewhat stabilised by the properties of the chamber itself. Another example of this principle is demonstrated by the Boyle's bottle, which utilised the high specific heat capacity of a water bath to provide thermostabilisation.

Temperature Compensation

Plenum vaporisers must also account for variations in temperature as would naturally be expected in the dynamic environment of an operating theatre or in different environments or settings around the world. Indeed, temperature must also be corrected for as a process of vaporising anaesthetic gases. The latent enthalpy of vaporisation of anaesthetic gases leads to evaporative cooling. As temperature falls due to this cooling, the saturated vapour pressure drops and the concentration in the vaporising chamber drops. This would lead to a lower concentration being delivered for a given setting. A temperature-sensitive value must respond to cooling and increase the relative proportion through the vaporising chamber.

To compensate, the vaporiser has built-in features to achieve this.

The most encountered correcting mechanism is bimetallic strips. These are two strips of metal with different coefficients of expansion that are adhered to each other. The metals typically used for this indication are copper and constantan, which is a copper and nickel alloy. As the temperature changes within the vaporiser, the metals expand and contract to differing degrees, causing the metal strip to bend. As the temperature cools the resistance to flow lessens, the reverse is true as the temperature rises.

Other commonly seen features for this temperature compensation are bellows valves or metal rods. In the bellows valves, gas or ether-filled bellows expand or contract with temperature and move a rod linked to an inlet valve. Similarly, in the metal rod, it expands and contracts with temperature variations and is linked to an inlet valve to control flow.

Some vaporisers avoid this issue altogether. The Siemens vaporiser injects measured amounts of volatile anaesthetic directly into the fresh gas flow through a fine nozzle, and the heated chamber vaporiser heats and pressurises the anaesthetic agent, which is then added to fresh gas flow in known quantities. We will expand upon these concepts further in the upcoming passages.

Flow Dependence

The greater the flow through the vaporising chamber, the less likely it is going to be fully saturated. Thus, the plenum vaporiser will tend to under-deliver at high flows. Flow dependence is countered by increasing the surface area in the vaporising chamber. Practically, this is achieved through inbuilt features in the chamber that maximally expose the gas flow to anaesthetic vapour. In the vaporiser, the gas passes over metal or fabric wicks soaked in the volatile agent. These wicks allow liquid anaesthetic agents to spread over a very large surface area. The fresh gas flow is directed over these wicks by baffles placed in the vaporising chamber. A historical alternative is to bubble the volatile through the liquid as in the copper kettle and Boyle's bottle.

Conversely, at low flows, the splitting ratio may also be affected by differences in the amount of turbulent and laminar flow. This is affected by the density and viscosity of the gases present. Theoretically, at very low flows, the output may vary depending on whether nitrous oxide or air is used.

Other Factors Affecting Variable Bypass Vaporisers

Hyperbaric Conditions

It is important to preface this section with some commentary regarding mean alveolar concentration (MAC) and the observed effects of volatile anaesthetic agents. MAC is described in terms of a percentage, but it is the partial pressure of the anaesthetic agents at its effect sites that determines its clinical effect. The saturated vapour pressure of the volatile anaesthetic agents is not impacted by ambient pressure, and as a result, the output of the agent also does not change with hyperbaric ambient environments (Fig. 5.2).

In contemporary variable bypass vaporisers with splitting control at the VC outlet, the vaporiser settings do not need to be adjusted. The 1% setting produces the same partial pressure during hyperbaric conditions as at one atmosphere. Although

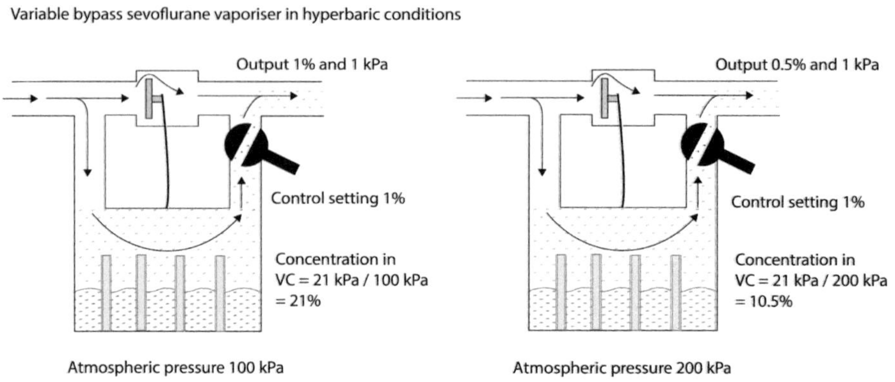

Fig. 5.2 Effect of hyperbaric conditions on sevoflurane variable bypass vaporiser

the concentration of volatile agent in the vaporising chamber is proportionately reduced, the mass of volatile agent added to the bypass flow is the same and the partial pressure delivered is unchanged.

In older vaporisers, with inlet splitting controls, the vaporiser may under-deliver partial pressure in hyperbaric conditions.

Pumping Effect

In older anaesthetic machines with gas-driven ventilators, fluctuating back pressure from the ventilator could cause increased pressure within the vapour chamber, causing back spill of vapour through the inlet channel into the bypass channel. This would lead to excess concentration leaving the vaporiser. The potential for increased concentrations of volatile anaesthetic also exists because of the recirculation of gases back into the vaporising chamber. This theoretical issue could only exist in inefficient systems whereby the gases in the vaporising chamber did not exit fully saturated. These issues can be prevented by the use of a downstream resistor or pressure-regulating valve. Physical features that may also help mitigate this effect are a vaporising chamber that is larger than the bypass channel, and a long inlet tube in the vaporising chamber.

Effect of Carrier Gases

The coadministration of certain gases may impact the performance of the vaporiser to variable effects. If nitrous oxide is in the carrier gas, a proportion will dissolve in the liquid volatile, reducing flow through the vaporiser and the quantity of anaesthetic vapour delivered back to the bypass flow. The output will be reduced until the liquid volatile is saturated with nitrous oxide. This factor would only be relevant in inlet splitting control valves.

The manufacturers of anaesthetic vaporisers calibrate the vaporisers using either air or 100% oxygen. When other carrier gases are used, the output may differ a little. The difference is magnified by extremes of flow rates.

Variation in carrier gas viscosity and density affects the nature of flow (laminar or turbulent) and the resistance to flow through the vaporising chamber. Air and, to a larger extent, nitrous oxide have lower viscosity than oxygen. This may affect the splitting ratio and the contact time between liquid and gas, with less flow through, and less output from, the vaporising chamber when using these less viscous gases. The effects, while modest under any conditions, are most marked at flows below 1 L/min.

Multiple Vaporisers

In older anaesthesia machines, it was possible to have more than one vaporiser on the back bar turned on at the same time. This could cause potentially lethal concentrations of volatile agent. At the very least, the downstream vaporisers could be contaminated by those upstream.

The least volatile agent should be placed furthest upstream and the most volatile downstream. If it was the reverse, highly volatile contaminant would be delivered at high MAC from the vaporisers calibrated for low-volatile agents.

Desflurane Vaporisers

The advent of desflurane created a unique situation whereby the traditional vaporiser technology was not suitable for the physical properties of this anaesthetic vapour. Desflurane's properties created unique indications for this agent, but also created a niche for novel vaporiser technology to emerge (Fig. 5.3).

The SVP of desflurane is 88.5 kPa with a boiling point of 22.8 °C. This is very close to room temperature so that, at normal operating temperatures, the SVP

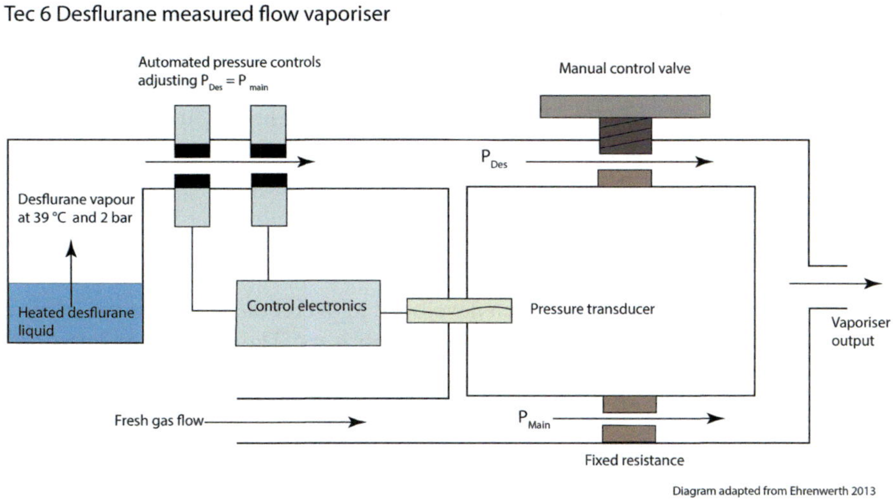

Fig. 5.3 Tec 6 desflurane vaporiser

changes greatly with only small changes in temperature. In addition, in a very warm OR, desflurane would boil, and very high concentrations might reach the patient. This variability could introduce a definite risk of harm; therefore, measures were required to allow the safe delivery of desflurane. These measures included artificial thermal and pressure control of the vaporising chamber to allow for known concentrations of vapour to be calculated.

Tec 6 Datex-Ohmeda

This vaporiser introduced new technology to account for the unique physical properties of desflurane and therefore is incompatible with other volatile anaesthetic agents. The vaporiser technology includes a measured flow vaporiser, an injector, and a dual-circuit gas-vapour blender, which will now be discussed in greater detail and visually displayed in the image above.

The operating principles of this vaporiser utilise two distinct circuits: one containing fresh gas flow, and the other a volatile anaesthetic-containing chamber with an injector. Within the chamber, desflurane is heated to 39 °C to produce vapour pressure of 2 bars. The vapour then leaves the chamber and enters a sump. The pressure in the sump is automatically adjusted to be the same as that in the fresh gas flow channel of the vaporiser. Thus, if the fresh gas flow is altered, the pressure in the fresh gas flow changes, and the pressure in the desflurane sump adjusts to match this automatically. Thus, if we reduce fresh gas flow, the pressure in the desflurane sump automatically reduces so that the amount injected into the fresh gas flow for a given concentration is proportionately reduced as well. The desflurane is injected into the fresh gas flow according to the user-controlled rotary dial.

Special Considerations

In hypobaric conditions, the Tec 6 delivers the dialled-up concentration but under-delivers in terms of partial pressure. In hyperbaric conditions, it over-delivers in terms of partial pressure. Dial settings must be adjusted.

Modern Advances in Vaporiser Technology

Newer vaporiser technology has been developed to overcome some sources of error and risk associated with traditional plenum vaporisers. The addition of microprocessors has allowed rapid corrections in gas flow rates, temperature, and pressure, and the ability to account and adjust for the use of differing carrier gases.

Aladin Cassette (GE Healthcare)

The Aladin cassette is the prototypical variable bypass vaporiser with electronic control. Physically, it is a stand-alone, microenvironment, vaporising chamber that is directly plugged into the bypass channel of the anaesthetic workstation. The cassettes are agent specific and prevent "wrong agent" insertion by utilising a series of magnetic tags located on the back of the cassette that correlate with a particular agent on the workstation. This vaporiser has a central processing unit that allows for rapid adjustments to the environment and to the demands of the user. In this unit, the vaporising chamber is high lamellated, greatly increasing the surface area for vaporisation. The bypass and chamber gases are throttled by the CPU, allowing very precise concentrations of vapour over a wide range of flows. Temperature and pressure in the vaporising chamber are closely monitored and controlled. With known temperatures and pressures in the chamber, the vapour pressure can be measured (as a percentage of total pressure), and the CPU can then adjust the amount of agent injected into the bypass flows providing accurate temperature compensation. Should the temperature in the unit fall below 18 °Celsius, the unit has warming fan which shifts heat from the anaesthetic workstation to the cassette. To manage the effects of carrier gases, the central processing unit adjusts, based on algorithm, for the different gases.

Dräger Diva (Dräger Zeus Anaesthetic Machine)

This is a measured flow vaporiser that utilises an anaesthetic agent injector to deliver the vapour into the fresh gas flow. In this device, volatile agent is housed in a storage tank and then flows by gravity from this tank into pump tank. The pump tank is pressurised to 2.4 bars, which drives the liquid anaesthetic agent into a metering tank.

Liquid is injected from metering tank into heated evaporation chamber to produce saturated vapour. Vapour is added to patient circuit and controlled by microprocessor-controlled valves linked to flow sensor regulator.

Safety Considerations for Plenum Vaporisers

Plenum vaporisers have a number of physical and mechanical safety features (Table 5.2). Broadly, these aim to prevent dosing errors and wrong drug errors and avoid failures of the integrity of the vaporising chamber.

Table 5.2 Safety considerations in plenum vaporisers (adapted from Boumphrey et al. 2011)

Safety considerations for plenum vaporisers
Calibration enables predictable concentrations
Keyed and colour-coded filling system
Methods to prevent the pumping effect
Control knobs always operate counterclockwise
Filling levels displayed
Mounting systems to prevent tandem operation
Machine checks to detect leaks
Anti-spill feature to prevent liquid from entering bypass channel when carrying vaporiser
Cannot be overfilled
Electronic alarms in desflurane vaporiser
MRI compatibility

Further Reading

Boumphrey S, Marshall N. Understanding vaporizers. Contin Educ Anaesth Crit Care Pain. 2011;11(6):199–203. https://doi.org/10.1093/bjaceaccp/mkr040.

Davis PD, Kenny GNC. Basic physics and measurement in anaesthesia. 5th ed. Oxford: Butterworth-Heinemann; 2003.

Ehrenwerth J, Eisenkraft JB, Berry JM. Anesthesia equipment: principles and applications. Philadelphia: Saunders; 2013.

Oxygen Production and Storage

6

Alan McLintic and Andrew Wong

Oxygen Production and Storage

Fractional Distillation

This is the most common commercial method of oxygen production. Oxygen is produced by separation of liquid mixtures. The liquid is heated to a point where one component vaporises. As different components of the liquid have different boiling points, they are able to be separated and collected.

Key Steps

- Air is compressed and liquified by cooling to –200 °C.
- CO_2 and water are solid at this temperature and are easily removed.
- Liquid air passes into a fractionating column where the temperature is warmer at the bottom than the top.
- Bottom (−185 °C):
  - Nitrogen is boiling vigorously and separating into bubbles of vapour.
  - Oxygen is still below its boiling point and remains as liquid at the bottom. The liquid oxygen is drawn off (Fig. 6.1).
- Top (−195 °C):
  - Nitrogen is still boiling at the temperature, and oxygen remains as liquid. Nitrogen vapour is removed from the top of the column. A little oxygen vapour may also be lost at the surface through evaporation.
- Argon has very similar BP to oxygen, so a second fractionating column may be added to separate argon from oxygen (Table 6.1).

A. McLintic · A. Wong (✉)
Epsom Anaesthesia, Auckland, New Zealand

C. Birch et al. (eds.), *Physics and Measurement for Anesthesia*,
https://doi.org/10.1007/978-3-031-65060-4_6

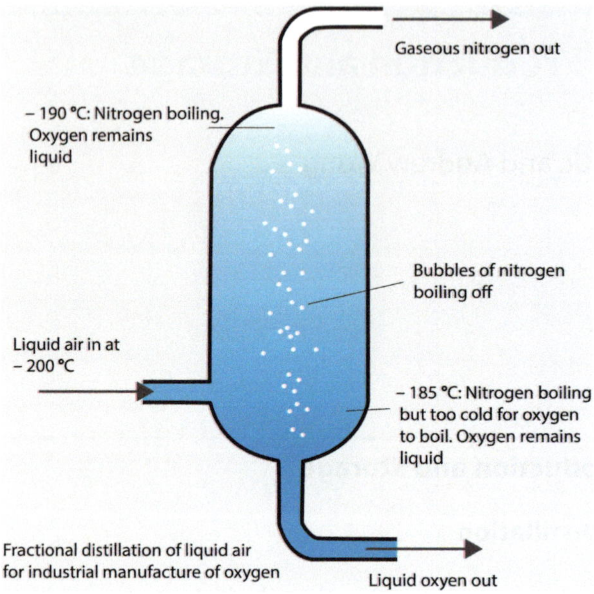

Fig. 6.1 Separating nitrogen from air

Table 6.1 Critical temperature/boiling point of some gases

	Critical temperature	Boiling point
Oxygen	−118 °C	−183 °C
Argon	−122 °C	−186 °C
Nitrogen	−147 °C	−196 °C

Oxygen Concentrators

Pressure Swing Adsorption

Oxygen concentrators work by absorption and removal of nitrogen. Nitrogen is extracted from air by differential adsorption in a zeolite molecular sieve.

What Is a Zeolite Sieve?

Crystalline aluminium silicates in a three-dimensional tetrahedral framework that contains entry pores and cavities. These are arranged in multiple columns to increase surface area. Under pressure, certain molecules (N_2) become trapped due to size and polarity, while others (O_2) pass through.

Key Steps

- Air is filtered and pressurised to ~137 kPa.
- Water is removed by aluminium silicates.
- The compressed air passes into the zeolite sieve.

- Under high pressure, the nitrogen is trapped in the zeolite while oxygen passes through to the patient (Fig. 6.2).
- The zeolite is arranged in two columns that are being used alternately in 20- to 30-s intervals:
  - One is under pressure and active in absorbing nitrogen from the air.
  - At the same time, the pressure is reduced to atmospheric level in the other, and this releases the nitrogen from the zeolite into the environment.
  - The columns are swapping around every 20–30 s.
- Thus, the zeolite sieve is being continuously regenerated, and a constant supply of oxygen is provided.

Delivery for Home Use

The maximum achievable oxygen concentration is around 95%, with argon around 2–5%. Depending on the unit size, flow rates of 5–10 L/min can be achieved.

Vacuum-Insulated Evaporator (VIE) for Bulk Liquid Oxygen Storage

Context

The major supply of oxygen to the hospital comes from liquid oxygen storage in a vacuum-insulated evaporator. The oxygen is then fed through the hospital pipeline network. In smaller facilities, it may be more economical to simply have a bank of cylinders attached to an oxygen manifold. Usually, there are two 'banks' of

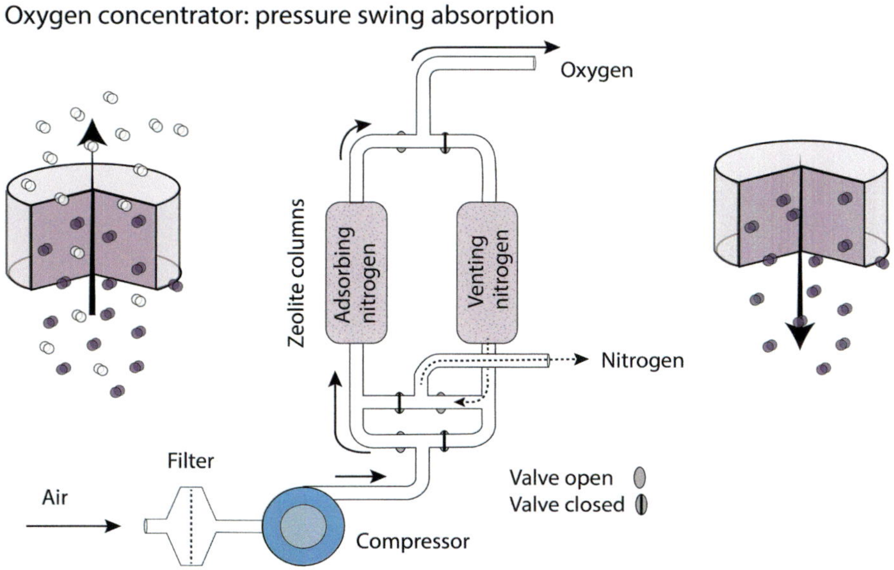

Fig. 6.2 Oxygen concentrator design

cylinders, enabling the facility to switch across to the other bank when one is exhausted.

Major Components

The most cost-effective way to supply large hospitals is to have stored oxygen in its liquid state. This requires that it is transported and stored in double-walled thermally insulated tanks, keeping it below its critical temperature. Pipeline pressure is maintained at around 420 kPa. In times of high demand, liquid oxygen is drawn off and passed through super-heaters before distribution in the pipeline network.

Principle

- The VIE stores oxygen in liquid form. The critical temperature of oxygen is −118 °C, so the liquid oxygen must be at a lower temperature than that (−150 to −170 °C).
- The evaporation of oxygen maintains temperature at around −160 °C through loss of latent heat as the oxygen evaporates (evaporative cooling).
- Pressure in the tank is the vapour pressure of oxygen at that temperature, 7–10 bars.
- Oxygen is drawn off the top of the liquid and passed through the super-heaters and then the pressure regulators.
- If demand is low for the hospital, the lack of evaporation will warm the tank and increase pressure. The safety valve relieves pressure at 1700 kPa.

International System of Units

7

Alan McLintic and Julian Dimech

Measurements and Units

The explosion of discoveries during the scientific revolution of the sixteenth and seventeenth centuries meant that scientists were making observations, measurements and calculations about a large number of hitherto unknown phenomena. With the development of the scientific method, the desire to replicate and peer review observations made by other scientists mandated standardisation of measurements and quantities. The metric system started in 1742 with Celsius's observations on the melting and boiling points of water.

In 1791, the French Academy of Sciences proposed a unified system of measures known as the système international d'unités, and although these measures were introduced, Napoleon ridiculed them and reintroduced traditional (non-metric) units. Today, the système international d'unités (the English abbreviation and translation being SI units) are commonplace in scientific observation and measurement and provide an internationally agreed system of metric units (metric system) for scientific measurement.

The System

The system contains base units and derived units. There are seven base units, from which all other units can be derived. There are 22 derived units, which have special names and symbols often pertaining to the person first describing the phenomenon

A. McLintic
Department of Anaesthesia and Pain Medicine, Counties Manukau Health, Auckland, New Zealand

J. Dimech (✉)
Anaesthesia & Pain Medicine, Middlemore Hospital, Auckland, New Zealand

C. Birch et al. (eds.), *Physics and Measurement for Anesthesia*,
https://doi.org/10.1007/978-3-031-65060-4_7

associated with the unit. Multiples or submultiple prefixes are also standardised and can be applied to any unit.

Base Units

Base units are displayed and defined in Table 7.1. It is worth noting that definitions of units have undergone several revisions over time. From the inception of international units up to 2019, various standardised prototypes or results of standardised experiments were used as unit references.

Examples of these references are the mass of platinum kept in Paris (kilogram), the force produced by current flowing between two parallel wires (ampere), the number of atoms in 12 g of 12C (mole) and the intensity of light emitted from a platinum electric wire (candela). The metre has had repeated redefinition, from 1/10,000,000th of the Earth's meridian through Paris to a multiple of wavelengths of krypton radiation.

In recent years, definitions of base units have moved away from prototypes and laboratory experiments to those where fundamental constants of nature are used to define units. Since 2019, SI units have been defined in terms of fundamental constants of nature (see Table 7.1). While there is scientific rigor in quantifying a unit

Table 7.1 Displays the seven base units of the international system of units (SI units, or metric system). Definitions have been refined over the years, and those in current use are presented in bold type. These descriptors attempt to define the base units in terms of 'fundamental constants' of nature

Unit		Current (simplified) definitions with previous definitions for comparison
Second	Historical	1/86,400 of a 24-h day
	Current	**Duration of 9,192,631,770 periods of radiation from caesium-133**
Metre	Historical	1/10,000,000 of the meridian through Paris
	Historical	Platinum prototypes
	Recent	1,650,763.73 wavelengths of the radiation krypton-86 atom
	Current	**Distance travelled by light in vacuum in 1/299,792,458 s**
Kilogram	Historical	Mass of a litre of fluid
	Recent	Prototypes of the kilogram made of a platinum alloy
	Current	**Defined by setting the [a]Planck constant exactly to 6.62607015 × 10^{-34} J·s (J = kg·m^2·s^{-2}). Given definitions of the metre and second**
Ampere	Recent	Current flowing in two parallel conductors, 1 m apart that would produce a force equal to 2 × 10^{-7} newtons per metre
	Current	**The flow of 1/1.602176634 × 10^{-19} times the elementary charge e per second**
Kelvin	Recent	1/273.16 of the thermodynamic temperature of the triple point of water
	Current	**Kelvin is defined according to the value of the Boltzmann constant 1.380 × 10^{-23} J·K^{-1}**
Mole	Recent	Amount of substance containing as many elementary entities as there are atoms in 12 g of carbon-12
	Current	**The amount of substance of exactly 6.022 × 10^{23} elementary entities**
Candela	Recent	Based on the intensity of a platinum electric light
	Current	**Luminous intensity of source emitting monochromatic radiation of frequency 5.4 × 10^{14} Hz**

[a] Broadly speaking, the Planck constant (J.s) relates the electromagnetic energy of light to its frequency

according to a constant of nature rather than according to a prototype in a Paris vault or an idealised experiment, it is not impossible that further refinement of these units may occur in the future.

Derived Units

There are 22 derived units which have special names and symbols. These are displayed and defined in Table 7.2. Examples of derived units with special names are the Newton, Joule or Watt. The units of measure of derived SI units are given in terms of base units; for example, the Newton has units of measure of kg.m.s^{-2}. Other derived units can be defined using base units. Area for example is defined as square meters (m^2). Additionally, derived units can also include those with special names. Measurement of torque (moment), for example, is measured in Newton metres (N.m).

Table 7.2 Displays the 22 derived international units, presented with their symbols, quantity and units of measure

Name	Symbol	Quantity	SI base units
Radian	rad	Plane angle	m/m
Steradian	sr	Solid angle	m^2/m^2
Hertz	Hz	Frequency	s^{-1}
Newton	N	Force	kg.m.s^{-2}
Pascal	Pa	Pressure	kg.m^{-1}.s^{-2}
Joule	J	Energy, work, heat	kg.m^2.s^{-2}
Watt	W	Power, radiant flux	kg.m^2.s^{-3}
Coulomb	C	Electric charge	s.A
Volt	V	Electrical potential difference, EMF	kg·m^2·s^{-3}·A^{-1}
Farad	F	Capacitance	kg^{-1}·m^{-2}·s^4·A^2
Ohm	Ω	Electrical resistance, impedance, reactance	kg·m^2·s^{-3}·A^{-2}
Siemens	S	Electrical conductance	kg^{-1}·m^{-2}·s^3·A^2
Weber	Wb	Magnetic flux	kg·m^2·s^{-2}·A^{-1}
Tesla	T	Magnetic flux density	kg·s^{-2}·A^{-1}
Henry	H	Inductance	kg·m^2·s^{-2}·A^{-2}
Degree Celsius	°C	Temperature	K
Lumen	lm	Luminous flux	cd.sr
Lux	lx	Illuminance	m^{-2}.cd
Becquerel	Bq	Radioactivity (decay per unit time)	s^{-1}
Gray	Gy	Absorbed dose of ionising radiation	m^2.s^{-2}
Sievert	Sv	Equivalent dose of ionising radiation	m^2.s^{-2}
Katal	kat	Catalytic decay	mol.s^{-1}

Expressing Derived Units

Deriving the joule, pascal, volt and ohm from base units is illustrated below. Other derived units can be expressed in a similar manner.

Example 1: Joule

- The joule is a unit of work.
- Work = Force × Distance.
- Force = Mass × Acceleration.
- 1 joule = 1 N.m.
- 1 N = 1 kg.m.s^{-2}.
- 1 Joule = 1 kg.m.s^{-2} × m.
- 1 Joule = 1 kg.m^2.s^{-2}.

Example 2: Pascal

- Pressure = Force/Area
- Force = Mass × Acceleration.
- 1 Pa = 1 N/m^2.
- 1 Pa = 1 kg.m.s^{-2}/m^2.
- 1 Pa = 1 kg.m^{-1}.s^{-2}.

Example 3: Volt

- 1 Volt = 1 joule per coulomb.
- 1 Joule = 1 N.m.
- 1 Joule = 1 kg.m.s^{-2} × m = 1 kg.m^2.s^{-2}.
- 1 Coulomb = 1 Amp × 1 s.
- 1 Volt = 1 kg.m^2.s^{-2}/ A.s.
- 1 Volt = 1 kg.m^2.s^{-3}.A^{-1}.

Example 4: Ohm

- V = IR and R = V/I.
- From the above, we arrived at V = 1 kg.m^2.s^{-3}.A^{-1}.
- Therefore, 1 ohm = 1 kg.m^2.s^{-3}.A^{-2}.

Prefixes

When describing very large or small measurements, prefixes to units are used. Prefixes between (and including) kilo and milli have been in use since the systems' introduction, while others have been added more recently. Table 7.3 provides an overview of prefixes used with SI units. In addition to the naming and descriptions of the prefixes, there are some rules pertaining to the use of prefixes.

Multiples are denoted with capital letter symbols (with the historical exceptions of deka (da), hecto (h) and kilo (k)). Submultiples are all denoted with lower case letters (with the exception of micro, denoted as the Greek letter mu, μ). Prefixes are combined with the base unit descriptor, e.g. kilowatt (kW), but cannot have more than one prefix ascribed to them.

Table 7.3 Displays multiple and submultiple metric prefixes for base and derived units. These are shown with their name, symbol, descriptor and base 10 factor multiplier

	Prefix name	Prefix symbol	Descriptor	Factor	Adopted
Multiples (larger quantities)	quetta	Q	Nonillion	10^{30}	2022
	ronna	R	Octillion	10^{27}	
	yotta	Y	Septillion	10^{24}	1991
	zetta	Z	Sextillion	10^{21}	
	exa	E	Quintillion	10^{18}	1975
	peta	P	Quadrillion	10^{15}	
	tera	T	Trillion	10^{12}	1960
	giga	G	Billion	10^{9}	
	mega	M	Million	10^{6}	1873
	kilo	k	Thousand	10^{3}	1795
	hecto	h	Hundred	10^{2}	
	deka	da	Ten	10^{1}	
			One	10^{0}	
Submultiples (smaller quantities)	deci	d	Tenth	10^{-1}	
	centi	c	Hundredth	10^{-2}	
	milli	m	Thousandth	10^{-3}	
	micro	μ	Millionth	10^{-6}	1873
	pico	p	Billionth	10^{-9}	1960
	nano	n	Trillionth	10^{-12}	
	atto	a	Quadrillionth	10^{-15}	1974
	femto	f	Quintillionth	10^{-18}	
	zepto	z	Sextillionth	10^{-21}	1991
	yocto	y	Septillionth	10^{-24}	
	ronto	r	Octillionth	10^{-27}	2022
	quecto	q	Nonillionth	10^{-30}	

Further Reading

International Union of Pure and Applied Chemistry. On the revision of the international system of units. 2018. https://iupac.org/on-the-revision-of-the-international-system-of-units/.
Metric prefix. Wikipedia. https://en.wikipedia.org/wiki/Metric_prefix. Accessed 23 May 2023.
Schmidt-Rohr K. Analysis of two definitions of the mole that are in simultaneous use, and their surprising consequences. J Chem Educ. 2020;97:597–602.

8 Oximetry

Alan McLintic and Andrew Wong

Pulse Oximetry

What Is a Pulse Oximeter?

Non-invasive device that estimates arterial haemoglobin oxygen saturation using light absorption (spectrophotometric) principles.

Fractional Saturation (FO_2Hb or $O_2Hb\%$)

Defined as the ratio of oxyhaemoglobin to all Hb species present.

This is most informative clinically because, if a large proportion of Hb is unable to combine with O_2, there will be hypoxia. The FO_2Hb reflects that. A multiwavelength pulse oximeter or laboratory CO-oximeter may be required to show FO_2Hb:

$$FO_2Hb = \left[(O_2Hb)/(O_2Hb + RHb + COHb + MetHb + SulphHb)\right]$$

RHb = reduced or deoxygenated Hb, COHb = carboxyhaemoglobin, MetHb = methaemoglobin, SulphHb = sulphaemoglobin.

Functional Saturation (S_aO_2)

Ratio of oxyhaemoglobin to all Hb capable of combining with O_2.

In a normal individual with negligible COHb and MetHb, the $FO_2Hb \cong SaO_2$ and the pulse oximeter reflects both. If there are high quantities of COHb or MetHb, a CO-oximeter will report the reduced FO_2Hb correctly, but the standard

A. McLintic · A. Wong (✉)
Epsom Anaesthesia, Auckland, New Zealand

C. Birch et al. (eds.), *Physics and Measurement for Anesthesia*,
https://doi.org/10.1007/978-3-031-65060-4_8

two-wavelength pulse oximeter will malfunction and cannot report FO_2Hb or SaO_2 accurately:

$$SaO_2 = \left[(O_2Hb)/(O_2Hb + RHb)\right]$$

Principles of Light Absorption

Lambert Law

Intensity of light transmitted through a solution of known concentration decreases exponentially with increasing length of the path that the light travels through.

Beer's Law

Intensity of light transmitted at a known distance through a solution decreases exponentially with increasing concentration of absorptive substance.

Beer-Lambert Equation

$$I_t = I_o e^{-Ecd}$$

I_o = Intensity of incident light, I_t = Intensity of transmitted light, c = Concentration, d = Length of path, E = Extinction coefficient. Quantifies the tendency of a given solute to absorb light.

Key Points in Design

Light Sources Are Usually Light-Emitting Diodes (LEDs)

LEDs are semiconductors containing electron 'holes'. Electrons from the flow of electrical current fill these 'holes' and release photons.

Light Shone at Two Wavelengths

- Red (660 nm). Reduced Hb (RHb) main absorber
- Infrared (940 nm). O_2Hb main absorber
  The wavelengths may vary a little between machines. Most pulse oximeters use only two wavelengths, but some have several and may include an isosbestic wavelength where absorption of O_2Hb and RHb is equal (~810 nm, Fig. 8.1).

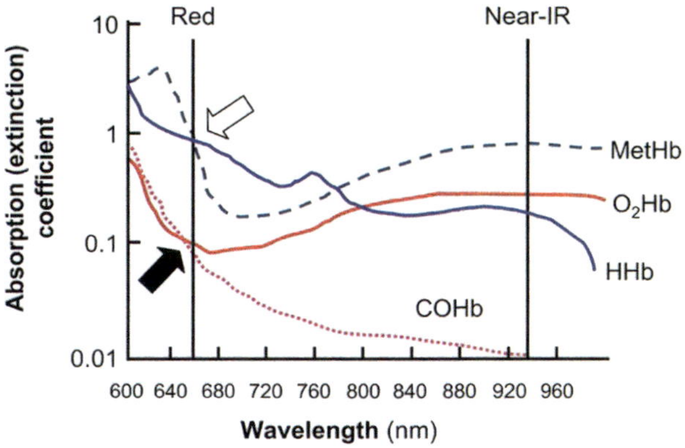

Fig. 8.1 Light absorption

LEDs Activated Sequentially

Sequential activation is followed by period off to measure ambient light component. The frequency of activation cycle varies between machines. Figures from 100 to 1000 Hz are quoted.

Intensity of Transmitted Light Measured by Photodetectors

- Photodiode detectors:
  - Photodiodes are semiconductors. A current is generated by photons being absorbed into the semiconductor.
- Thermopile photodetector:
  - Mass of tiny thermocouples on a small pad with the measuring junctions all pointing in the same direction. The transmitted light warms the junction and creates a measurable voltage across the thermocouples.

In both types of detectors, the greater the absorbance, the lower their output.

Processing the Signal: AC and DC Absorption

- AC refers to the absorbance of light by the pulsatile arterial component. This is what we are mostly interested in (Fig. 8.2).
- DC refers to the non-pulsatile absorbance by venous blood and tissues.
- The AC component is usually no more than 1% of DC component, so functionality is easily disrupted by poor peripheral perfusion.

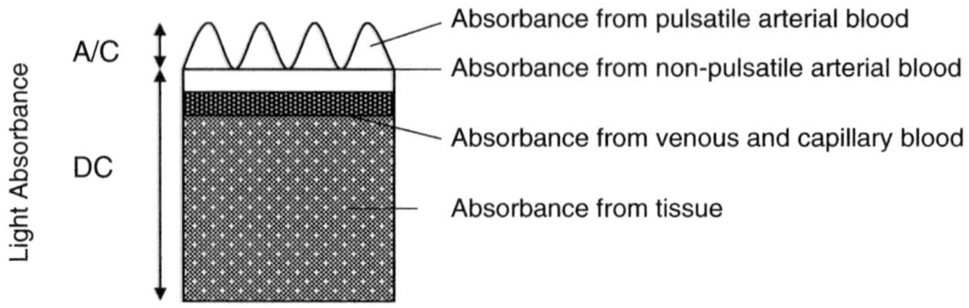

Note: Diagram not to scale. In reality the AC component is ~ 1% of the DC component.

Fig. 8.2 AC and DC Signal Components

Fig. 8.3 *R* value and SpO2

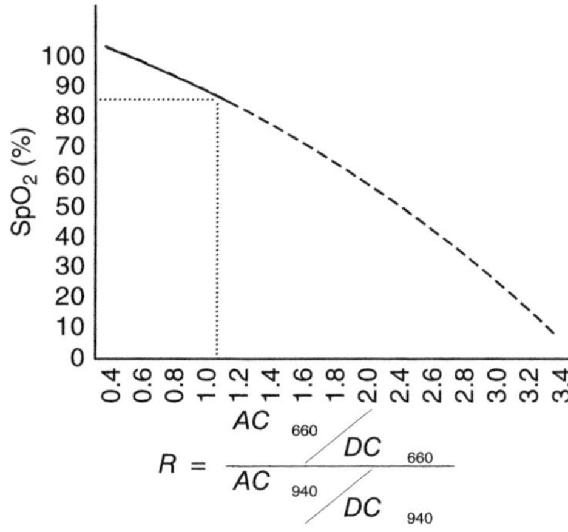

Processing the Signal: AC/DC Ratio

The AC component is the most important, but it is the scaled ratios of AC/DC for each wavelength that are used in the calculation. Scaling accounts for variation in the intensity of the LED output

Calculation of the R Value

$$R = \frac{ac660 / dc660}{ac940 / dc940}$$

The *R* value is used to determine the SpO2. The *R* value has a curvilinear relationship with a calibration curve based on experimental data from healthy human volunteers. Most experimental calibration points are between 80 and 100%. Values below that are extrapolated from the higher readings and are subject to error.

When the absorbance is equal at 660 nm and 940 nm, the R value becomes 1.0 and the estimated SaO_2 is 85% (Fig. 8.3).

In a normal individual with <1% RHb, the absorption by HbO_2 of 940 nm light dominates. This means that R is towards its lower values, where SaO_2 is the highest. As desaturation occurs, the proportion of RHb increases and absorption of light at 660 nm by RHb increases. This increases the R value and decreases the estimated value of SaO_2.

Types of Oximeters

Transmission Pulse Oximeters

Light passes through finger or earlobe and is picked up on the other side. Most are designed as above, but some may have multiple wavelengths and the ability to detect COHb and MetHb. The Masimo Rad-57 emits eight wavelengths.

Reflection Oximetry

The light source and detector are on the same side. Scattering results in weaker, less accurate signal, countered by the surrounding light sources by detectors and/or using multiple wavelengths.

Pulmonary artery mixed venous oximetry and neonatal oximeters are often this type.

CO-Oximeters

CO-oximeters are laboratory devices using multiple wavelengths and have the capability to detect several haemoglobin species.

Problems and Inaccuracies with Pulse Oximeters

Intrinsic Accuracy

- ±2% above 70%
- ±5% between 50 and 70% SaO_2
- Most very inaccurate below 70%.

Delay

Delay due to signal averaging and processing. This delay can be significant and can be up to 20–30 s in some monitoring units.

Patient Factors

Poor Peripheral Perfusion, Movement

This may occur with vasoconstriction, elderly or patients with peripheral vascular disease. Loss of AC component tends to force *R* value towards 1.0 and the saturation towards 85%. Similar effects are seen with movement or shivering.

Venous Engorgement

This may result in the underestimation of SaO_2.

Tricuspid incompetence causes peripheral venous pulsation and can cause underestimation of SaO_2.

Carboxyhaemoglobin

Overestimation of SaO_2.

CO has 250 times the affinity for RHb as O_2. This results in reduced O_2Hb and reduced RHb.

COHb absorbs identically to O_2Hb at 660 nm, so the *R* value is maintained despite hypoxia, thus overreading.

Because of the high affinity of CO for RHb, RHb is quantitatively reduced as well, and this reduces RHb absorption at 660 nm. This can decrease the numerator of the *R* value, contributing to overreading.

Methaemoglobin

Usually underestimation of SaO_2 but more correctly drives the value towards 85%.

Methaemoglobin absorbs strongly at both 600 nm and 940 nm resulting in an R value that trends towards 1.0.

Sulphaemogobin

This has a similar effect to methaemoglobin but milder. May occur with dapsone, sulphonamides, nitrates and metoclopramide.

Foetal Hb

Absorbances of red and near-IR light by HbF are the same as adult Hb, so pulse oximeter measurements are as reliable in newborn as in adults.

HbF may be misread as COHb by older CO-oximeters, thus spuriously lowering foetal O_2Hb.

Hyperbilirubinaemia

Pulse oximeter is unaffected.

Some CO-oximeters may artefactually elevate MetHb and COHb in the presence of hyperbilirubinaemia. Their estimation of fractional SaO_2 is thus artefactually reduced.

Sickle Haemoglobin

Should have little effect on pulse oximetry but difficult to confirm experimentally.

Methylene Blue

Underestimation of SaO_2.

Absorbs strongly at ~660 nm (668 nm) resulting in increase in R value mimicking hypoxia.

Indocyanine Green

Less absorption than above. Minor reduction in reading.

Nail Polish

Variable effect but may produce falsely low readings with dark opaque polishes.

Reduction of Signal/Noise Ratio

- Reduced peripheral perfusion.
- Probe malpositioning particularly if the emitted light just grazes fingertip (penumbra effect).
- *R* value tends towards 1.0.
- Ambient light is absorbed by photodetectors; hence, LED has off period to measure background component.
- Electrosurgery: Electromagnetic radiation from ESU may be picked up by the oximetry cabling and cause severe artefact.
- Severe anaemia may reduce S/N ratio or complete loss of signal.

Near-Infrared Cerebral Oximetry

What Is it?

Emerging technology to determine the regional haemoglobin oxygen saturation in the sub-surface cerebral tissue.

Principle

Two wavelengths of infrared light (~730 and 810 nm).

Two surface detectors positioned to detect shallow and deeper signals.

The shallow data is subtracted from the deeper to leave only deeper signals.

This spatial resolution allows the ability to localise the deeper areas of interest.

Absorbance data is from both venous and arterial blood in a 3:1 ratio.

Inferences

- Provides data about the balance or imbalance of oxygen supply and demand.
- Reflects venous oxygen reserve.
- Oxygen remaining after extraction by tissues and vital organs.
- Thus, early detection of regional ischaemia.
- rSO_2 baseline about 75%.
- Alarm limits may be set (if <55%, may indicate regional ischaemia).
- Clinical applications are increasing including cardiac surgery, coronary bypass, hypothermic arrest, vascular (carotid) surgery and neonatal paediatrics.

Gas Analysis

9

Alan McLintic and Julian Dimech

Gas Analysis in Anaesthetic Breathing Systems

In clinical anaesthesia, it is imperative to measure both the fraction of inspired oxygen present in patient breathing systems (see chapter on oxygen analysis) and a variety of other inspired and expired gas elements. Aside from oxygen, gases of particular clinical interest are carbon dioxide, nitrous oxide, volatile anaesthetic gases and carbon monoxide. The majority of gas analysers in anaesthetic breathing systems exploit physical principles of infrared absorption in order to perform measurements of patient gas mixtures.

Infrared and Infrared Gas Analysis

Infrared (IR) (sometimes referred to as infrared light) is an electromagnetic radiation with wavelengths longer than those of visible light, typically ~780 nm–1 mm. As such, IR is not visible to the human eye. Within this broad wavelength range, three sub-ranges are also recognised: near IR (~780 nm–2.5 μm), mid-IR (~2.5–50 μm) and far IR (~50–1000 μm).

The key physical principle behind infrared gas analysis is the fact that infrared is absorbed by polyatomic molecules with dissimilar atoms. Molecules with an asymmetrical configuration vibrate, producing a changing dipole (charge distribution) across the molecule making it susceptible to the absorption of infrared.

A. McLintic
Department of Anaesthesia and Pain Medicine, Counties Manukau Health, Auckland, New Zealand

J. Dimech (✉)
Anaesthesia & Pain Medicine, Middlemore Hospital, Auckland, New Zealand

C. Birch et al. (eds.), *Physics and Measurement for Anesthesia*,
https://doi.org/10.1007/978-3-031-65060-4_9

Table 9.1 Wavelength of IR absorption by gases of anaesthetic interest

Gas	Wavelength of peak IR absorption
CO_2	4.28 μm
N_2O	4.5 μm
Volatile anaesthetic gases	3.3–12 μm
CO	4.7 μm

The precise wavelength of IR absorbed by any molecule is specific to the characteristics of the molecular structure and its vibration frequency; see Table 9.1. It is this molecular quality which is exploited in IR analysis and identification of anaesthetic gases. Additionally, total light absorption is a function of the number of molecules encountered by the light, and, since the number of molecules present determines the partial pressure of a particular gas, the IR analyser measures partial pressure.

Wavelengths of IR are absorbed by some gases of particular anaesthetic interest. All wavelengths fall within the 'mid-IR' range.

Physical Principles of Light Absorption

Light attenuates as it traverses a medium. The amount of attenuation which occurs is described by two laws (Lambert's law and Beer's law), which are often combined and referred to as the Beer-Lambert law.

Lambert's Law

This states that the intensity of light transmitted through a solution of known concentration decreases exponentially with **length** of the light path.

Beer's Law

Beer's law states that the intensity of light transmitted at a known distance through a solution decreases exponentially with the **concentration** of the solution.

The Beer-Lambert Equation

When combined, the above laws can be given as the Beer-Lambert equation:

The Beer-Lambert equation:

$$I_t = I_o e^{-Ecd} \tag{9.1}$$

where I_o = intensity of incident light, I_t = intensity of transmitted light, c = concentration of solution, d = length of light path through medium and E = extinction coefficient. The extinction coefficient quantifies the tendency of a given solute to absorb light.

The majority of anaesthetic gas analysis is performed using machines which employ this equation in their analytical process. The equation is not valid for all circumstances however, and there are a number of conditions or assumptions made when using this equation:

- The attenuating factors must act independently; there should be no electromagnetic coupling. In solutions of high concentration, solute particles interact with each other and interfere with light absorption.
- The Beer-Lambert law also assumes that no fluorescence occurs and that the attenuating medium should be homogenous in nature.
- All light traversing the medium should have parallel rays, which travel the same length through the sample, and the sample medium should not cause scattering of light.

Practical Measurement Issues

When wanting to analyse patient gas samples, there are two practical issues to consider: obtaining a sample of gas for analysis, and obtaining IR of sufficiently large and specific number of wavelengths to be confident of component identification in a mixed gas sample.

Gas samples for analysis can be obtained from the 'main stream' (main stream analysers) of gas from which the patient is breathing or from a sample drawn down a side channel off the main stream, hence called 'side stream' analysers.

In order to provide IR with several discrete wavelengths with which to interrogate gas samples, analysers use dispersive or non-dispersive techniques.

Mainstream Versus Side Stream Analysis

Main Stream Analysers

Main stream analysers are placed within the breathing circuit, as close as possible to the patient (e.g. Capnostat 5). Historically, these devices were limited to the measurement of carbon dioxide only, since the analysis device must be small and light enough to sit within the main gas stream of the breathing circuit. Newer devices are, however, able to use micro-spinning disc technology to achieve the analysis of nitrous oxide, anaesthetic volatile agents as well as carbon dioxide (IRMA, Phasein).

Since the analysis device is present in the breathing circuit and not located distantly, there is no sample transfer delay and analysis occurs very quickly. The response time is entirely 'rise time' (see below) and is typically <60 ms for the Capnostat 5 device. However, being located in this position does require additional connections to be made within the circuit, increasing disconnection risks, and also subjects these devices to interference from water vapour. To combat the latter issue, the cuvette window used for analysis can be coated with water-repellent material or heated. Typically, the sample cuvettes are disposable in order to separate patient gases from the analyser per se. A calibration with air is required prior to use.

Side Stream Analysers

Side stream analysers are located remotely from the patient, and so a sample of gas needs to be drawn to the analyser. The sample line is usually 1.2 mm diameter

Teflon tubing, which is impervious to CO_2. The flow of gas drawn from the patient circuit to the analyser is approximately 200 mL/min. With the analysis occurring remotely from the patient, size and weight are less critical. Side stream analysers typically possess multi-gas analysis capability and undergo self-calibration.

The total response time of side stream analysers to a change in gas concentration at the patient end is typically 3–4 s and is composed of two delays.

Total response time = transit time + rise time:

- The transit time (sometimes referred to as 'lag time') is the time taken for the sample to reach the analyser, which depends on the tubing length, diameter and flow rate. Typically, the transit time is the more significant component of the total response time for side stream analysers (~3 s).
- Rise time: This is the time the analyser takes to interrogate the sample and is in the order of 300–500 ms.

Disadvantages of side stream analysers include the response delay, potential for sampling line obstruction, leaks, loss of ~200 mL/min of gas from the circuit and requirement for scavenging or return to circuit of the sample gas volume. The sampling rate may also limit closed-flow circuit use. Furthermore, in paediatric cases where an infant's flow rate is close to the sampling rate, the expired gas may be contaminated by inspiratory gases.

Non-dispersive Versus Dispersive Analysers

Non-dispersive Analysers

Most anaesthetic gas analysers are non-dispersive side stream analysers. IR is selectively filtered into multiple discrete wavelengths, each carefully selected to correspond to the absorption band of a gas of interest. Figure 9.1 illustrates the key structural elements of a non-dispersive analyser.

Dispersive Analysers

Instead of filtering to specific wavelengths, IR is diffracted into a spectrum and the full spectrum is analysed. The spectrum produced by this technique will contain absorption bands characteristic of all gases present. Analysis occurs at multiple points along the spectrum and is compared with a built-in algorithm. This technique is less common in anaesthetic practice but is used in the Andros/Luma Sense 4800 analyser.

Key Elements of a Typical Anaesthetic IR Gas Analyser

Most commonly used gas analysers are side stream, non-dispersive, multi-gas IR analysers. They are used for monitoring CO_2, N_2O and volatile anaesthetic agents. Usually, there are no moving parts. The IR beam is divided and passes through fixed optical filters. An alternative design has multiple filters on a spinning disc. The single beam is interrupted by this disc and is sequentially filtered into different wavelengths as the disc spins.

The following outline is based on a typical non-dispersive, multi-gas IR analyser such as the Datex TPX.

Infrared Source

A light-emitting diode (see oximetry) or heated tungsten wire is used as a source of IR as these are able to emit IR with a wide range of wavelengths. The light is pulsed rather than continuous as this prevents the sensor from heating up, which could result in base line drift.

Sample Chamber

The gas sample, drawn from the circuit, passes through a small analysis chamber with sapphire windows (glass absorbs IR, so cannot be used). The mixture of gases present in the sample chamber absorbs IR, each gas absorbing a specific wavelength of IR according to its unique molecular properties. Some models have a second air-filled reference chamber.

Filters

The light emerging from the chamber is filtered into several wavelengths (seven in the Datex TPX analyser) by optical filters, which may be placed between the IR source and sample chamber or between the analysis chamber and detector depending on design. There is at least one filter that produces a reference wavelength where there is little or no absorption. (See Table 9.1 for the wavelengths of peak IR absorption by different gases of interest.)

Detectors

A detector for each of the filtered wavelengths is present at the sensor end of the device. Photodiodes or thermopiles (see section on oximetry) are often used for

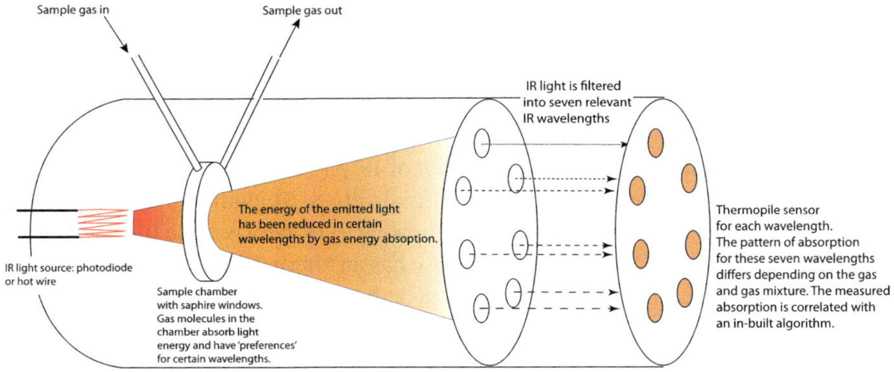

Fig. 9.1 A schematic representation of a non-dispersive side stream analyser. See text below for a more detailed description of how a typical non-dispersive, multi-gas IR analyser such as the Datex TPX works

detection, although a variety of different types of detectors can also be used. These include lead selenide photodetectors which are semiconductors whose electrical resistance decreases with incident photons from IR light. Older techniques utilise the Luft cell detector where transmitted light warms a gas-filled cell, raising its pressure. Because the light is pulsed, pressure rises and falls creating an oscillation which can be picked up by microphone.

Analysis

It is important to remember that the energy reaching the detector is the energy remaining after absorption by gases in the sample chamber. The more gas molecules present, the greater the absorption will occur, and output from detectors falls. Each gas absorbs light with a characteristic absorption spectrum (see Table 9.1), and the relative absorption at each of the seven wavelengths is correlated with expected data for each gas in an in-built algorithm.

Variations of IR Gas Analysis Techniques

A variety of alternate configurations exist in the design of multi-gas analysers. One variation used by Dräger (Dräger ILCA IR monitor) is based on the use of a pulsed infrared source and multispectral detector as described above. The design variation is that IR passes through the sample chamber, and emerging IR is reflected into four beams travelling in different directions, as illustrated in Fig. 9.2.

The four IR beams pass through filters with very narrow wavelength filters, specific to maximum absorption patterns for CO_2, N_2O and volatiles (a reference module is also included). These filters allow transmission of a specific wavelength IR to reach a pyroelectric detector. The sample flow rate needed for this device is 200 mL/min, and there are no moving parts. This analysis method does not suffer from interference from the presence of water vapour, ethanol or acetone, which can be issues in other analysers (ethanol absorbs IR with wavelengths of 1.4–10 μm).

Another variation on gas analyser design uses a rotational filter wheel to interrupt the IR beam (see Fig. 9.3). Although less common in Australasia, examples of this type of analyser are the PHASEIN ISA and Artema AION (both side stream analysers), and the PHASEIN IRMA which is a main stream analyser with micro-discs.

In these rotational devices, a single beam of IR passes through a rapidly rotating wheel containing a large number of filters (typically 8–9), with one or two of these being reference filters. The rotating disc is opaque to IR between the filter windows, and so the IR emerging from the rotating disc has an alternating wavelength with the reference filters absorbing little, if any IR. The beam then passes through a sample chamber and on to a single detector, with the reference filter beam enabling the detector to return to baseline/reference levels frequently. The IR absorption at each wavelength is determined and correlated with inbuilt algorithm.

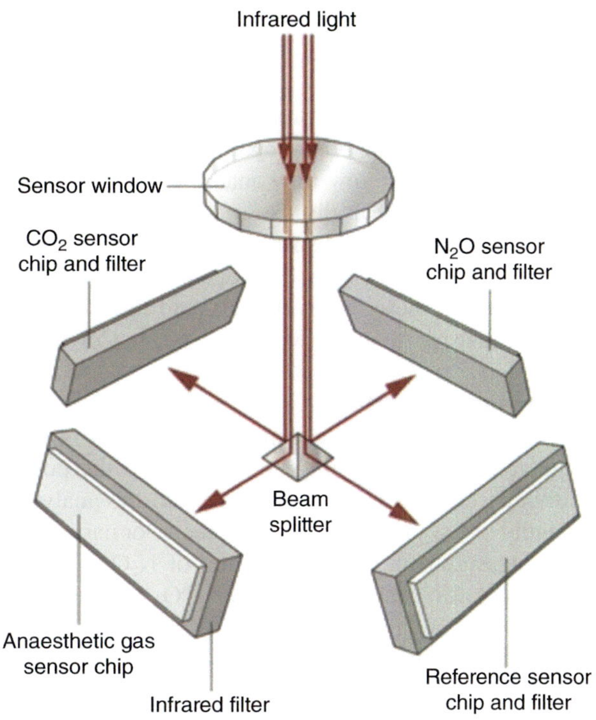

Fig. 9.2 A schematic representation of how the Dräger ILA IR gas analyser works

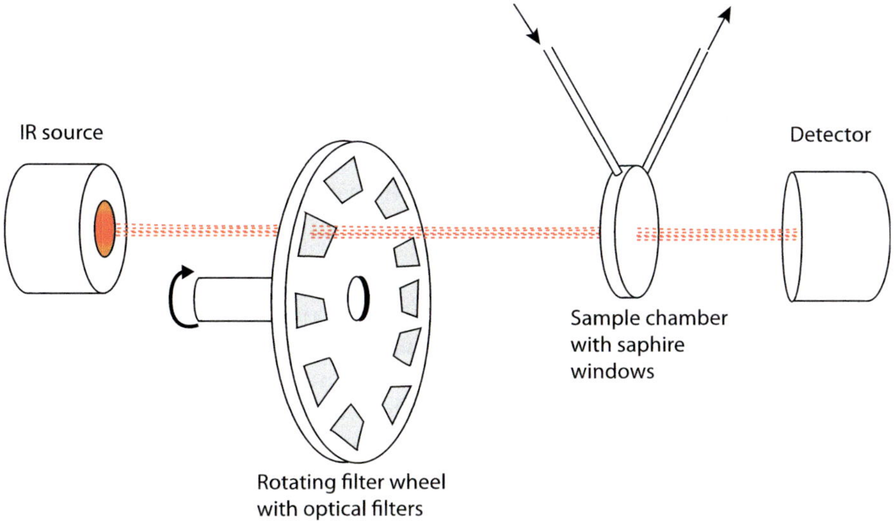

Fig. 9.3 Diagrammatic representation of a gas analyser which uses a rotational disc filter system (e.g. PHASEIN ISA)

Technical Challenges with Conventional Side Stream Gas Analysers

Side stream analysers are prone to a time delay in response to signal step changes at the patient end of the breathing circuit, as outlined above. The additional issues of sample flow rate on low-flow anaesthesia and potential impact on paediatric practice have already been discussed above. The general risks of sample tubing problems (disconnections, obstructions, leaks, scavenging/return of sample gas) have also been discussed above. The technical challenges with side stream analysers are not limited to these issues though, and there are some potential sources of error worth noting, particularly with reference to CO_2 analysis.

Wavelength Overlap

N_2O and CO_2 absorb IR at similar wavelengths (4.28 μm and 4.5 μm, respectively). Thus, a sample containing both gases has the potential to cause analysis errors. Although only an issue if N_2O is used, the analyser displays an artificially high quantity of CO_2. Using extremely precise or narrow-band IR filters will help prevent this. Measurement of concentration of N_2O with the introduction of a correction factor will also enable more precise CO_2 analysis.

Collision Broadening

The IR absorption spectrum of CO_2 can be broadened over a wider range of wavelengths than should normally be the case simply by the presence of other gases in the sample mixture. This occurs because *intermolecular* forces are able to alter the internal energy and dipole of the CO_2 molecule. A variety of other gases are able to exert this effect, including many which may be in the patients' breathing circuit, e.g. O_2, N_2 and N_2O. The magnitude of this effect can be reasonably significant, with CO_2 readings increasing by 10% when in the presence of 50% N_2O. This can be a difficult problem to resolve, although measuring the background gases independently and then compensating for them in the analysis should prevent large errors.

Water Vapour

Water and secretions absorb IR and may falsely increase reading CO_2 as well as damaging the instrument; this is an issue since most sample line tubing is Teflon (which is impermeable to carbon dioxide) and can result in condensation within the sample lumen. Water traps and/or filters may help to overcome this issue. An alternative semipermeable tubing which allows water to evaporate to the surrounding air is also available (NormoLine tubing, Masimo).

Atmospheric Pressure (Adjustment for ATPS Back to BTPS)

Side stream analysers measure dry samples which are usually reported as ambient temperature, pressure and dry (ATPD). At BTPS (body temperature, pressure, water vapour saturated), the alveolar PCO_2 is approximately 2.5 mmHg (~0.33 kPa) lower and can be calculated from the following equation:

To adjust the analysed pCO_2 (ATPD) back to alveolar value (kPa):

$$pCO_{2(BTPS)} = pCO_{2(ATPD)} \times \left(P_{ATM} - 6.3\right) / P_{ATM}$$

Photoacoustic Spectrometry

Although this technique uses IR for gas analysis, its practical use is in atmosphere trace gas analysis and not in contemporary anaesthetic gas monitoring. Only an overview of the technique is given here. The incident IR is divided into separate beams, which are directed through a filter wheel, creating beams of specific wavelengths. These beams are then pulsed, such that beams with different wavelengths also have different pulse frequencies. The pulsed beams enter the sample chamber, and gases absorb differing amounts of IR. The gases absorb IR and become warmer and increase in pressure. Because the light is pulsed at wavelength-specific frequencies, the chamber vibrates at a mixture of frequencies depending on the gas identities which are picked up by microphone and amplified. The frequency of vibration identifies the gas, and the amplitude is inversely related to concentration. A simple analogy would be that this is like listening to an orchestra and picking out the pitches and volumes of different instruments.

Non-infrared Methods of Gas Analysis

Chemical Colourimetry

This simple technique is used by devices such as the Covidien Easy Cap II for confirmation of tracheal intubation. Colourimetry relies on the fact that CO_2 is acidic in solution, so pH-sensitive dyes can be used to detect and measure its presence. pH paper impregnated with metacresol purple changes colour from purple to yellow in the presence of dissolved CO_2, with the degree of colour change related to CO_2 concentration. The colour change reverses back to purple on inspiration. Observing the variation with the respiratory cycle is important when distinguishing from malfunction or contamination. This is a lightweight, main stream (rapid response) device. It is only semi-quantitative as the colour change can be calibrated to an approximate pH value. Neither numerical display of CO_2 concentration nor display of CO_2 waveforms is possible. Additionally, it has the potential for false positives if gastric distension with air prior to intubation is achieved. Reflux of gastric contents may also limit functionality due to the acidity of gastric secretions.

Mass Spectrometry

A mass spectrometer separates components of a gas mixture according to their mass/charge (m/z) ratio. Mass spectrometers are typically large, heavy and expensive devices. Although smaller more portable devices are available, accuracy of analysis is compromised a little, and while larger units can be used as a central multiplexed analyser for a theatre suite, they will not provide continuous capnometry. They are not widely used in clinical anaesthesia.

There are four key components to mass spectrometry: ionisation, acceleration, deflection and collection/detection. Figure 9.4 illustrates the schematic design and function of a mass spectrometer.

During ionisation, a small portion of the gas sample is sucked into the analyser and passes through an ionising beam of electrons. The ionising (high energy) electrons knock electrons off the sample molecules, causing the sample molecules to become positively charged (usually +1).

- An oxygen molecule with a molecular mass of 32 having had one electron removed would therefore have an m/z ratio of 32/1 = 32.
- If two electrons were knocked off the oxygen molecule, the m/z ratio would be 32/2 = 16.

The ions formed in this manner are then accelerated forwards using positively charged plates. As the ions accelerate, they traverse a magnetic field, causing them to change direction (deflect) in accordance to their mass/charge (m/z) ratio. As ions

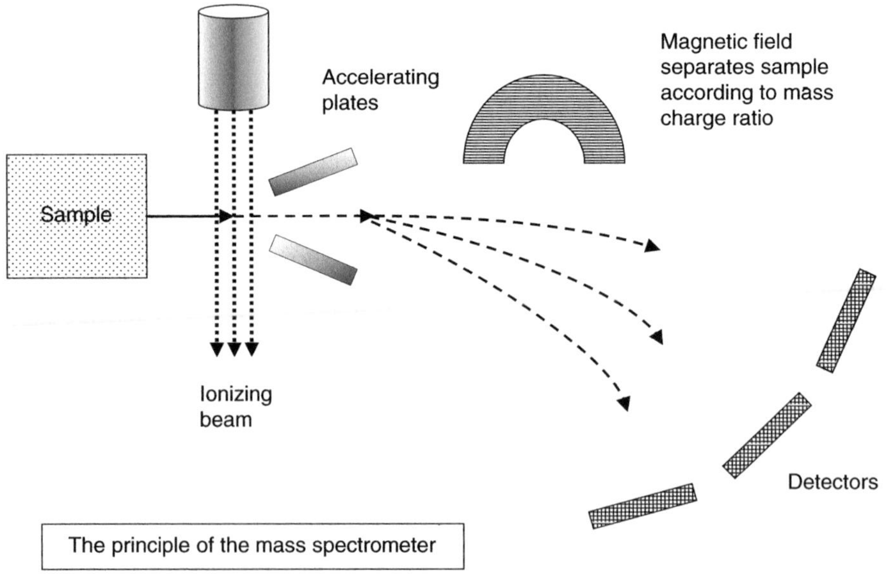

Fig. 9.4 Schematic diagram to illustrate how a mass spectrometer works

are relatively unstable, there will also be a breakdown of large parent molecules into smaller ion fragments.

Most ions produced have a + 1 charge so they are principally deflected according to mass rather than charge. Gas emerging from the magnetic field will therefore form several rays; those with ions of smaller mass will have greater deflection, while those with the heavier ions will be deflected least.

The positively charged ions hit metal plates specific to each mass/charge ratio and create a voltage on that detection plate. The voltage generated is proportional to the quantity of ions striking the detection plate. The total voltage produced is assumed to be 100% of the gas mixture. Each individual voltage collected at a particular plate is a fraction of that total which, if multiplied by atmospheric pressure, is the partial pressure of that component gas. Strictly speaking therefore, the mass spectrometer measures volumes per cent (vol%) rather than partial pressure although the latter can be deduced.

Technical Challenges with Mass Spectrometry

Molecules with the Same Molecular Weight

Ionisation of the sample molecules can result in fragmentation of some gases. The 'parent' gas often fragments in a particular manner, producing characteristic fragmentation patterns, which helps to identify the parent molecule and to distinguish it from molecules which have the same molecular weight. If a collector detects an ion that has exactly half the mass/charge ratio of another, it is probable that it is the same molecule or molecule fragment but with a + 2 charge.

Other Limitations on Use

These are large, expensive machines and when used for gas analysis are located some way from individual patient equipment. This means that they are subject to significant delays that are not suitable for breath-by-breath analysis. Furthermore, some knowledge of the gas mixture is required in order to identify individual components as the device will only identify molecules it has been set for. Lastly, the ionised gases must be discarded safely.

There are four key components to mass spectrometry: ionisation, acceleration, deflection and collection/detection (Fig. 9.4).

Quadrupole Mass Filter

A quadrupole mass filter is broadly similar to a mass spectrometer, but the ionised beam passes through a quadrupole mass filter which has four rods carrying electrical charges alternating at specific radiofrequencies. By alternating the frequency and charge on these rods, ions can be allowed to pass through to the detector, while others undergo increasing oscillation, hit the rods and lose their charge. Molecules with different mass can therefore be separated in this manner.

Gas-Liquid Chromatography

Gas-liquid chromatography (GLC) is an analytic technique used to measure blood anaesthetic concentrations in the lab, or atmospheric concentrations of gases. It is not used for monitoring anaesthetic gas concentrations in clinical practice.

The principle of GLC is that solute (gas) molecules will separate or partition out between two solvents according to the balance of attractive and repulsive forces between the solute and solvents.

Sample mixtures are vaporised and carried in an inert phase, usually helium or argon. This mobile phase is then passed over a stationary phase, typically a column of silica-alumina covered in silicone oil. Separation of the gas (solute) molecules depends on the partition coefficients between mobile and stationary phases.

Molecules with poor solubility and high volatility pass through the column rapidly and appear at the outlet first, while highly soluble components of the mixture appear last. While separation of gases within mixtures is possible, the technique does not per se identify the individual components; an additional process, usually mass spectrometry or thermal conductivity detection (see below), is required to so.

Katharometer

This technique, illustrated in Fig. 9.5, is often combined with GLC and provides identification of the separated solutes from the output of GLC. It is based on the observation that thermal conductivity (TC), a measure of a substance's ability to conduct heat, is specific to the substance. Katharometry is often used with GLC since the thermal conductivity of the carrier gas helium is very high, meaning that other gases in the mixture are easily detectable as they have TC less than the carrier gas.

The diagram illustrates the key features of a katharometer. Reference and sample chambers contain heated wires connected to a Wheatstone bridge measuring their electrical resistance. The reference chamber usually contains helium only, with the analysis chamber containing both helium and sample gas. Gases with high thermal conductivity will cool a heated wire to a greater degree than a gas with low thermal

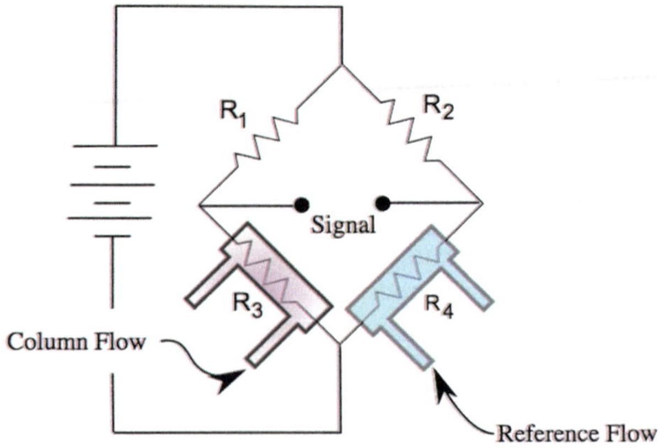

Fig. 9.5 Schematic design of the key elements of a katharometric device

conductivity, and the higher the concentration of gas, the greater the cooling effect. The cooling effect results in a lower electrical resistance across the wire, and this is measured with a Wheatstone bridge. Temperature and gas flow are controlled, so that differences in electrical resistance between the chambers are due to helium concentration differences. Applications include measurement of inert gases such as helium and xenon, diving and anaesthesia.

Ultrasound Gas Analyser

The speed of sound through a gas depends on the temperature of the sample and the concentration of gas molecules present (see chapter on ultrasound for more details on the speed of sound in different media). In a mixture of two gases, the concentration of both gases is relevant. If the composition of one gas changes, the speed of sound will also change. These analysers are therefore ideal to use where binary mixtures of gases are concerned and where the nature of gases is known, so that devices can be calibrated for the relevant speed of sound through each component gas. Temperature and pressure must be controlled. Ultrasound waves pass through a fixed length column, which has a detection chamber at the other end. Time is recorded, and the difference in time taken for sound to traverse the sample chamber is dependent on the variable component gas concentration.

Laser Analysers

Using a similar principle to infrared analysis, the intensity of helium-argon light can be measured after absorption by a gas. Devices can be used for CO_2 and alcohol detection.

Nitrogen Meter

Using a gas discharge tube (a gas-filled tube containing two electrodes), the detection and measurement of nitrogen are possible using the principle of emission of electromagnetic radiation. This may be of clinical interest when anatomic dead space in the lung is measured using Fowler's method (nitrogen washout).

A sample of gas is drawn through a discharge tube between the ionising electrodes. The gas glows, with the specific wavelength of the emitted radiation being characteristic of the gas. For nitrogen, this gas sample glows purple. Using a photocell detector, the intensity of emitted radiation is measured and is related to concentration. The detection method is specific and fast but not suitable for gas mixtures.

Nitric Oxide Sensors

Therapeutic inhaled nitric oxide is used in intensive care units, particularly for neonatal respiratory support. Very small amounts are needed for therapeutic benefit (0–40 parts per million), so nitric oxide measurement is critical. Fuel cell analysers or chemiluminescence techniques are commonly used.

Nitric Oxide Fuel Cell

These fuel cells follow the same principles used in an oxygen fuel cell. Electrochemical changes in the cell are detected and displayed using amperometry. Nitric oxide passes over a nanoporous electrode and loses electrons to it, creating a current through an electrolyte to a reference electrode with the resulting current directly proportional to the concentration of nitric oxide.

Chemiluminescence

Luminescence occurs when molecules or atoms are excited to higher energies and, on returning to their ground state, lose energy by emitting photons of light.

Fluorescence occurs when molecules are excited to higher energies by absorbing light or other electromagnetic radiation. The emitted light usually has a lower energy and longer wavelength than the absorbed energy.

Where a chemical reaction rather than electromagnetic radiation transfers energy to molecules and results in light emission, the process is termed chemiluminescence.

When trying to measure nitric oxide, a chemical reaction with ozone occurs producing an energised form of nitrogen dioxide according to the following equation:

$$NO + O_3 \rightarrow O_2 + NO_2 [\Diamond]$$

where NO = nitric oxide, O_3 = ozone, O_2 = oxygen and NO_2 [$\diamond$] = energised nitric oxide.

The energised nitric oxide releases photons of light with wavelengths of between 590 and 2600 nm[9] with the photons being released in proportion to the concentration of nitric oxide present. A photodetector measures the intensity of the light emitted.

Raman Spectroscopy

This technique can also be used to identify molecules and requires a high-intensity monochromatic light source such as an argon or helium-neon laser. Devices using this technique have historically been used as anaesthetic agent monitors (Ohmeda Rascal anaesthetic agent monitor). They are portable and able to provide accurate, rapid, breath-to-breath analysis of multi-gas samples. They are, however, expensive and unsuitable for monoatomic gases and have a high energy requirement.

Raman Scattering

When a photon of light penetrates a particle that is much smaller than the wavelength of the incident photon, the kinetic energy (and wavelength) of the photon is conserved, but its direction changes. This is a type of elastic scattering referred to as Rayleigh scattering and accounts for the overwhelming majority of scattering interactions between photons and particles.

Raman scattering is a type of inelastic scattering where a photon of light penetrates a particle, putting it temporarily into an excited state before being emitted. The photon is emitted with reduced energy and a longer wavelength. The wavelength shift is specific to the molecule, and the number of photons hitting the detector is a function of the concentration of the sample molecule. Only a very small number, maybe as few as 1 per 10^7 molecules in a sample, will scatter light in this way.

Although asymmetrical (e.g. CO_2) and symmetrical (e.g. O_2) molecules produce Raman scattering, monoatomic gases (e.g. He, Xe, Ar) do not. Raman scattered light is of very low intensity, and detectors must be placed perpendicular to the light beam for recording purposes.

Piezoelectric Gas Analyser

This technique has been used to measure volatile anaesthetic agent concentration (Engstrom Emma gas analyser). The technique is no longer in general use, and so only a brief outline of the concept is included here.

An electrical current is applied across two piezoelectric crystals causing them to resonate (see chapter on ultrasound). One crystal is covered in silicone oil, which causes the two crystals to resonate at different frequencies. When exposed to an anaesthetic agent, the volatile is absorbed into the oil causing the frequency of the oiled crystal to change. The frequency shift is dependent on the volatile concentration.

Ultraviolet Light Absorption

All gases absorb ultraviolet light, so this absorption technique may be used for those which do not absorb in the IR spectrum, e.g. N_2, O_2 and H_2. Historically, this technique was used in anaesthesia (Penlon Halothane monitor), but halothane exposed to UV brakes down into bromide and hydrochloric acid, and these compounds cannot be returned to the patient breathing circuit. This technique is no longer widely used in anaesthesia, but is of commercial interest in atmospheric or other gas analysis.

Interferometry/Riken Refractometer

Superimposing waves (of any kind) will cause interference. Interferometry is a technique where deliberately superimposed waves are analysed and information about them is extracted. Interferometry was famously used to try and detect alterations in the speed of light in the Michelson-Morley experiments and more recently to detect gravitational waves.

The principle of interferometry is that the velocity of light through a gas is dependent on the number of gas molecules present. Consider the refractive index of light, which is defined as the ratio of the speed of light in a vacuum divided by the velocity of light in the medium:

Refractive index of X = Velocity of light through vacuum / Velocity of light through X

Note that the denominator is dependent on the number of molecules of gas X and therefore the temperature and pressure of X.

The Riken refractometer has been used to check the calibration of vaporisers and is a device which exploits this principle. In a Riken refractometer, two beams of light from the same source are focused onto a screen and allowed to overlap. The result is a fringe pattern of light with both light and dark bands. Light bands occur where the two beams are in phase; in these bands, light has travelled the same distance or is out of phase by whole wavelength. Dark bands are where the beams are out of phase by 180° (see Figs. 9.6 and 9.7).

The refractometer has both a reference and sample chamber, with a beam passing through each chamber. The interference pattern is calibrated by noting the pattern of air occurring in both chambers. The gas to be analysed is then aspirated into the sample chamber causing the velocity of light in this chamber to reduce and the interference fringe to shift. The degree of the shift is related to the concentration of the gas and is read from a previously calibrated scale.

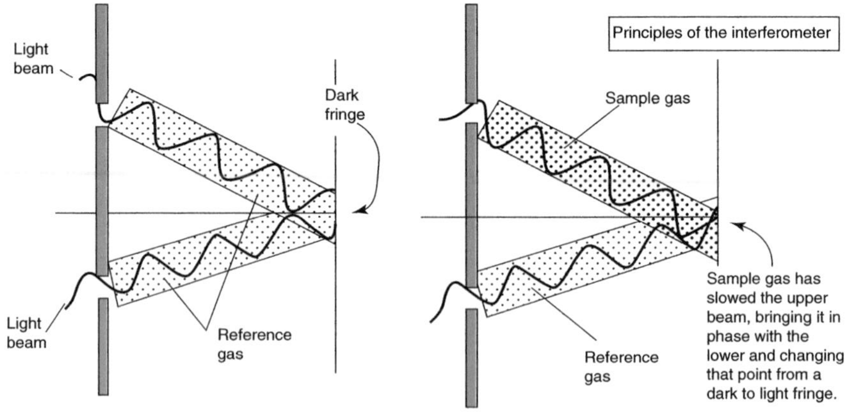

Fig. 9.6 ScheSchematic to represent the principle of interferometry as used in a Riken refractometer

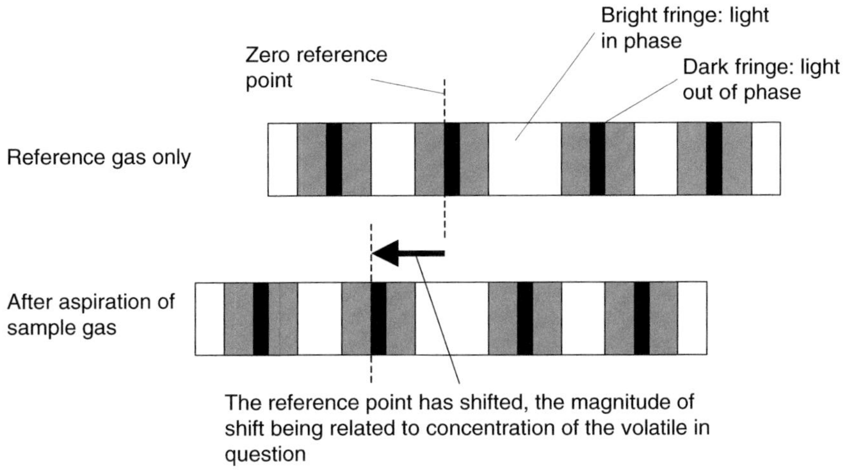

Fig. 9.7 A characteristic image of the light and dark interference bands created by interference

Further Reading

Davey AJ, Diba A. Ward's anaesthetic equipment. 6th ed. Edinburgh: Elsevier; 2012.

Ehrenwerth J, Eisenkraft JB. Anesthesia equipment: principles and applications. Philadelphia: Saunders; 2013.

King R, Bretland M, Wilkes A, Dingley J. Xenon measurement in breathing systems: a comparison of ultrasonic and thermal conductivity methods. Anaesthesia. 2005;60(12):1226–30.

Oxygen Measurement

10

Alan McLintic and Julian Dimech

Oxygen Measurement

Do Clinical Devices Measure Partial Pressure or Concentration of O_2?

When quantifying oxygen in patient breathing or anaesthetic systems, devices are mostly concerned with oxygen concentration (expressed as % volume). However, the measurement of amount of oxygen present in most of the devices mentioned below is dependent on the number of oxygen molecules present. Thus, the measurement relates to partial pressure of O_2, rather than the number of molecules per given volume. It is therefore more correct to acknowledge that oxygen analysis devices measure partial pressure but are calibrated to read concentration.

There are three techniques (some with subcategories) that are commonly used in the measurement of oxygen partial pressure within anaesthesia: paramagnetic analysis, electrochemical analysis and ultrasound. Older 'dumbbell on filament' type paramagnetic analysers are no longer used in contemporary anaesthesia.

Paramagnetic Analysis

The differential pressure paramagnetic analyser is the standard method of measuring the partial pressure of oxygen in anaesthetic breathing systems. Typically, the sample gas is drawn from a circle breathing system via a side stream sample line from the circle system.

A. McLintic
Department of Anaesthesia and Pain Medicine, Counties Manukau Health, Auckland, New Zealand

J. Dimech (✉)
Anaesthesia & Pain Medicine, Middlemore Hospital, Auckland, New Zealand

C. Birch et al. (eds.), *Physics and Measurement for Anesthesia*,
https://doi.org/10.1007/978-3-031-65060-4_10

Paramagnetic and Diamagnetic Substances

Paramagnetic substances are those which contain unpaired electrons in the outer shell of their atom or molecules. The presence of an unpaired electron results in an unopposed spin and magnetic moment (torque produced in a magnetic field) across the atom/molecule, and the molecule is therefore able to orientate with an externally applied magnetic field. Many substances including oxygen and nitric oxide are paramagnetic.

In diamagnetic substances, all electrons are paired in the atom or molecule. Paired electrons spin in opposing orientations, such that when spinning within their shells, their magnetic moments cancel each other out. Thus, diamagnetic substances repel magnetic fields. Nitrous oxide and nitrogen are diamagnetic.

Differential Pressure Paramagnetic Analyser

A schematic diagram of a paramagnetic gas analyser is shown in Fig. 10.1. In these analysers, a sample gas and reference (air; 21% oxygen) are drawn into the analyser in two separate channels separated by a diaphragm pressure transducer, which measures the difference in pressure between the two channels. Both these channels also pass through an electromagnet that switches on and off at very high frequency (~150 Hz).

When the electromagnet is on, the oxygen molecules in the channels are immediately attracted into the magnetic field. This creates a pressure drop behind onrushing molecules, and, if there is a difference in oxygen partial pressure between the two channels, the pressure transducer registers a pressure difference that is proportional to the oxygen partial pressure difference between the sample and reference gases.

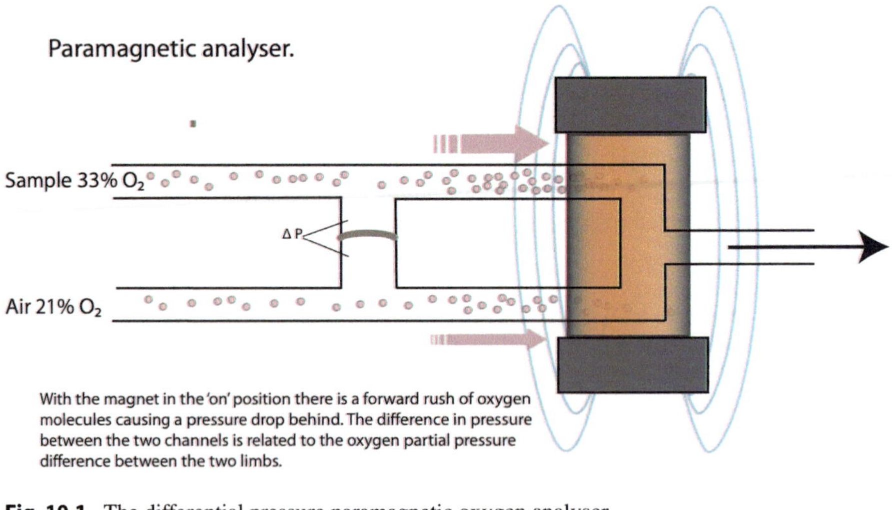

Fig. 10.1 The differential pressure paramagnetic oxygen analyser

The system pressures reset when the magnet is switched off, and as this is happening at very high frequency, the transducer registers an oscillating pressure whose magnitude is related to the oxygen partial pressure difference between sample and air. Although the device is sensitive to partial pressure oxygen differences, for practical reasons, the readout is recalibrated to volume per cent.

The differential pressure paramagnetic oxygen analyser is the standard method of measuring the partial pressure of oxygen in anaesthetic breathing systems. Its response time of around 150 ms enables breath-to-breath analyses for clinical applications and has the advantage of providing a linear response to the sample and is not affected by vibration (unlike older 'dumbbell on filament' design analysers). It does however require regular calibration.

The trans-diaphragmatic pressure changes are sensitive to temperature and water vapour changes, so the sample gas must be dry and temperature must be held constant.

If the analysed gas is returned to a closed or near-closed circuit, the reference air component will add nitrogen to the circuit. In contemporary side-stream modules (e.g. in Dräger Zeus), the analysed gas is often scavenged rather than returned. Since nitric oxide is also paramagnetic, this could theoretically cause over-reading, but therapeutic concentrations (~40 ppm) are far too low to make any impact.

Thermo-Paramagnetic Analysis

A variation or alternative to the above technique, based on thermal conductivity, is used by some oxygen analysers. These thermo-paramagnetic oxygen devices can be found on the Dräger Zeus, PIA and PATO machine. Figure 10.2 shows how these analysers work.

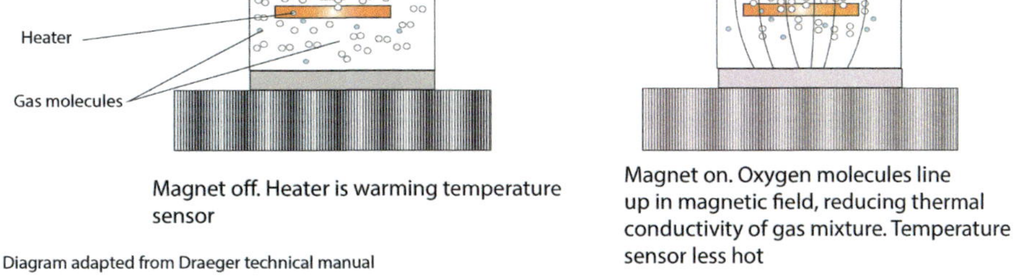

Fig. 10.2 The thermo-paramagnetic pressure oxygen analyser

A sample of gas is presented to a chamber, in which both a heating element and a temperature sensor lie in close proximity. A magnetic field is applied externally to the gas sample, which results in the redistribution of oxygen molecules in accordance with their paramagnetic behaviour. The movement of the oxygen molecules, lining up in the magnetic field, reduces the thermal conductivity of the gas mixture. The temperature sensor gains less heat when the magnet is on, compared to when the magnetic is off due to the reduction in thermal conductivity. The difference in thermal conductivity is proportional to the partial pressure of oxygen in the sample. This type of analyser also has a fast response rate, enabling breath-to-breath analysis, and has the added advantage of being self-calibrating using air, so there is no need for a reference sample. Both pressure and humidity need to be measured and controlled in order for proper calibration.

Electrochemical Cells

There are two common types of electrochemical cells used for the measurement of oxygen partial pressure, galvanic/voltaic cells and electrolytic cells.

Galvanic/voltaic cells are those in which a spontaneous chemical reaction occurs and generates electricity. They are often referred to as a fuel cell or battery. A diagram illustrating the electrochemical reactions occurring within the fuel cell is shown in Fig. 10.3.

Electrolytic cells require an electrical current to generate a chemical reaction.

Fuel Cell/Galvanic Cell

The spontaneous chemical reaction occurring in a fuel cell results in the generation of electrons at the anode. Oxygen captures the electrons at the cathode, and the

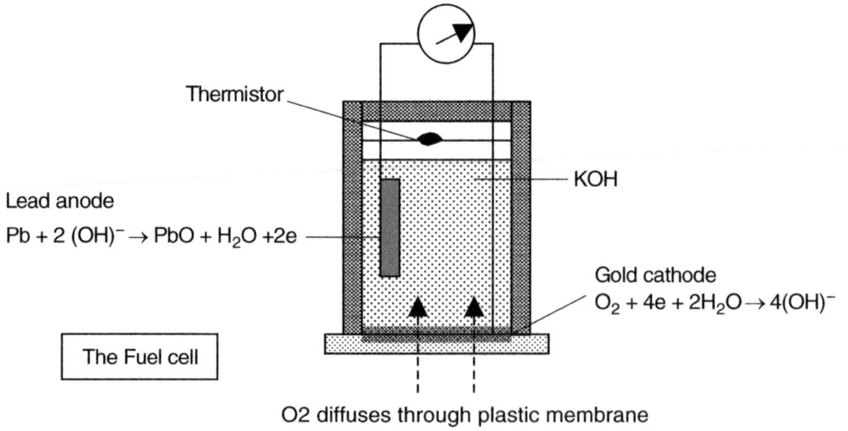

Fig. 10.3 The chemical reactions of a fuel cell used for oxygen analysis

resulting ionisation completes an electrical circuit, producing a current which is detectable. The magnitude of the current generated is proportional to the partial pressure of oxygen.

The standard fuel cell's response time is too slow for breath-to-breath oxygen monitoring of the patient breathing system gases although fuel cells are present in some ventilators for system gas analysis. Of note, the GE Aisys anaesthetic machine has a fuel cell behind the connection of the inspiratory limb of the circle, and some Dräger Zeus models have an internal fuel cell of a non-standard type (see below).

The fuel cell is a spontaneous oxidation/reduction ('redox') reaction, and devices usually measure current or occasionally voltage (potentiometry). At the lead anode, spontaneous oxidation occurs, with the electrons generated travelling to the gold cathode via an ammeter:

$$Pb + 2(OH)^- \rightarrow PbO + H_2O + 2e$$

At the cathode, the electrons reduce oxygen which has entered the fuel cell:

$$O_2 + 4e + 2H_2O \rightarrow 4(OH)^-$$

The more oxygen that enters, the more electrons are able to leave the cathode and generate greater current flow. The current produced is directly proportional to the partial pressure of oxygen at the gold cathode. Gold is not part of the chemical reaction; it merely acts as a 'springboard' for the electrons. The potassium hydroxide solution allows the hydroxide ions to complete the circuit by returning to the lead anode. A thermistor is required to control the temperature of the reaction, since chemical reactions are temperature dependant.

The main clinical issue with these devices is the slow (approximately 30 s) response time preventing breath-to-breath analysis. Additionally, the lead anode is slowly consumed over time, and (depending on the duration and amount of oxygen being used) replacement is usually required after a period of approximately 6 months.

Oxygen Electrode/Clark Electrode/Polarographic Electrode

The oxygen electrode (or Clark electrode, named after the American chemist Leyland Clark) is also sometimes referred to as a polarographic electrode. It finds applications in blood gas machine analysers and transcutaneous, intra-vascular and conjunctival sensors and was the basis for the first generation of glucose biosensors. Figure 10.4 illustrates the electrochemical reactions occurring in the oxygen electrode (see below).

Physical Principles

As an electrolytic cell, the functioning of this device requires an electric current to be applied before analysis is possible. While redox reactions do occur in these devices, they do not occur spontaneously.

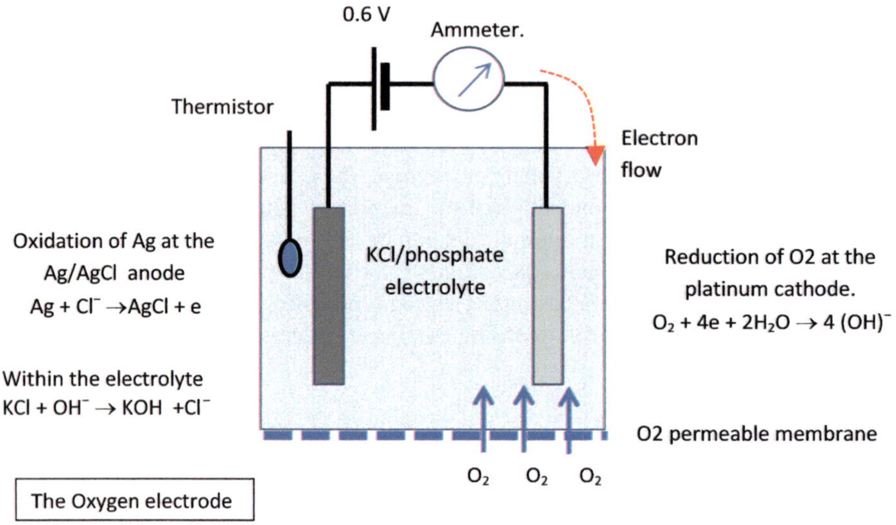

Fig. 10.4 The chemical reactions of the oxygen electrode/Clark electrode

A polarising voltage of between 0.6 and 0.8 V is typically applied, and consequently electrons move from the power source to a platinum cathode where oxygen diffusing into the cell is reduced.

At the cathode, oxygen is reduced producing hydroxyl ions:

$$O_2 + 4e + 2H_2O \rightarrow 4(OH)^-$$

which are able to disperse within the potassium chloride electrolyte and according to the equation below release free chloride ions which migrate to the anode.

Within the electrolyte, the following reaction occurs:

$$4KCl + 4OH^- \rightarrow 4KOH + 4Cl^-$$

While at the anode, electrons are provided by the oxidation of a silver anode, according to the simplified equation below:

$$4Ag + 4Cl^- \rightarrow 4AgCl + 4e^-$$

The resulting current flow is linear and proportional to oxygen partial pressure at the cathode.

The oxygen electrode has a response time faster than that of a fuel cell (around 10–20 s) but still too slow for breath-to-breath analysis in anaesthetic breathing systems. The chemical reaction is temperature dependant and must therefore be controlled. The electrode requires regular maintenance and calibration and must be kept clean of protein deposits; to this end, the electrode compartment is separated from blood or other tissues by the presence of a thin plastic membrane covering the platinum electrode.

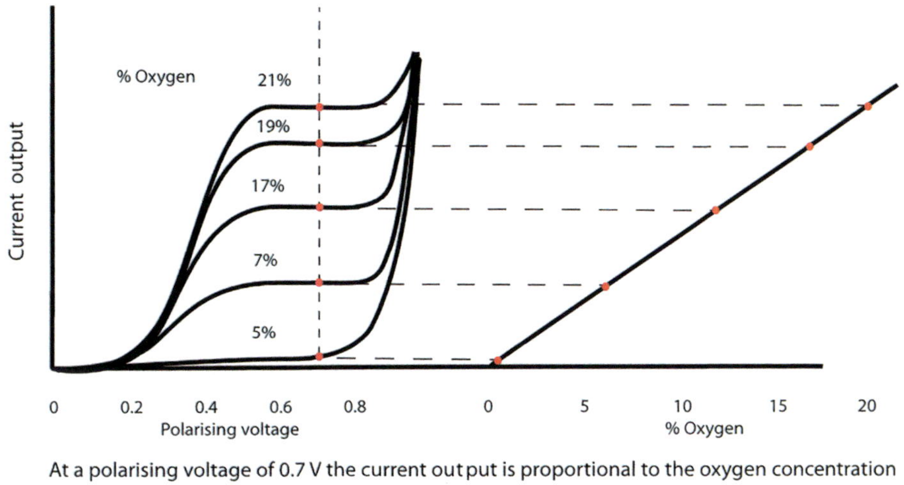

Fig. 10.5 Current output plotted against polarising voltages in an oxygen electrode with a selection of samples containing different oxygen concentrations

A potential of between 0.6 and 0.8 V is used by the electrode because in this range all oxygen molecules reaching the cathode are reduced meaning that the current which results is proportional to the oxygen tension at the cathode. See Fig. 10.5.

Oxygen Pump Electrochemical Cell

This is an additional type of electrochemical cell, used on some Dräger model anaesthetic machines to measure oxygen levels in the inspiratory limb (*OxyTrace A* sensor used in Dräger Zeus). It uses three electrodes, a cathode and anode as well as a reference electrode.

A controlled voltage is applied across the cathode and reference electrodes to facilitate the reduction of oxygen as it enters the cell. As oxygen diffuses in, it is reduced at the cathode according to the equation

$$O_2 + 4H^+ + 4e- \rightarrow 2H_2O$$

Electrolysis of water occurs at the anode which releases H^+ ions:

$$2H_2O \rightarrow 4H^+ + O_2 + 4e-$$

These are able to move through an electrolyte and across a gas-impermeable membrane to be consumed at the cathode.

The movement of electrons from anode to cathode in the external circuit is measured as current, and its magnitude is related to the oxygen partial pressure at the cathode. Oxygen formed at the anode is vented from the cell, hence the term O_2 pump. This type of analyser is faster than both fuel cell and oxygen electrode, with response times of less than 1 s possible.

Ultrasound Measurement of Oxygen Concentration

This is an uncommonly used technique for oxygen analysis, and it is only practicable when the identity of a single gas or binary gas mixtures under examination is known, for example, air/O_2, N_2O/O_2, He/O_2 and Xe/O_2 mixtures. The Maquet Servo-i ventilator utilises this technique in the inspiratory limb as did the Gem 9100 anaesthesia machine.

The use of ultrasound for oxygen analysis is possible since, at a given temperature, the speed of sound through a gas is dependant on the combined molecular weight and heat capacity of the gas. In a varying binary gas mixture of oxygen and nitrogen (air + oxygen), each mixture ratio has its own unique speed of sound without overlap. Thus, changing the amount of oxygen in the mixture alters the speed of sound through the sample in a predictable manner.

The analysis is conducted in a side channel measurement chamber with two ultrasound transducers: a transmitter and a receiver. The time measured for an ultrasonic pulse to travel over a given distance in the air/oxygen mixture is recorded, and the speed of sound can be calculated. Knowing the molecular weight and heat capacity of oxygen enables the conversion of this time measurement to an oxygen concentration.

Further Reading

Davey AJ, Diba A. Ward's anaesthetic equipment, 6th ed. Edinburgh: Elsevier; 2012.

pH and CO_2 Electrodes

11

Alan McLintic and Matthew Taylor

What Is pH?

The "potential" or "power of hydrogen" (pH) is a dimensionless measure of the acidity or alkalinity of a solution. pH is dependent on the H^+ activity, which itself is dependent on the hydrogen ion concentration and temperature:

$$pH = -\log_{10}\left[H^+\right]$$

The pH scale is an inverse logarithmic representation of $[H^+]$. In a neutral solution with a pH of 7, there are 10 million (10^7) fewer hydrogen ions than there would be in a solution with pH 1. Whilst pH is typically referred to having a range from 0 to 14, extremely strong acids and alkali can have values outside of this.

At 25 °C, aqueous solutions with a pH <7 are considered acidic and those with pH >7 are considered basic (alkaline). The pH decreases as temperature increases due to the increased dissociation of H_2O into H^+ and OH^-. As these are balanced, it does not actually change the overall "acidity" of the solution as the pOH changes in proportion to the pH and thus there is no excess of $[H^+]$ over $[OH^-]$.

A solution's pH can be measured using colour or potentiometric methods. Colour-based systems utilise organic pigments that alter colour in response to pH change. These may be "read" visually to a reference chart or through a photometric process using transmitted light.

A. McLintic · M. Taylor (✉)
Department of Anaesthesia and Pain Medicine, Counties Manukau Health, Auckland, New Zealand
e-mail: Matthew.Taylor@middlemore.com

C. Birch et al. (eds.), *Physics and Measurement for Anesthesia*,
https://doi.org/10.1007/978-3-031-65060-4_11

pH Electrode

The pH electrode is a device that utilises a redox reaction to transduce the [H^+] into a voltage change, hence "potentiometric". A "pH-sensitive glass filter" on an electrode is placed in contact with a solution and compared with a non-selective reference electrode also in the solution. H^+ ions will effectively travel across this glass down their concentration gradient until balanced by the electrical potential generated that resists the movement. The voltmeter measuring this potential is designed to have very high impedance to increase its sensitivity to H^+ interactions at the glass. As seen in cell membranes, this process is described by the Nernst equation. Typically made of a Ag/AgCl half cell, the electrode ion concentrations and electrical potential are kept constant by having the metal in contact with its saturated chloride salt (AgCl) which is, in turn, in contact with a chloride solution (HCl). The HCl also buffers H^+ concentration between the electrode and the glass (Fig. 11.1).

The reference electrode is a salt bridge electrode connection used to complete the circuit. This enables us to measure the potential generated across the pH-sensitive glass. This reference electrode is in essence an advanced version of sticking a wire into the solution. A bare wire is impractical as doing this would result in unstable ionic reactions, thereby introducing significant error into the measurement. The reference electrode is Hg/Hg_2Cl_2 ("calomel") or Ag/AgCl metal in contact with its saturated chloride salt (Hg_2Cl_2 or AgCl) which is, in turn, in contact with a chloride solution (KCl). This makes indirect electrical contact with the blood via a porous plug containing KCl.

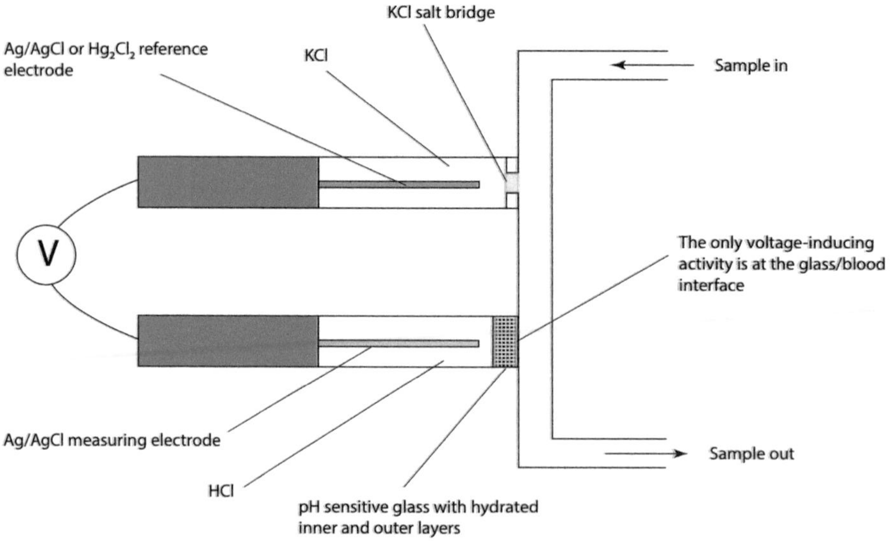

Fig. 11.1 Schematic of the pH electrode

pH-sensitive glass is typically silicon dioxide (SiO_2) that has been "doped" with metal ions such as lithium or sodium. The glass has an outer hydrated layer but is otherwise dry. The metal ions are free to move within both the wet and dry glass matrix by binding to free O^-. Hydrogen ions, on the other hand, can enter the hydrated layer but are unable to move within the dry glass component. Having entered the wet glass, the hydrogen ions bind to the oxygen of SiO_2. Na^+ then diffuses out of the dry glass into the wet glass in ion exchange. The difference in H^+ activity on each side of the glass causes a net movement of Na^+ across the glass, thereby transmitting the charge. Technically, it is therefore misleading to describe the glass as semi-permeable to H^+ ions. It is ion exchange and the net movement of Na^+ that is creating the voltage.

There are numerous variations in the above facts, particularly in the electrolyte solutions and electrode metals. The system is additionally sensitive to temperature as the dissociation of acids and bases increases with temperature. The electrode temperature is therefore kept constant at 37 °C. If a sample is taken from a hypothermic patient and analysed at 37 °C, there will be more dissociation in vitro than in vivo, and a correction factor (Rosenthal's correction factor) is required to adjust back to the patient's true temperature:

$$\mathrm{pH} = \mathrm{pH}_{(37^\circ\mathrm{C})} - 0.015 \times (\text{Body temp} - 37^\circ\mathrm{C})$$

The pH electrode, utilising redox ½ cell systems, is like a battery and runs down with time and use. Calibration with buffers of different pH is required on a regular basis. One buffer has a pH of 6.841, which is the pH of the measuring electrode buffer. This calibration provides an arbitrary zero. The other buffer, with pH of 7.383, establishes a calibration curve. At 37 °C, there is approximately 61.5 mV change per pH unit.

Other methods of measuring pH exist. The chemical colourimetry methods are often used in "test strip" lab or point-of-care situations but are also used in anaesthetic practice for $ETCO_2$ detection. There are a variety of indicators with differing reversible colour responses. Covidien Easy Cap II uses metacresol purple. Colour changes reversibly from purple to yellow with the reduced pH seen during exhalation and can confirm endotracheal tube placement. Colourimetry methods have also been developed for intravascular use.

Ion-sensitive field-effect transistor is a transistor in which the flow of current is controlled by a voltage applied across it. The voltage can be applied by a chemical reaction, and if that chemical reaction is pH dependent, the device can be used to measure pH. This is an alternative method to measure pH and was mentioned in an ANZCA examiner's SAQ report.

CO_2 Electrode (Severinghaus Electrode)

The Severinghaus electrode is used in blood gas machines to measure CO_2 tension and is a modification of the pH electrode. The electrodes used follow the same principles as outlined, but an additional component allows CO_2 from the blood to drive

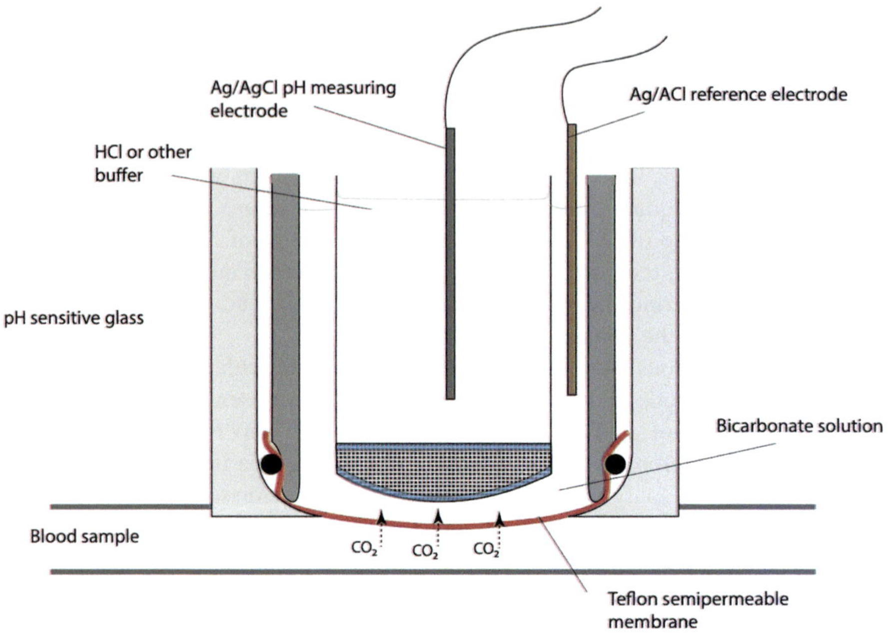

Fig. 11.2 Schematic of the CO_2/Severinghaus electrode

a pH change that is in turn detected by the electrode. This is achieved by immersing the pH-measuring electrode with its pH-sensitive glass in a solution of sodium bicarbonate, which is then separated from the blood sample by a Teflon membrane. The Teflon is permeable to CO_2 but not to water, H^+ or electrolytes. CO_2 moves across the membrane and dissolves in the bicarbonate solution, pushing the equilibrium to free up H^+ ions:

$$CO_2 + H_2O \Leftrightarrow H_2CO_3 \Leftrightarrow H^+ + HCO_3^-$$

The H+ ions react with the glass of the pH electrode producing a voltage. pH is linearly related to log PCO_2 allowing determination of the PCO_2.

As the reference electrode (incorporated in the electrode housing) is detecting the potential difference of [H+], it is referencing against (and therefore sits in) the bicarbonate solution. It is commonly an Ag/AgCl electrode. The electrode is regularly calibrated against CO_2 solutions and is maintained at 37 °C (Fig. 11.2).

Other Methods to Estimate PCO_2 in Blood

Estimation from $ETCO_2$

The difference is approximately 0.7 kPa in the normal lung but increases as dead space increases.

Rebreathing Technique

Patient rebreathes until gas in a bag is in equilibrium with mixed venous blood. Normally, the difference between arterial and venous PCO_2 is about 0.8 kPa, and this is subtracted from the bag PCO_2. Cardiac output must be normal.

Astrup Interpolation

There is a linear relationship between pH and log PCO_2. PCO_2 can, therefore, be estimated from pH if differences in buffer activity are accounted for. This was the method used to measure PCO_2 before the Severinghaus electrode became widely available. A sample of arterial blood is taken and divided into three aliquots, A, B and C. Samples A and B are equilibrated with two gases of different CO_2 concentrations. The pH of the two samples is then measured and plotted on the Siggaard-Andersen nomogram and a line drawn between them. The position and slope of the line are affected by the patient's organic and inorganic buffer activity. The pH of sample C is then measured and plotted on the line. The PCO_2 of that sample can then be read from the nomogram (Fig. 11.3).

What Determines the Position and Slope of the Buffering Line?

The slope is determined by the haemoglobin concentration. Increased [Hb] increases overall buffering capacity and steepens the slope. The lateral positioning of the line

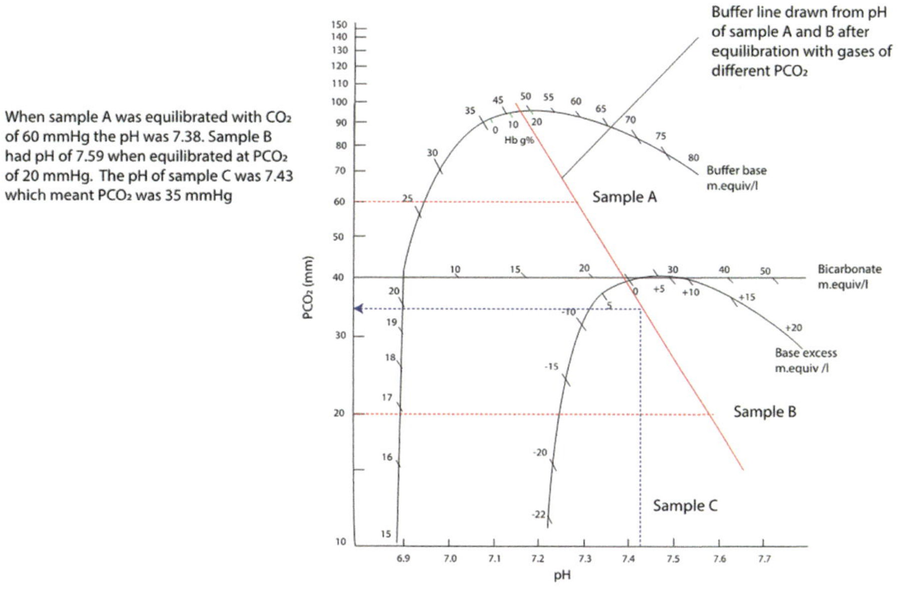

Fig. 11.3 Astrup interpolation of the Siggaard-Andersen nomogram

is determined by the metabolic component. Metabolic acidosis shifts line to the left, and metabolic alkalosis shifts the line to the right.

pH-Stat and Alpha-Stat

As described above, the dissociation of water into H^+ and OH^- varies with temperature. Similarly, many other biochemical processes including formation of HCO_3^- are temperature sensitive, which will result in a variation of pH and pH-sensitive reactions with body temperature. This is a consideration when managing deep hypothermia in paediatric and adult cardiac and aortic arch surgery. There remains debate about whether a pH-stat or alpha-stat strategy to manage blood gases during hypothermia is the optimal approach in preventing perioperative morbidity.

Blood gases of "normal" blood at 28 °C		
	In vivo values	Uncorrected values after warming to 37 °C in BG analyser
pH	7.5	7.4
pCO_2	28 mmHg	40 mmHg

Blood Gases During Hypothermia

The physiological changes in hypothermia are complex, and those that affect blood gases include:

- Decreased oxygen consumption.
- The solubility of gases increases, lowering their partial pressure.
- The dissociation of weak acids decreases, pK_a increases and there is alkalosis.
- The oxyhaemoglobin dissociation curve shifts to the left.
- CO_2 binding to Hb increases.

The net effect is that "normal" blood that is cooled to 28 °C has a pH and pCO_2 of around 7.5 and 28 mmHg, respectively. However, blood gas machines analyse blood samples at 37 °C, so an uncorrected read-out will show a pH and CO_2 of 7.4 mmHg and 40 mmHg, respectively. The question is do you accept the patient's alkalosis and pCO_2 status at hypothermia (alpha-stat) with the rationale that the physiological processes are changing in synchrony or do you ask for CO_2 to be added to the bypass pump to try and produce normal pH and pCO_2 in the hypothermic state (pH stat).

pH-Stat Strategy

Here, the pH is managed on temperature-corrected blood gases. CO_2 is added to the pump to maintain a pCO_2 of 40 mmHg during hypothermia. This is justified on the principle that post-bypass cerebral injury in infants is related to hypoperfusion rather than embolic phenomenon. Cerebral blood flow (CBF), perfusion and homogeneity of brain cooling are improved with the higher pCO_2 of pH-stat.

Alpha-Stat Strategy

Those adhering to alpha-stat do not add more CO_2. In mammals, the ionisation and function of protein buffers remain constant as temperature falls. This is due to the pKa of the α-imidazole group of histidine changing in synch with the rising pH as temperature drops. Protein function is, thus, optimum if the acid-base balance is allowed to vary naturally as temperature falls. This strategy is thought to best preserve adult perioperative myocardial function and reduce incidents of ventricular fibrillation. Additionally, the increased cerebral blood flow of pH-stat is not necessarily an advantage in adults, as stroke following CBP is embolic not ischaemic and increased CBF will not protect against emboli and may even worsen the embolic load. CBF should match cerebral oxygen consumption, which is reduced in hypothermia, and cerebral autoregulation is better preserved with an alpha-stat approach.

Numerous studies lend support to all the above without coming down definitively on one side or the other. As a general rule, pH-stat is more commonly employed in paediatric cardiac anaesthesia and alpha-stat in adult anaesthesia.

Measuring Temperature 12

Alan McLintic and Stacey Byers

What Is Temperature?

Temperature is the measure of the thermal energy of a substance. It is an indication of the kinetic energy possessed by the molecules.

Three scales of temperature measurement are in common use:

Celsius (°C)

- Most common scale
- Devised from the freezing and boiling points of water (at 1 atmosphere) with 100 intervening increments, called degrees:
  - Freezing point = 0 °C
  - Boiling point = 100 °C

Kelvin (K)

- A scale of temperature which starts at an absolute zero where matter contains no thermal energy and molecular movement stops.
- The Kelvin is one of the SI base units.
- One Kelvin has the same magnitude as one degree Celsius.
- The offset between Kelvin and Celsius is 273.15 °C:
  - Absolute zero = 0 K = −273.15 °C
  - Freezing point of water = 273.15 K = 0 °C

A. McLintic · S. Byers (✉)
Department of Anaesthesia and Pain Medicine, Counties Manukau Health, Auckland, New Zealand
e-mail: Stacey.Byers@middlemore.co.nz

C. Birch et al. (eds.), *Physics and Measurement for Anesthesia*,
https://doi.org/10.1007/978-3-031-65060-4_12

- It was calculated from the established direct relationship between the expansion of gas volume and increasing temperature. Once the coefficient of the relationship was established experimentally, it was possible to extrapolate down to the temperature at which all motion ceased.

Fahrenheit (°F)

- A scale initially devised from taking the temperature at which ice melts, and approximate body temperature, and dividing the intervening temperatures by 64 increments (degrees). A zero point was defined by the freezing temperature of a mixture of ice, water and ammonium chloride (0 °F).
- Hence:
  - Melting point of ice water = 32 °F
  - Approximate body temperature = 96 °F
  - Boiling point of water = 212 °F
- It is still in use today as the official temperature scale in the United States.

Classification of Devices

Devices which measure temperature can be broadly classified as non-electrical and electrical (see Table 12.1):

Non-electrical/Direct Reading

Liquid-Filled Manometers

- Liquid-filled columns with a vacuum above them for the liquid to expand into.
- Simple, linear.
- Mercury thermometers. Mercury freezes at −38.7 °C and boils at 357 °C.

Table 12.1 Classification of temperature measurement devices

Non-electrical/direct reading	
Liquid manometers	Mercury
	Alcohol
Bimetallic strip	
Bourdon gauge	
Chemical	
Electrical	
Resistance wire	
Thermistor	
Thermocouple	Including infrared via a thermopile
Diodes and transistors	

- Alcohol thermometers for lower temperatures. Alcohol freezes at −117 °C and boils at 78.5 °C.

Bimetallic Strip

- Two metals with different coefficients of expansion are stuck together. As temperature changes, the differing expansions cause the strip to bend and move a dial as per the diagram below (see Fig. 12.1).
- Remain in common use in numerous settings such as circuit breakers and thermostats.

Bourdon Gauge

- A steel coiled tube filled with gas.
- As temperature increases, the pressure rises internally (third gas law) and the coil straightens somewhat, thus driving a pointer (see Fig. 12.1).
- Modern applications remain common, e.g. industrial thermometers.

Chemical Methods

- Involve a 'change of state' of varying types:
- Melting dye strips—a strip that contains rolls of cells containing dye, which melts at a certain temperature. The higher the temperature, the more cells melt and the more dye is released.

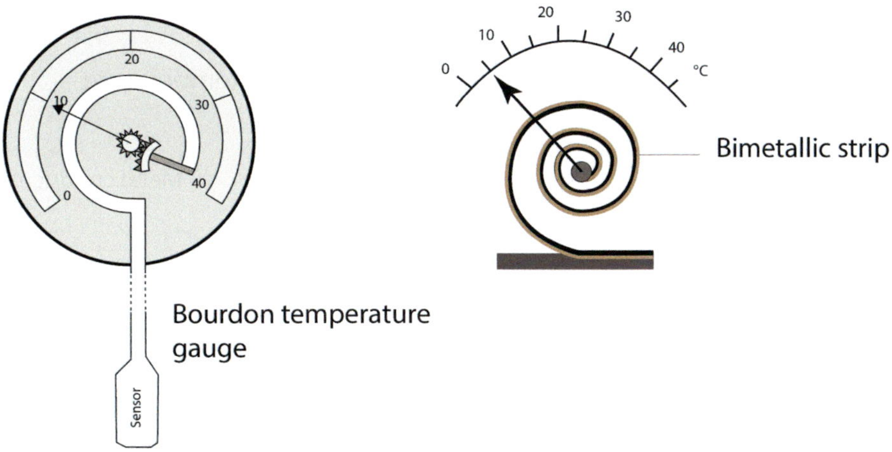

Fig. 12.1 The bourdon gauge (left) and bimetallic strip (right)

- Long-chain polymers—cells of different long-chain polymers whose optical properties (and therefore colour) change with temperature.
- Liquid crystal thermometers—cholesteric liquid crystals alter their 3D arrangement (and therefore their optical properties) in a temperature-dependent way.

Electrical Methods

Resistance Temperature Detectors (RTDs)

- A length of metal wire conductor whose electrical resistance varies almost linearly with temperature as per the diagram below (see Fig. 12.2).
- Usual metal is platinum but may also be nickel or copper.
- Resistance is then measured via Wheatstone bridge (see 'Electrical Principles').
- Very narrow diameter to improve response time but slower response time than thermistor or thermocouple.
- Range of industrial applications including infant incubators and dialysis machines.

Thermistor

- A metal oxide semiconductor (often in the form of a bead) whose resistance decreases exponentially with increasing temperature as per the diagram above. This is called a negative temperature coefficient thermistor (NTC thermistor) because of the curve's negative gradient.
- Oxide may be of cobalt, manganese, mercury, zinc or nickel.
- Greater change in resistance per unit change in temperature means more sensitive and rapid than the RTD and therefore ideal for measuring small changes in temperature rapidly, as required for continuous body temperature measurement.

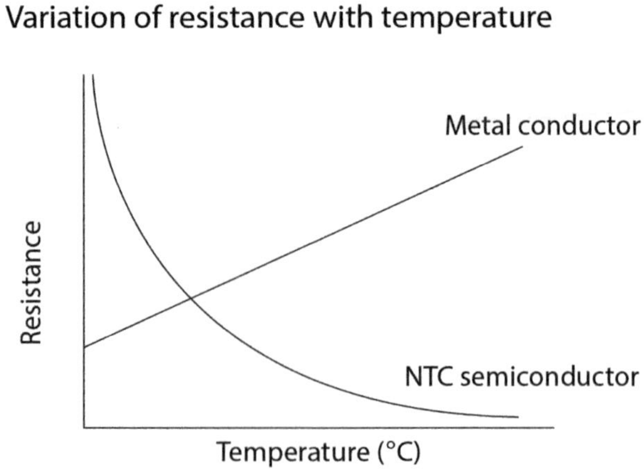

Fig. 12.2 Variation of resistance with temperature in metal and negative temperature coefficient (NTC) semiconductors

- Small and inexpensive.
- May exhibit some hysteresis but irrelevant over clinical range of temperatures.
- Resistance measured via Wheatstone bridge (see 'Electrical Principles').
- Most common technology in skin, bladder, rectal, intravascular and nasopharyngeal temperature sensors.

Thermocouple

- An electrical method of measuring temperature utilising the Seebeck effect.
- The Seebeck effect is the generation of an electromotive force from a temperature gradient in a conductor. This was originally demonstrated by an experiment involving two strips of dissimilar metals joined at both ends. When one junction was heated, magnetism could be detected, later found to be due to a current flowing in the circuit.
- Thermocouples vary in their design but have the following common features:
- Two dissimilar metals are joined at the ends, creating two junctions: the measuring junction and the reference junction (see Fig. 12.3).
- The measuring junction is the sensing tip of the probe.
- The reference junction must be kept at a constant temperature, e.g. by attaching to a heat sink (see 'Heat'), or alternatively, the temperature at the reference junction is monitored and appropriate compensation made in the calibration.
- A typical combination of metals is copper joined to a nickel alloy such as constantan (copper-nickel).
- At the junction between any two dissimilar metals, there is a flow of electrons from one metal to the other, and the flow varies with temperature. Thus, at the measuring junction, electrons flow from one metal to the other because of a potential difference between the two that is temperature dependent.
- If the reference junction is kept at constant temperature, a voltmeter can be placed across it and any change in voltage will be proportional to the temperature changes at the measuring junction (see diagram below).

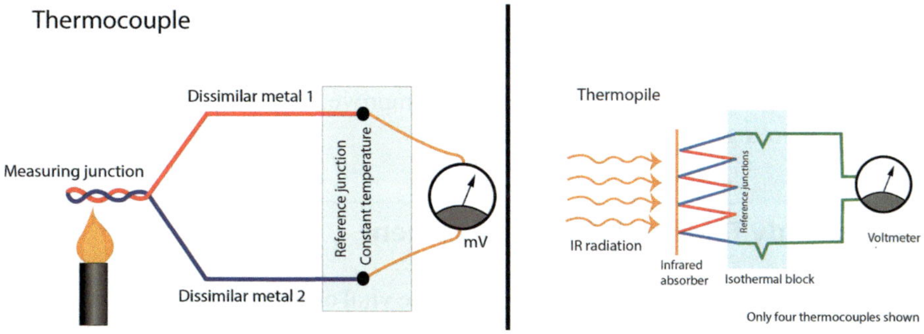

Fig. 12.3 Diagram of thermocouple (left) and thermopile (right)

- The voltage/temperature relationship is not necessarily linear, but near-linear over the required range.
- Thermocouples have a large range of industrial applications, suitable for measuring over large temperature ranges. Less suitable for measuring smaller temperature changes with accuracy.

Infrared Thermometers and Thermopiles

- Infrared thermometers measure infrared energy radiating from the tympanic membrane or skin. A laser dot is used to aim the instrument but is not, otherwise, involved in the measurement. The energy is detected by a thermopile.
- A thermopile detector is a mass of hundreds of thermocouples incorporated into a small mat of several square millimetres (see Fig. 12.3).
- The measuring junctions all point outwards and are warmed by the infrared energy emitted by the tympanic membrane.
- The reference junctions are connected to heat sinks.
- The electrical signal is then processed and displayed.
- The thermopile principle is also used in oximeters (see 'Pulse Oximetry') and infrared gas analysers (see 'Anaesthetic Vapour Analysis').

Diodes and Transistors

- Diodes are an electrical component through which current passes primarily in one direction between two terminals. They are generally made of semiconductors such as silicon or germanium.
- Silicon diodes can be used as temperature sensors because the current flowing across them varies with temperature.
- Transistors are semiconductor devices used to amplify or switch electronic signals within an electric circuit. Transistors can be added into the circuitry of a silicone diode to help convert the non-linear voltage–temperature relationship to a linear appearance.
- Silicone diode thermometers are less sensitive than thermistors and operate over a limited temperature range, traditionally limiting their applications (e.g. temperature sensors within small electrical appliances/computers). However, their low cost and advances in their circuitry to improve sensitivity and accuracy have seen their range of applications increase.

Site of Body Temperature Measurement

Core body temperature is the temperature of the vital organs (e.g. heart, brain, liver), but its estimate varies according to measurement site (see Table 12.2):

Table 12.2 Comparison of body temperature measurement site with core temperature

Measurement site	Temperature compared with core	Notes
Buccal	−0.2 to 0.4 °C	
Nasopharyngeal	≅Brain	Close to hypothalamus when sited posterior to soft palate
Tympanic membrane	≅Brain	Wax and obstructions decrease accuracy. Large variability in studies of correlation
Skin	−2 to 4 °C	Most studies show poor correlation with core
Axilla	−0.4 to 0.7 °C	
Lower oesophagus	−0.5 °C	
Rectum	≅ Core	Slow to equilibrate during anaesthesia
Pulmonary artery	≅Core	
Bladder	≅Core	

Further Reading

Dorsch J, Dorsch S. Chapter 24. Temperature monitoring and control. A practical approach to anesthesia equipment; 2010.

Guruswamy J, Omosule AJ. Chapter 13. Temperature monitoring. In: Ehrenwerth J, Eisenkraft J, Berry J, editors. Anesthesia equipment: principles and applications, 3rd ed. 2020. pp. 287–303. https://doi.org/10.1016/B978-0-323-67279-5.00013-3.

Measuring Humidity

13

Alan McLintic and Stacey Byers

What Is Absolute Humidity?

The mass of water vapour present in a given volume.

Usual units are either mg L^{-1} or g m^{-3} (values are the same).

Humidity at Saturation

The maximum amount of water vapour that can be carried in a cubic metre at a given temperature. In other words, the absolute humidity when saturated vapour pressure (SVP) is reached.Increases with temperature.The amount of water vapour that can exist in a given space is virtually independent of the other oxygen, nitrogen, etc. molecules of air present. A cubic metre vacuum will hold virtually the same amount of water vapour as a cubic metre of air at the same temperature. The determinant is the saturated vapour pressure which is, in turn, dependent on temperature (see Table 13.1 and Fig. 13.1).

A. McLintic · S. Byers (✉)
Department of Anaesthesia and Pain Medicine, Counties Manukau Health,
Auckland, New Zealand
e-mail: Stacey.Byers@middlemore.co.nz

C. Birch et al. (eds.), *Physics and Measurement for Anesthesia*,
https://doi.org/10.1007/978-3-031-65060-4_13

Table 13.1 Change in humidity and saturated vapour pressure with temperature

Temperature (°C)	Condition	Humidity at saturation ($g\ m^{-3}$)	SVP	
			mmHg	kPa
0	Freezing point	4.9	4.6	0.6
20	Room temperature	17	17.5	2.3
34	Trachea	38	40	5.3
37	Lung	44	47	6.3
99	Just below boiling at 1 atmosphere	570	734	97.8

Values can be checked at this website: https://www.aqua-calc.com/calculate/humidity

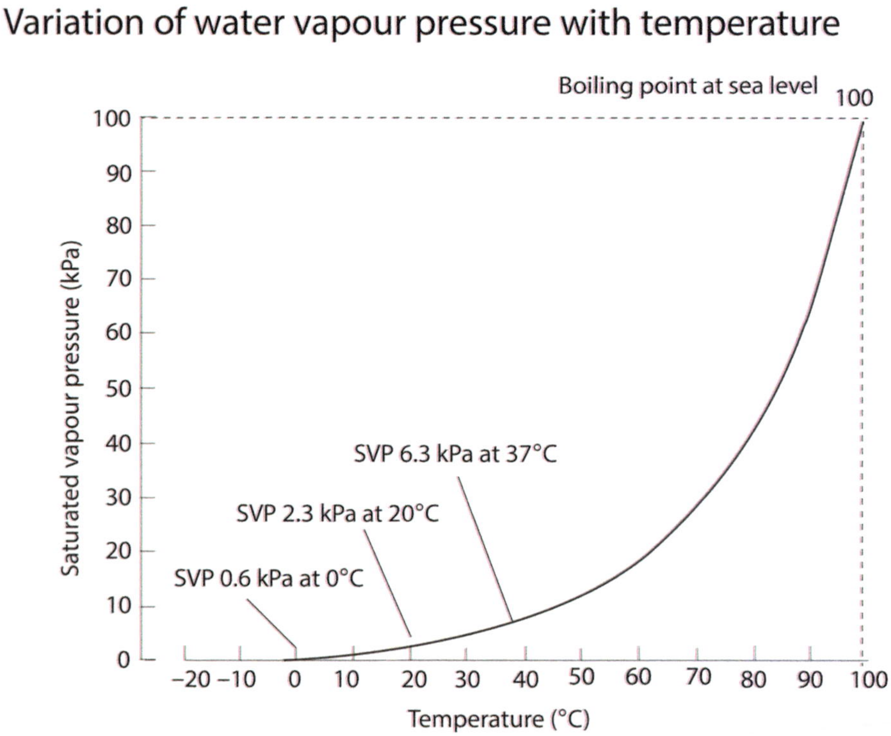

Fig. 13.1 Graph showing change in saturated vapour pressure (SVP) with temperature

What Is Relative Humidity?

The ratio of mass of water vapour in a given volume of air to the mass required to saturate it at the same temperature and pressure:

$$\text{Relative humidity} = \frac{\text{Mass present}}{\text{Mass to saturate}}$$

Because the pressure of a volume of gas or vapour at a given temperature is determined by the number of molecules, this relationship may also be expressed as the ratio of partial pressure of the water vapour to the saturated vapour pressure:

$$\text{Relative humidity} = \frac{\text{Vapour pressure}}{\text{Saturated vapour pressure}}$$

Relative humidity decreases with increasing temperature (because SVP increases with increasing temperature).

Relative humidity would also increase with increasing pressure if the system were closed and could be kept at a constant temperature; for example, if a fixed volume of air-water vapour at 50% humidity is gradually compressed, the partial pressure of vapour will rise until it reaches saturated vapour pressure (when relative humidity =100%), at which point the vapour will start to liquefy.

Devices for Measuring Humidity

Hair Hygrometer

- As relative humidity increases, hair lengthens and moves a lever. A synthetic fibre or membrane may be used instead of a hair (see Fig. 13.2).
- Remains in wide use.
- Accuracy ± 2%.

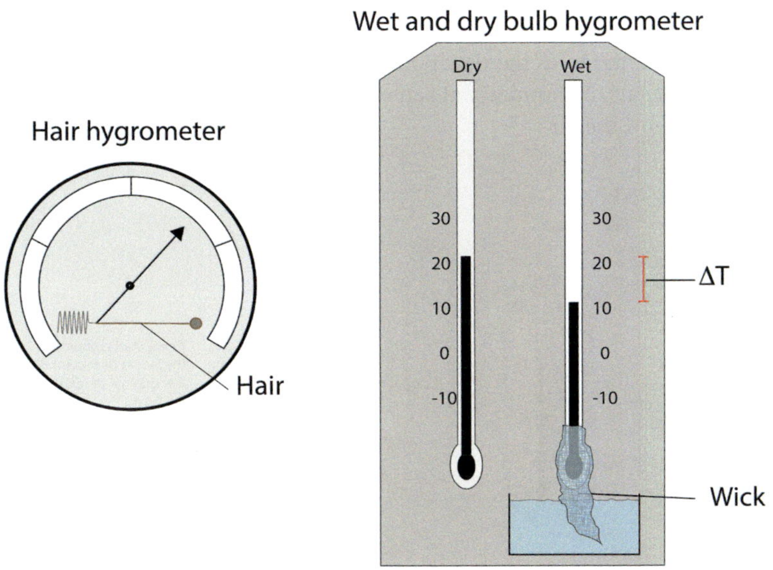

Fig. 13.2 Diagram of the hair hygrometer (left) and wet and dry bulb hygrometer (right)

Wet and Dry Bulb

- Standard instrument for measuring climatic relative humidity.
- Instrument contains two thermometers (see Fig. 13.2):
  - Dry thermometer reads ambient temperature.
  - Wet thermometer is surrounded by wet wick. This cools the thermometer as water evaporates.
- Evaporation causes the water surrounding the wet thermometer to cool through loss of latent heat.
- The degree of evaporation from the wet wick is dependent on the relative humidity. The lower the relative humidity, the faster the evaporation, and the lower the wet bulb temperature.
- The difference in temperature between the two thermometers is recorded and related to the relative humidity via tables.
- If there is no temperature difference between the thermometers, the relative humidity is 100%.

Condensation Methods

Regnault's Hygrometer

- Air is blown through a silver tube containing ether. This results in cooling of the tube due to vaporisation of ether. The air surrounding the tube is therefore also cooled (see Fig. 13.3).
- Cooling of the air reduces the amount of water vapour that can be held in the air so that, eventually, the air becomes saturated and SVP is reached.
- At this temperature, dew starts forming on the surface of the tube, and this temperature is referred to as the dew point.
- Tables will tell us the humidity at saturation at this temperature. This is the absolute humidity of the air.

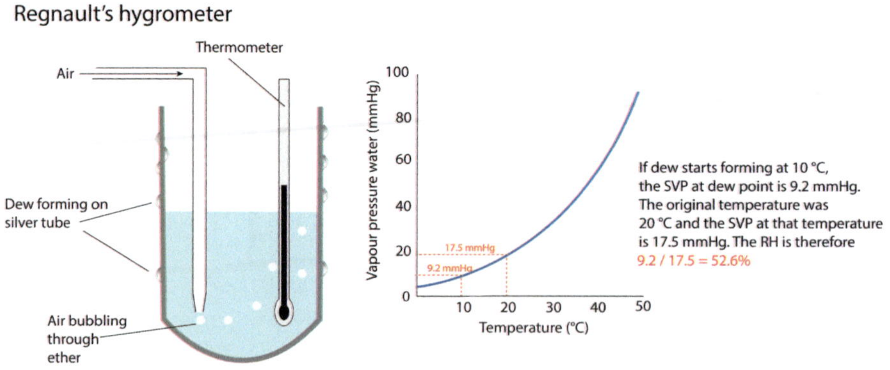

Fig. 13.3 Diagram of Regnault's hygrometer (left) and correlation with the graph of vapour pressure against temperature

- To calculate the relative humidity, one then needs to find out the maximum amount of water that could be held in air at the original ambient temperature. This is obtained from tables.
- The relative humidity is therefore:

$$\text{Relative humidity} = \frac{\text{Absolute humidity at saturation}\left(\text{dew point temperature}\right)}{\text{Absolute humidity at saturation}\left(\text{original temperature}\right)}$$

- As noted previously, the relative humidity ratio is also equivalent to the corresponding saturated vapour pressures at the given temperatures:

$$\text{Relative humidity} = \frac{\text{SVP}\left(\text{dew point temperature}\right)}{\text{SVP}\left(\text{original temperature}\right)}$$

Chilled Mirror Hygrometer

- A contemporary version of Regnault's hygrometer.
- Air is passed through a sample chamber that contains a coolable mirror and an optical system that measures reflectivity.
- The mirror is cooled to dew point, and this is detected by a change in reflectivity and optical output.

Electrical Methods

- Resistance—resistance of a substance (e.g. a salt) decreases with increasing absolute humidity.
- Capacitance—capacitance increases with absolute humidity.
- Thermal conductivity—the thermal conductivity of humid air is greater than dry air. The thermal conductivity of the sample is compared with a sample of dry reference gas.

Weighing/Absorption

- Water vapour is absorbed in silica gel or anhydrous calcium chloride and change in weight measured.

Mass Spectrometry

- Measures the amount of water vapour in volume of gas (see chapter).

Ultraviolet and Infrared Absorption

- Water vapour absorbs UV and IR radiation (see chapter).

Humidification

- Typical comfortable room humidity (and therefore inspired gas under normal breathing conditions) is 50–60% at 20 °C.
- This inspired air is then warmed and humidified by the nose, nasopharynx, oropharynx and trachea and finally reaches 100% saturation at 37 °C at a point just distal to the carina (the isothermic saturation boundary).
- If inspired gas is relatively cool and dry (e.g. standard medical gases), this point moves distally into the smaller airways. This effect is compounded further if an endotracheal tube bypasses the upper airways.

Problems from Lack of Humidification

See Table 13.2.

Further Calculations

- Tracheal air is at 34 °C and, if RH is 100%, will contain ~38 mg L^{-1} water.
- The humidity deficit between dry and tracheal gases is therefore 38 mg L^{-1}. The air entering trachea will be warmed to 34 °C, and evaporation will continue from the respiratory tract until RH = 100% and will entail 38 mg L^{-1} being added.
- If they are breathing 7 L min^{-1}, they will therefore be losing 0.266 g min^{-1}.
- The latent heat of vaporisation is 2.4 kJ g^{-1}.
- Energy lost = 2.4 kJ g^{-1} × 0.238 g min^{-1} = 638 J.min^{-1} = 10.6 W.

Table 13.2 Table of problems caused by lack of humidification in the clinical setting

Problem	
Cooling	Loss of latent heat from water evaporating into dry gases. Particular problem in neonates
Dehydration	
Decreased ciliary function (impaired mucociliary elevator)	Decreased mucus flow
	Mucosal degeneration
	Squamous metaplasia
	Tracheobronchitis
	Broncho-pulmonary dysplasia
	Infection/mucus plugs/collapse
	General increase in post-op pulmonary complications
Increased risk sparks and explosions	

Methods of Humidification

What Is the Difference Between a Humidifier and a Nebuliser?

Humidifier produces vapour (molecular water), and a nebuliser produces an aerosol (droplets).

Humidifiers

Heat and Moisture Exchanger (HME)

- A device that retains a proportion of a patient's expired moisture and heat and returns it to the patient during inspiration.
- Warm expired air meets cool interface and condenses.
- Inspired gases pick up the water on HME and carry it back into the patient (see Fig. 13.4).
- A temperature difference is essential. Material with low thermal conductivity helps maintain this interface.
- May achieve an RH of 60–80%.
- Maximum efficiency is ~80%. Thus, if expired air contains 38 g m^{-3}, the inspired air might achieve 30 g m^{-3} absolute humidity.

- Interfaces:
  - Hygroscopic (moisture retaining):
    Paper, foam or other material impregnated with moisture-retaining salt, e.g. $CaCl_2$
    May also incorporate an electrostatic filter layer
    More efficient humidifier but more flow resistance when wet

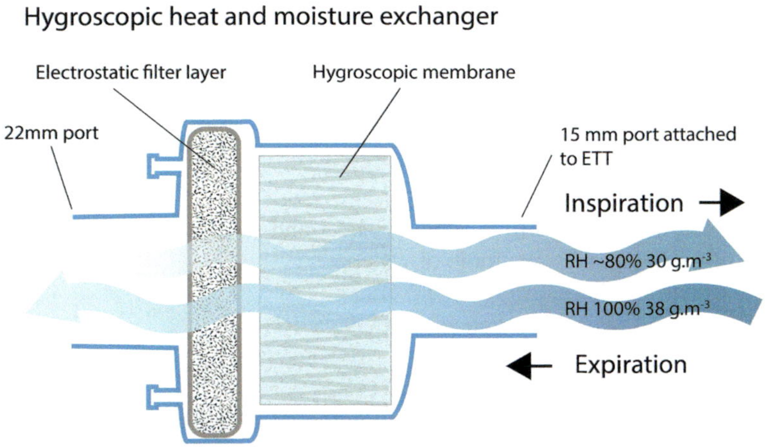

Fig. 13.4 Diagram showing relative humidity (RH) achieved with inspiration and expiration through hygroscopic heat and moisture exchanger (HME)

- Hydrophobic (repels moisture):
  Pleated membranes with much smaller pores
  Small pores of 0.2 μm acting as microbial filter
  Less efficient humidifier but less flow resistance when wet
- Factors decreasing efficiency:
  - Dry inspired air
  - Large V_T or high flow rate
  - Hot climate
  - Not placed directly on ETT
  - Hydrophobic interface less efficient than hydroscopic
- Potential problems:
  - Increased dead space
  - Increased resistance
  - Potential obstruction with moisture, vomit
  - Decreased efficiency in conditions above
  - Reservoir for infective colonisation

Active Heated Humidifiers

- Water bath with a thermostatically controlled heating element
- Heated tubing with water traps
- 100% Humidity at room temperature will be <100% at 37 °C, overcome by warming inspired gases ± supersaturation (adding mist of water droplets that vaporise when temperature increases and RH decreases)
- Efficiency:
  - Capable of fully saturating and heating inspired gases to 37 °C at high flows
  - Far superior to HME
  - Heated delivery hose prevents cooling and loss of humidity in the inspiratory limb of the circuit
- Potential problems:
  - Cost
  - Circuit complexity
  - Water rain-out leading to monitor malfunction or tubing occlusion
  - Infection hazard
  - Potential for burns and drowning

Circle System and Absorber

- CO_2 absorption by soda lime produces heat and moisture. The removal of one mole of CO_2 generates one mole of water.
- Start of anaesthesia: ~30% RH.
- With low flow, anaesthesia can achieve ~93% RH.

Nebulisers

Produce an aerosol of water droplets with potential for several hundred grams per cubic metre of water. Unless there is a heating component, this may cool the patient.

Gas-Driven Nebulisers

- These use the Bernoulli principle to entrain water into a high-flow gas stream. An anvil in the gas flow breaks the droplets into smaller ones.
- Droplet size 2–4 μm diameter. Mainly deposited between upper airway and bronchial level.

Ultrasound Nebulisers

- Water is dropped onto a plate that is vibrating secondary to a piezo-electric crystal. The droplets are broken up by the vibration.
- Droplet size down to ~1 μm and can reach alveoli.
- Risk of overhydration in children.

Further Reading

Al-Shaikh B, Stacey S. Essentials of equipment in anaesthesia, critical care and perioperative medicine. In: Chapter 9: Humidification and filtration. 5th ed; 2018. p. 137–46.

Davey A, Diba A. Ward's anaesthesia equipment. Chapter 11: Breathing filters, humidifiers and nebulisers. 6th ed; 2003. p. 275–87. (Wilkes A)

Ehrenwerth J, Eisenkraft J, Berry J. Anesthesia equipment: principles and applications. In: Hyers B, Spencer C, Eisenkraft J, editors. Chapter 7: Humidification and filtration. 3rd ed; 2020. p. 183–92. https://doi.org/10.1016/B978-0-323-67279-5.00013-3.

Filters

14

Alan McLintic and Craig Birch

Filtration Mechanisms

Direct interception:

- Particle impacts a fibre because of its size.
- Dust and large bacteria >1 μm.

Inertial impaction:

- Particle impacts fibre because it cannot follow the path of least resistance of the flow.
- 0.5–1.0 μm.

Gravitational settling:

- Large particles separate from the gas flow due to gravity.
- Particles of >5 μm usually settle before reaching the filter.

Brownian motion/diffusion:

- Small particles' motion is influenced by surrounding particles , thus increasing their apparent size.
- Very small particles such as viruses (<0.5 μm).

A. McLintic · C. Birch (✉)
Department of Anaesthesia and Pain Medicine, Counties Manukau Health,
Auckland, New Zealand

C. Birch et al. (eds.), *Physics and Measurement for Anesthesia*,
https://doi.org/10.1007/978-3-031-65060-4_14

Electrostatic attraction:

- Particle deviates from gas stream through electrostatic attraction with oppositely charged fibres.

Electrostatic Filters

The filtration element consists of two types of fibres that are selected such that positive and negative static charge develops on them:

- Filtration efficiency ~99.99%.
- Fibre density is less than with hydrophobic filters, so there is less resistance to flow.
- May be combined with an HME hygroscopic layer.
- Charge decreases with time and with humidity/"wetting".

Hydrophobic Filters

Rely on a much finer mesh structure with finer pore size to mechanically trap particles:

- Various materials including glass fibre, paper and aluminium forming large pleated surface area
- Cohesive forces of water > adhesive forces so water accumulates on the fibres
- More efficient filters of microbes ~99.999%
- Higher resistance to flow

HMEF: Heat and Moisture Exchange Filter

HMEs add heat and moisture to cool dry inspired gases. They are passive humidifiers as they do not require external energy to function. The HME is used in anaesthesia and intensive care to prevent cool dry gases from damaging the mucociliary clearance of sputum and secretions in the distal airways. They also prevent heat loss. HMEs can be combined with electrostatic microbial filters (HMEF) so that they protect the ventilated patient and equipment from particulate matter, including some bacteria. They recover and retain heat and moisture during expiration and then return it to the cool, dry gas that passes in the opposite direction on inspiration. They contain hygroscopic, hydrophobic and electrostatic material in order to function optimally.

Epidural Filters

Epidural filters prevent the injection of contaminants that may damage the central nervous system, e.g. infection by bacteria or inflammation. They are low-volume hydrophilic filters, approximately 0.5 ml. They increase resistance to fluid flow, but do not retain drugs, and prevent contamination by bacteria and endotoxins.

Blood Filters

Blood products (RBCs, platelets, cryoprecipitate and fresh frozen plasma) should be given through a blood giving set with a 170–200 μm filter to filter particulate matter and thrombi from donor blood products during infusion.

Human albumin, immunoglobulin and stem cells require a 15 μm filter (found on standard intravenous giving sets).

A standard blood giving set has a double-chambered reservoir with an in-line mesh filter (170–200 μm pore size). This removes large clots and aggregates.

Ideal Filter

- Efficient
- Provides some humidification
- Minimal dead space and flow resistance
- Effective wet and dry
- Lightweight, small, non-traumatic
- Disposable and cheap

Further Reading

Wilkes AR. Heat and moisture exchangers and breathing system filters: their use in anaesthesia and intensive care. Part 1: History, principles and efficiency. Anaesthesia. 2011;66:31–51.

Wilkes AR. Heat and moisture exchangers and breathing system filters: their use in anaesthesia and intensive care. Part 2: Practical use, including problems, and their use with paediatric patients. Anaesthesia. 2011;66(1):31–51.

Ultrasound

15

Alan McLintic and Julian Dimech

Ultrasound

Physical Principles of Ultrasound

What Is Ultrasound?

Sound and ultrasound are acoustic waves and possess the same physical properties, differing only in respect to their frequency (see below). Humans can receive and perceive acoustic waves as sound when their frequencies lie between approximately 20 Hz and 20 kHz. Sound waves with frequencies of >20 kHz are beyond the normal range of human hearing and are referred to as ultrasound. Sound waves with frequencies below the lower range of hearing are termed infrasound. There is some interpersonal variability in the cut-offs for these frequency ranges, as well as a loss in perception of high-frequency waves with increasing age. Other animals can perceive sound waves with frequencies >20 kHz.

Ultrasound is a longitudinal pressure wave, which propagates through a medium (gas, liquid or solid) by passing kinetic energy on to neighbouring particles. It is generated by, and originates from, a source. As the pressure wave moves forward, it alters the molecular density of the transmission medium, creating areas of increased molecular density (compression) as well as areas of reduced molecular density (rarefaction). It can be considered to be a moving vibration.

A. McLintic
Department of Anaesthesia and Pain Medicine, Counties Manukau Health,
Auckland, New Zealand

J. Dimech (✉)
Anaesthesia & Pain Medicine, Middlemore Hospital,
Auckland, New Zealand

C. Birch et al. (eds.), *Physics and Measurement for Anesthesia*,
https://doi.org/10.1007/978-3-031-65060-4_15

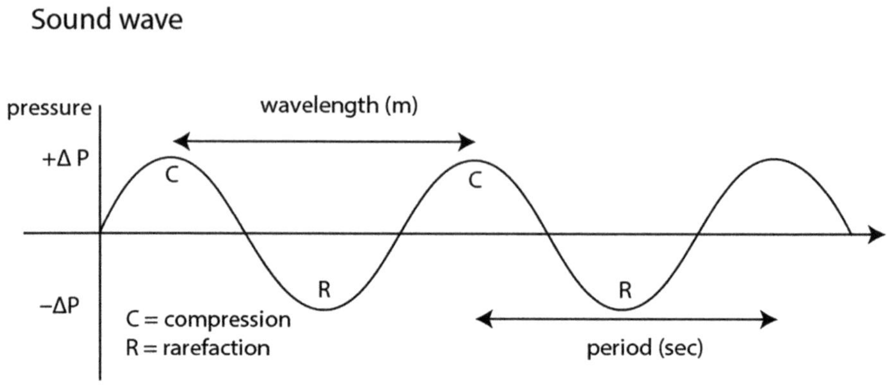

Fig. 15.1 Representation of a sound wave. Change in pressure around a neutral point, plotted against time

Frequency

The frequency (f) of a sound (or ultrasound) wave is the number of cycles per second. 1 MHz = 1 million cycles per second. In clinical use, most ultrasound probes generate waves with frequencies in the range of 2–15 MHz.

The period is the time taken to complete one cycle, e.g. the time taken for the wave to travel from the peak of one compression point to the next peak compression point (see Fig. 15.1).

The frequency of a sound wave is set by the source and is primarily a function of the source element's thickness. The thinner/finer the element, the higher its resonant frequency.

Wavelength

The wavelength is the distance travelled in one cycle and is inversely proportional to the frequency. It is usually assigned the Greek letter lambda (λ).

The wavelength of a sound wave will depend on the medium through which it travels, e.g. vacuum, air or water. It is a function of the speed of sound through a medium and the frequency of the wave generated by the source.

Equation 15.1: Calculating the wavelength of sound waves:

$$\lambda = c/f \tag{15.1}$$

where λ = wavelength, c = speed of sound and f = frequency.

In clinical use, ultrasound with short wavelengths generates images with greater resolution than those with longer wavelengths, albeit with a loss in tissue penetration (see below).

Acoustic Velocity

The speed of sound through a medium depends on the nature of that medium. The fundamental properties of the material (density and rigidity) influence the acoustic velocity of waves traversing through it.

The mediums' rigidity (elastic bulk modulus) is defined as the tendency of an object to deform (in all directions) when uniformly loaded (in all directions).

Equation 15.2: The Newton-Laplace equation used to calculate acoustic velocity:

$$\text{Speed of sound}(c) \propto \sqrt{\text{Rigidity}(K) \big/ \text{Density}(\rho)} \tag{15.2}$$

Thus, the velocity of sound through a medium is proportional to the rigidity (the elastic bulk modulus, *K*) of the material and inversely proportional to the density of the material.

These concepts can be illustrated by considering a string of weights or beads connected to each other with springs. In this model illustrated in Fig. 15.2, the molecules of the transmission medium are the beads, and the springs represent the rigidity of the medium.

If a force was applied to one end of the string, initiating a wave, the speed of transmission of the wave along the string would be determined by the stiffness of the springs and the mass of the beads. The waveform would be transmitted fastest with stiff springs and beads of low mass.

Density 'Paradox'

The speed of sound varies inversely with density, yet dense materials tend to transmit sound at high velocity. This occurs since with increasing density, rigidity tends to increase proportionately more. As a general rule, the elastic properties of a medium tend to have a greater influence on acoustic velocity than density. However, if two materials have similar rigidity, the one with the lower molecular mass will transmit sound fastest. This is because large molecules require more energy to move them. For example:

- Aluminium and gold have similar elastic properties, but aluminium transmits sound at higher velocity due to its lower atomic mass.
- Nickel and bronze have similar densities, but nickel transmits sound faster because it is more rigid.

Acoustic Velocity in States of Matter

The acoustic velocities of solids are greater than those of liquids, which are in turn greater than those of gases.

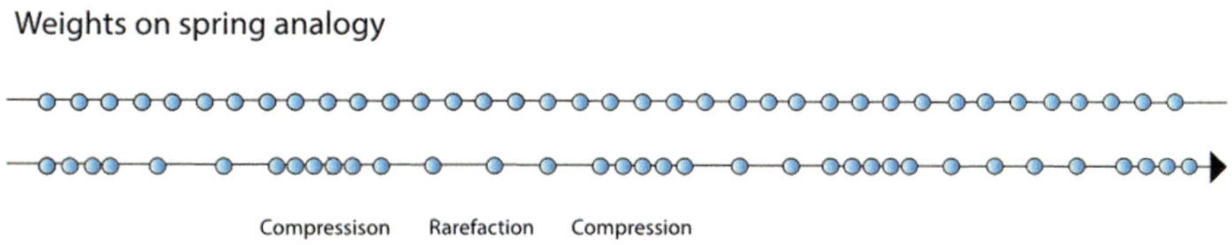

Fig. 15.2 Weights on a spring analogy used to illustrate how sound waves are transmitted through materials

Intermolecular bonds between solid molecules are strong and provide a rigid, minimally deformable framework for the material. Thus, sound propagates fastest in solid material due to its poor elasticity/high rigidity.

In liquids, where the intermolecular bonds are weaker, the resulting increase in compressibility/deformation of the material means that they transmit sound at lower velocity than solids.

The speed of sound through gases is low as there are negligible bonds between molecules. Gases with lower molecular mass transmit sound faster, and, for a given gas, the acoustic velocity increases with increasing temperature because the molecules have more energy and vibrate faster. This is despite gas density being lower at higher temperature.

In the clinical context, this means that ultrasound has different acoustic velocities in tissues such as bone, soft tissue/blood, and air as shown in Table 15.1.

Pressure, Energy, Power and Intensity

Sound Pressure and Decibels

Sound pressure is the average pressure in the wave over time. It is a gauge pressure and must be referenced to the average local pressure (e.g. atmospheric pressure). It is therefore the difference between average local pressure and the pressure in the sound wave, measured in pascals.

The decibel is also often used in acoustics as a unit of sound pressure.

- The decibel is a measure of power relative to a reference value on a logarithmic scale. Since the measure is compared to a reference value, it is a power ratio.
- The power ratio is expressed as a log (base 10) and then multiplied by 10.
- Thus, consider a pressure that is 1000 times a reference pressure:
  $1000 = \log_{10}3$; thus, $10 \times 3 = 30$ dB.
- In circumstances where the squared pressure is of interest, the log to the base 10 is multiplied by 20 rather than 10.

Sound Energy

Sound energy in a medium is the sum of the potential energy of the pressure oscillations and the kinetic energy in displacing the medium or tissue mass. It is measured in joules (J). The greater the energy, the greater the heating effect of the beam. The energy is greatest within the centre of the beam.

Table 15.1 A comparison of the differing acoustic velocities within different biological tissues

Tissue	Acoustic velocity
Air	330–340 m s^{-1}
Soft tissues	1460–1630 m s^{-1} (Average is ~1540 m s^{-1})
Bone	2700–4100 m s^{-1}

Sound Power

The rate at which sound energy is emitted and received (or even reflected or transmitted) per unit time is referred to as sound power and carries units of watt (W). Sound pressure is a property of the wave located at a point in space, while sound power is a property of a sound source and is the total power emitted by that source in all directions. It is independent of the room and distance from source, unlike sound pressure.

Sound Intensity

Sound intensity is the rate at which an acoustic wave transmits energy to a unit area and carries the units of (W cm^{-2}).

Tissue Interactions: Reflection, Interfaces and Acoustic Impedance

Reflection

Reflection of sound waves is the change in direction of a wave at an interface between two different media/tissue types. The wave direction is returned into the medium from which it originated. If the interface is perfectly smooth, the reflection is described as specular (mirror like); if the reflecting surface is not smooth, reflection is diffuse and the reflected wave is scattered in a variety of directions.

In specular reflection, the angle of the incident waveform which the wave makes with the normal is equal to the angle which the reflected wave makes to the same normal. The incident and reflected waves are on the opposite sides of the normal as shown in Fig. 15.3. Reflected sound waves will result in echoes or reverberations.

Tissue Interfaces

An interface is created at the junction of two tissues, which possess different acoustic impedances. This might be bone and muscle, or muscle and vascular tissue. The ultrasound signal is reflected at the tissue interface, and the reflected wave is returned to the receiver where it is converted to an electrical signal by the piezoelectric

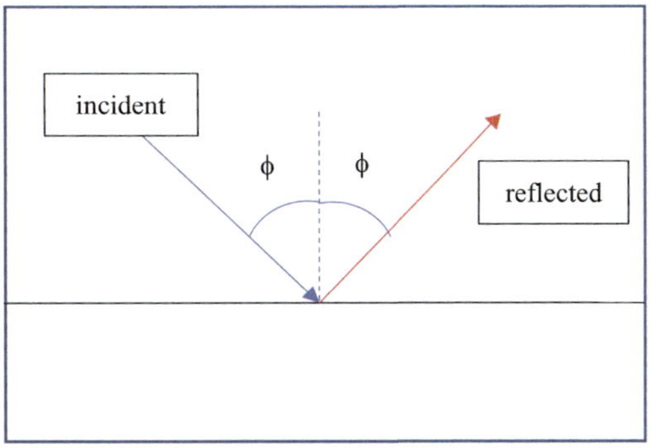

Fig. 15.3 Schematic diagram to represent specular reflection. The incident wave (blue) makes an angle Φ, with the normal (dotted line) at a specular reflective surface (solid line). The reflected wave (red) makes the same angle Φ on the opposite side of the normal

crystal (see later). This signal is displayed as a dot whose brightness indicates the intensity of the returning signal.

Acoustic Impedance

Acoustic impedance is a measure of the opposition that the transmission medium provides against forward sound progression. The greater the mismatch in acoustic impedance between tissues at an interface, the greater the proportion of signal reflected (and therefore received) and the less the proportion that is transmitted onward.

Calculating Acoustic Impedance

The acoustic impedance is the product of tissue density and acoustic velocity of that tissue.

Equation 15.3: Calculating acoustic impedance.

$$\text{Acoustic impedance}(z) = \text{tissue density}(\rho) \times \text{acoustic velocity}(c) \quad (15.3)$$

Note that the acoustic velocity of the tissue type under examination is specific to that tissue.

It is the mismatch between the acoustic impedances created by tissue interfaces that determines the proportion of energy reflected, not the sequence of the different tissue types. For example, the fraction of sound energy reflected at a concrete-water interface is exactly the same as at a water-concrete interface (49%). This may not sound intuitive but is illustrated in Fig. 15.4.

The reason lies in the conditions which allow transfer of pressure energy and momentum across a boundary of materials. Energy that is traveling fast in a high-density medium (high *Z*) has high momentum and cannot readily be transferred to a medium that conveys energy with low momentum (low speed and low density [low *Z*]). The opposite is true as well. Energy with low momentum that is traveling slowly

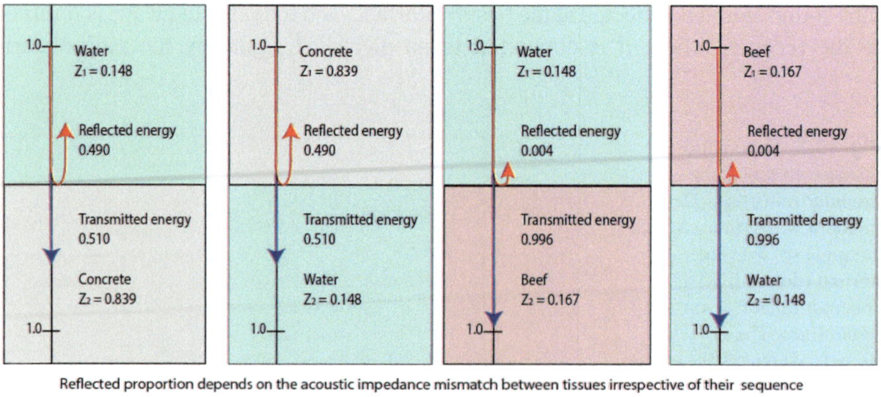

Fig. 15.4 The mismatch, not the sequence of two different tissue types, determines the proportion of reflected sound

in a low-density medium (low Z) cannot readily be transferred to a medium that conveys energy with high momentum (high density and high speed [high Z]). The law of conservation of momentum means that, in both cases, because there is mismatch in acoustic impedance, the energy transmitted across the boundary is reduced and the surplus reflected.

Importance of Coupling Gel

In clinical applications, an ultrasound transducer is placed on a patients' body part (typically skin). Air between the transducer and skin creates transducer-air and air-skin interfaces, both of which have high acoustic impedance mismatch and would result in the reflection of almost all sound with very little transmitted. Coupling gel eradicates these extra interfaces.

Depth of the Interface

Since both the emitting and receiving elements are present in an ultrasound transducer probe, the depth of a tissue interface from the probe on the surface of the patient is estimated from the length of time it has taken for the sound wave to return back to the probe. The assumption is that the speed of sound through typical soft tissues is ~1540 m s^{-1}. This is an average acoustic velocity of sound travelling through a variety of soft tissue types, so it provides a reasonable estimate, but not exact measurement of the depth of the interface.

Equation 15.4: The depth of a tissue interface can be calculated as follows:

$$\text{Depth} = \left(\frac{\text{Time for signal to return}}{2}\right) \times \text{Assumed velocity}\left(1540\,\text{m.sec}^{-1}\right) \quad (15.4)$$

Note that the time for signal to return is halved, as the sound beam has travelled both to and from the probe (transmitter/receiver).

One consequence of the assumption of velocity is that if the signal passes through a tissue with slower acoustic velocity, structures beneath it will be incorrectly positioned at an overly deep point. This is termed propagation speed error.

Attenuation

As sound waves progress through biological tissue, their amplitude and intensity reduce. This phenomenon is known as attenuation and is a measure of the absorption of sound energy by tissues. The loss of energy is exponential in homogenous tissue. The principal way in which this occurs is due to frictional loss of energy as heat. The intrinsic propensity of a material or tissue to attenuate sound waves is termed the attenuation coefficient (α), and this is measured in dB/[mHz × cm].

From this description, it is apparent that for a given propagation distance, attenuation in biological tissues affects high-frequency waveforms to a much greater extent than low-frequency waveforms. This phenomenon therefore dictates the use of lower frequency ultrasound transducers for clinical examination of areas deep within body tissues albeit at the expense of image resolution. Clinically used ultrasound devices generate waves which have frequencies in the order of 2–15 MHz, which represents the best compromise between penetration and resolution.

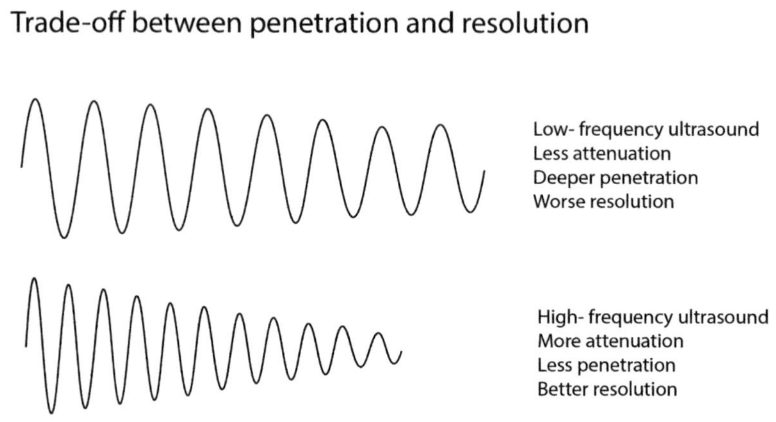

Fig. 15.5 Diagrammatic representation of how waves of differing frequencies are disproportionately affected by attenuation with consequent effects on image resolution and tissue penetration

Equation 15.5: The summary equation for attenuation:

$$I_x = I_o e^{-\alpha x} \tag{15.5}$$

where I_x is the intensity after distance x, I_o is the intensity at start,

α is the attenuation coefficient expressed as fractional change in intensity per unit distance and x is the distance traversed.

It is important to remember that attenuation does not alter frequency, wavelength or velocity of the ultrasound, but reduces the penetration and the ability to detect deep and weakly reflecting structures as shown in Fig. 15.5.

- The distance to target of interest, with attenuation increasing with increasing distance traversed by the ultrasound beam.
- The frequency of ultrasound wave. Since frictional energy losses increase with increasing molecular motion, high-frequency ultrasound is disproportionately affected by attenuation. This results in poorer tissue penetration. Lower frequency waves penetrate further but with correspondingly less resolution.
- Individual tissue types. Viscous tissues and those which relax more slowly offer greater attenuation. The attenuation coefficient quantifies the fractional decrease in energy of a 1 MHz ultrasound signal per unit distance travelled in different tissues. Aerated lung or pockets of air have very high attenuation coefficients, as does cortical bone. Vascular tissue or water-filled tissues have very low attenuation coefficients.
- Different tissue types have intrinsic attenuation coefficients, and these are displayed in Table 15.2.

Loss of Intensity Due to Redirection of Energy

In addition to frictional energy losses, the energy of an ultrasound beam propagating through biological tissue can be redirected in a number of additional albeit

Table 15.2 A comparison of the attenuation coefficients for a variety of tissue types

Attenuation coefficient (m) for 1 MHz beam	
Blood	20 dB m^{-1}
Fat	60 dB m^{-1}
Soft tissue	70 dB m^{-1}
Liver	90 dB m^{-1}
Muscle	180 dB m^{-1}

generally less clinically significant ways such as scatter, reflection, divergence, diffraction and interference.

Reflection, Specular and Scattered

Specular (mirror-like) reflection occurs when the interface surface is very smooth. A large, smooth surface will ensure that a significant proportion of the sound wave is reflected, and consequently, less forward transmission will ensue.

Where there is tissue heterogeneity or imperfectly smooth tissue interfaces, or small objects with high acoustic impedance (particularly structures which have a smaller diameter than the wavelength of the incident sound beam—red blood cells are a problem), a diffuse reflection occurs. This results in scattering of ultrasound waves in a variety of directions creating multiple echoes propagating from numerous tiny structures as well as the echoes themselves interfering with the primary propagating wave.

Beam Divergence

As an ultrasound beam leaves the transducer, its form is restricted, typically in a cylindrical shape. As the beam spreads through the tissue, it diverges and loses its configuration with sound pulses spreading out as they move away from the probe source.

Refraction

When a sound wave meets an interface at an angle, part of the beam is reflected off at the same angle and part is transmitted on at a different angle. A schematic diagram of the phenomenon of refraction is shown in Fig. 15.6. The onwardly transmitted wave is said to be refracted or bent, as the trajectory of the incident wave has changed. The amount of refraction (angle of refraction) which occurs is dependent on the relative acoustic velocities of the two tissue types present at the interface. Refraction is always accompanied by a wavelength and speed change.

The refraction or bending of the wave path occurs because, when the front of the sound wave is travelling at an angle through the interface, one part of the front starts moving at a different velocity from the other. Refraction has minimal effect in medical ultrasound because soft tissues have similar acoustic velocities, but the ultrasound beam should, nevertheless, be directed as perpendicular as possible.

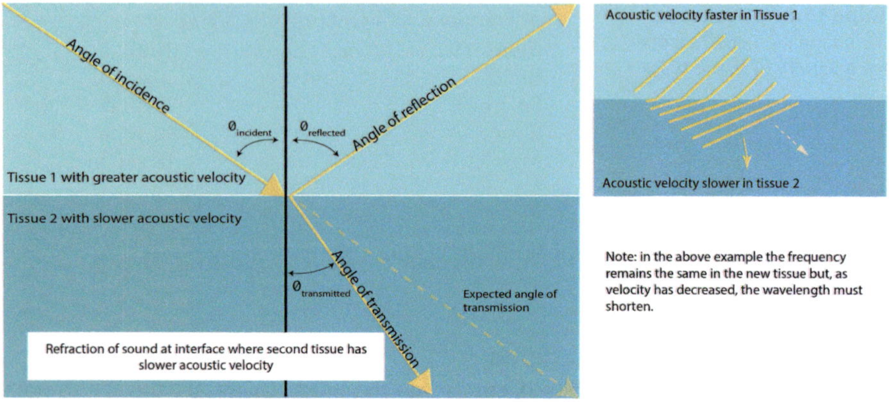

Fig. 15.6 Schematic diagram illustrating the phenomenon of refraction, which occurs when an ultrasound beam meets a tissue interface at an angle

Fig. 15.7 Diffraction occurring as waves pass through a narrow opening which results in a change in direction

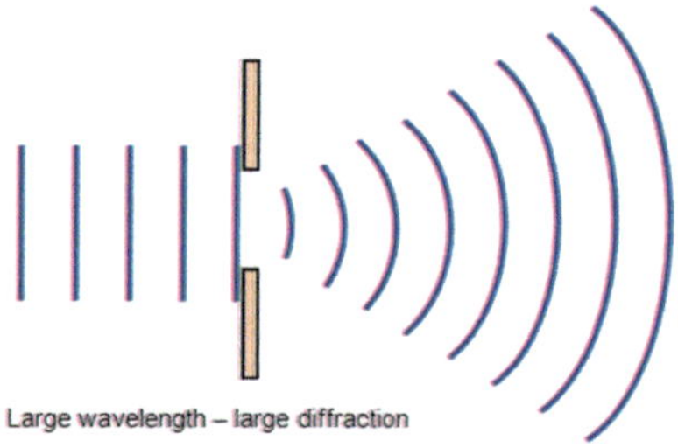

Diffraction

Diffraction involves a change in direction of waves as they pass through a small opening or around a barrier in their path. Long-wavelength waves need to flex through the narrow opening (or round an object in their path), and in so doing, their direction is changed (see Fig. 15.7). Shorter wavelength waves are able to pass through without needing to deform, so their trajectory is not disturbed and they continue travelling along their original path, undergoing little or no diffraction. Consequently, diffraction increases, increasing wavelength.

Transducers, Signal and Beam Shape

Piezoelectric Effect

Certain crystals, ceramics and some biological materials such as bone and DNA can, when a mechanical stress is applied to them, develop an electrical charge. This reversible phenomenon is known as the piezoelectric effect and was first described by Pierre and Marie Curie in 1880.

The phenomenon arises because when there is no applied stress, the positive and negative charges across a piezoelectric element's structural lattice are evenly

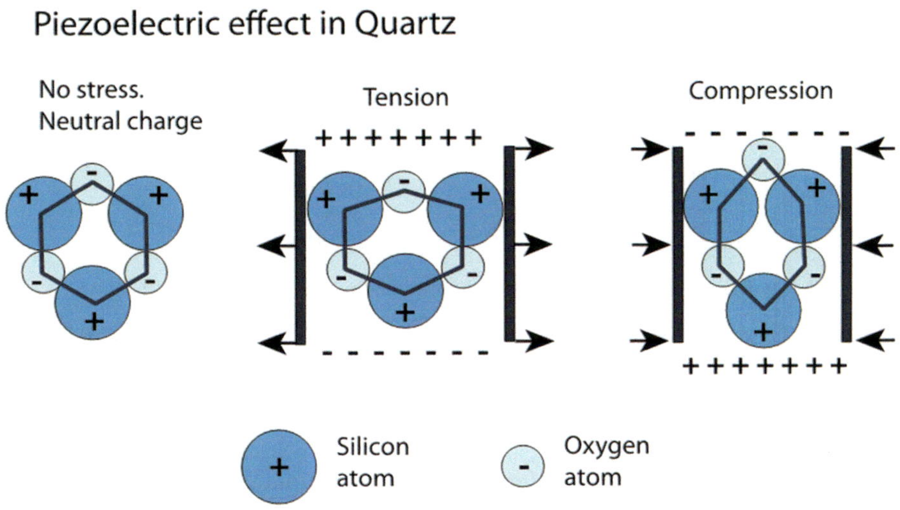

Fig. 15.8 Schematic representation of the piezoelectric effect in a quartz crystal

distributed. If stress is applied to the structure, the charge balance is disturbed and a voltage occurs across it. This effect is illustrated in Fig. 15.8.

These materials also exhibit the reverse piezoelectric effect: a change in shape when an electric change is applied across them. If the charge applied to the piezoelectric material has alternating polarity, the crystal structure expands and contracts in response to this alternating charge.

Piezoelectric Crystals

Ultrasound is generated by activating piezoelectric elements and detected when the element is impacted by the returning pressure wave. Each crystal has its own natural frequency, and if 'struck' with a voltage pulse, it will vibrate ('ring') at its natural frequency. The thinner the crystal, the higher the frequency. Quartz was used initially, but contemporary transducers use ceramic materials such as lead zirconate titanate (PZT).

Pulsed Signal

A voltage pulse is applied across the element causing it to vibrate ('ring') at its resonant frequency. The frequency remains the same throughout its course into and back out of tissues. The transducer probes have inbuilt electronic damping that inhibits the ultrasound oscillations after 2–4 cycles. The ultrasound signal is thus pulsed in short bursts of 2–4 cycles. A diagram of a pulsed ultrasound signal is illustrated in Fig. 15.9.

The pulse repetition frequency (PRF) is the number of times the element is pulsed per second and is typically between 1 and 12 kHz.

The spatial pulse length (SPL) is the length of each pulse and is calculated by multiplying the number of cycles per pulse by the wavelength (λ).

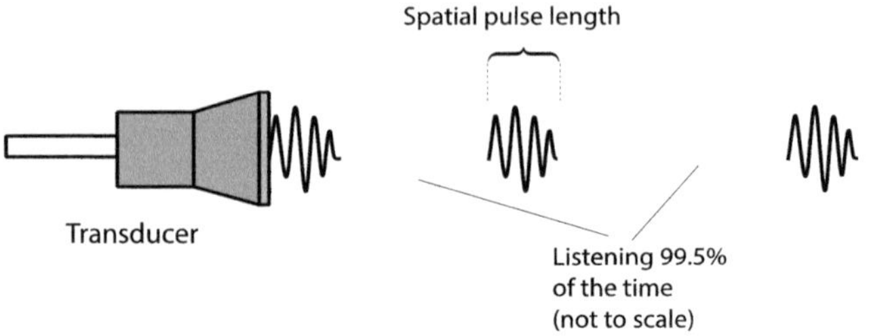

Fig. 15.9 An illustration of how pulsed signal ultrasound probes emit and receive signals

Between pulses, the transducer elements are receiving the returning echoes and are in this 'listening mode' ~99.5% of the time.

Resolution

This usually refers to spatial resolution which is the minimal separation that close-together objects can be distinguished as distinct entities. A general rule is that the higher the frequency, the better the resolution. High-frequency waves, however, have poor tissue penetration, so high-quality image resolution for clinical interpretation is usually only possible for superficial structures.

Axial Resolution

When a pulse encounters two objects that are close together along the beam axis, the echoes generated must return as two separate pulses for them to be seen separately in the image. The minimum separation whereby this can occur is half the spatial pulse length (SPL), so the shorter the wavelength, the better. The higher the frequency, the better the axial resolution. Hence, axial resolution is dependent on frequency and is illustrated in Fig. 15.10.

Equation 15.6: Calculation of axial resolution:

$$\text{Axial resolution} = \frac{\text{Number of cycles} \times \text{Wavelength}}{2} \tag{15.6}$$

Lateral Resolution

This is the minimum side-by-side distance between two objects that can be distinguished. The narrower the beam width at the focal zone, the better the resolution. The width is a function of several issues but, in a single-element transducer, the higher the frequency, the narrower the focal zone. The difference between axial and lateral resolution is illustrated in Fig. 15.10.

Temporal Resolution

The rate at which an image is updated to give the appearance of movement. Usually at least 25 frame updates per second are required for the eye to see smooth movement.

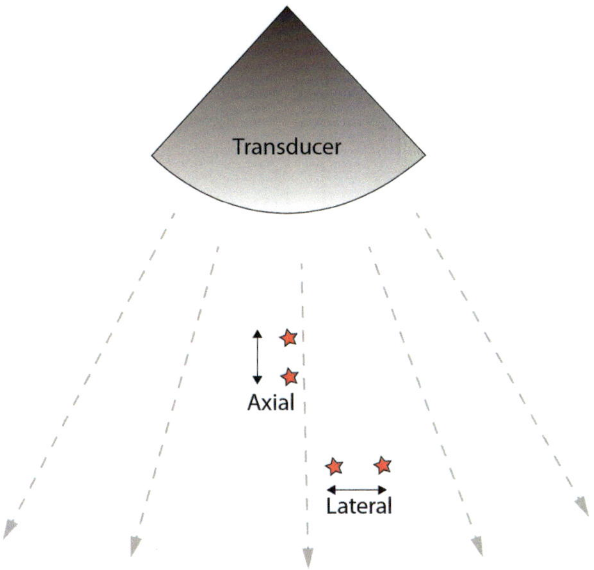

Fig. 15.10 An illustration of the difference between axial and lateral resolution

Time Gain Compensation

With increasing tissue penetration and depth of the ultrasound beam, the energy of the beam decreases and resolution deteriorates. Time gain compensation selectively increases the gain of the deeper signals; however, this function will also increase the 'noise' component of these signals.

Single-Element Transducers

A single-element transducer has one large piezoelectric element. The shape of a single-element beam is represented schematically in Fig. 15.11 and has the following characteristics:

Near Field (Fresnel Zone)

The beam extends out with narrowing diameter before diverging into the far field. The larger the element diameter and the higher the frequency, the longer the near field depth (NFD).

Far Field (Fraunhofer Zone)

The zone beyond the near field where the beam begins to diverge is the far field or Fraunhofer zone. The larger the element diameter and the higher the frequency, the less the angle of divergence.

Focal Zone

The focal zone is the transition between zones. The focal *point* within the focal zone is the narrowest point of the beam, and this is where the greatest lateral resolution is found. Before the focal point is the near field (Fresnel zone), where beams converge,

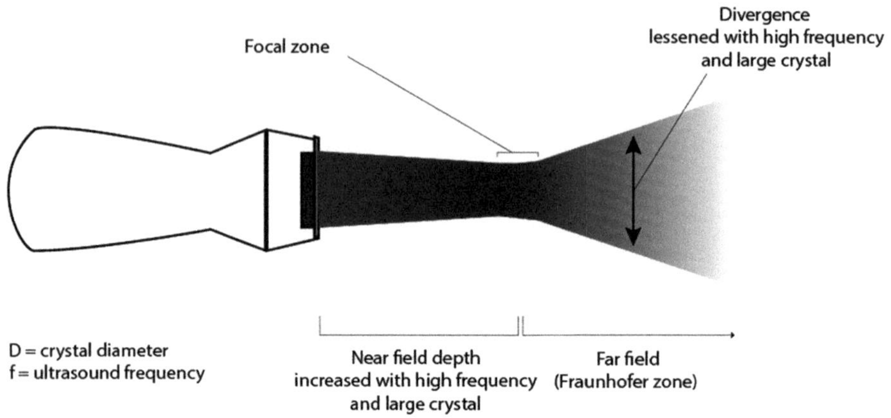

Fig. 15.11 The component areas of the ultrasound beam

and distal to the focal point is the far field or Fraunhofer zone where the beams diverge. The longer and narrower the focal zone, the better the resolution.

Both near-field depth and focal zone length are increased with large-diameter crystals and short wavelength. Thus, increasing the frequency allows lateral resolution to be maintained at increased depth. The trade-off is that increasing the frequency means penetration is decreased. In single-element transducers, the ultrasound beam can be focused by using either acoustic or mechanical lenses.

Acoustic lenses (polystyrene, aluminium or nylon) can be placed in front of the piezoelectric element to focus the beam. Acoustic lenses have an acoustic velocity greater than the element so that sound refracts towards the centre.

Alternatively, the piezoelectric crystal can be designed with a concave face which ensures that sound waves are directed inwards, thus focussing the beam mechanically.

Linear Array Multiple-Element Transducers

Contemporary medical transducers have multiple (150–500) rectangular piezoelectric elements arranged in a row along the face of the probe. Activation occurs sequentially in blocks along the face with a pause between activation so that the block can receive its echoes.

The complete set of images from the 500 or so elements makes up one frame, and this is updated at least 25 times per second to give a 2-dimensional sector in which tissue has the appearance of movement (see Fig. 15.12).

Focusing in Multiple-Element Transducers

The near-field depth, focal length and shape of the sector are modified using electronic focussing. The sound wave pattern from each crystal interferes with the adjacent crystals in its group, so by offsetting the timing of activation of each crystal, the delay can be used to shape the overall wave pattern from the block.

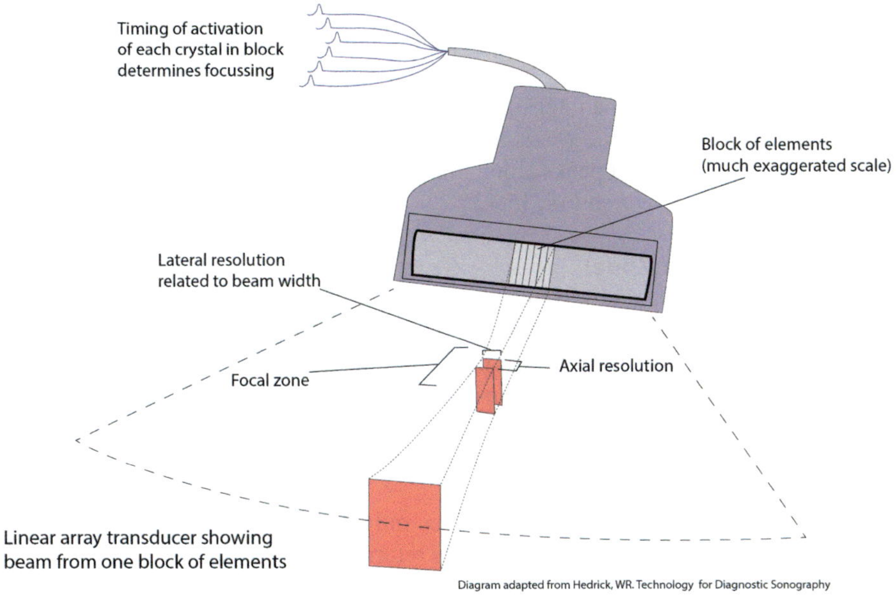

Fig. 15.12 An illustration of how a linear array, multiple-element ultrasound transducer probe builds images and addresses resolution within a scanned sector

- Lateral resolution depends on the beam width from each block at the focal zone which, in turn, depends on the number of elements in each block and electronic focussing of their emissions.
- Axial resolution is determined by spatial pulse length.

Image Modes

General Principles

Pulsed signals are sent out from the ultrasound transducer probe, and the reflected waves return along the same path. The pause between pulses is sufficient for the deepest signals to get back before the next pulse is transmitted. The echoes strike the crystal in listening mode and generate an electrical signal. This signal is then amplified.

Amplitude and Brightness Mode

Amplitude mode (A mode) and brightness (B mode) are different methods of depicting the strength of the signal returning to the transducer. A mode is the original form of echo display, but has few applications in contemporary medicine. All ultrasound imaging in anaesthetic clinical practice is B mode.

Amplitude (A Mode)

A single-element stationary beam is pulsed through the tissue, and its echoes return along the same path. Only the echoes in this one line are imaged at any given moment on the display. The intensity of the returning signals is displayed as amplitude on the *y*-axis, while the *x*-axis represents the length of path through which the beam is passing. Different peaks along that path represent echoes from interfaces at different depths as shown in Fig. 15.13.

Brightness Mode (B Mode)

All conventional clinical ultrasound imaging is B mode. In this mode, the returning echo is displayed as a dot, and the greater the intensity of the signal, the brighter the dot. The longer the time delay from transmission, the deeper the interface is positioned in the image. It can be confusing, but 2-D and M-mode imaging are both B-mode ultrasound.

2-D Imaging

A stationary single beam produces echoes only from that beam's direction. If a beam moves rapidly back and forth, echoes return and enable the formation of a 2-D sector. If the scan speed is fast enough (25 frames/s), tissues appear to move within the image display. Originally, mechanical sector scanners contained a motor that moved the crystal back and forth collecting echoes from multiple lines of ultrasonic interrogation. Contemporary ultrasound imaging uses linear array transducers containing multiple elements, which are activated sequentially in blocks to sweep across a sector of tissue. This is done so rapidly that the tissue movement is reproduced in real time (see Fig. 15.12).

Phased Arrays

Linear arrays produce a rectangular field of view because the elements are laid out in a straight row. The length of this row can prevent access of narrow apertures such

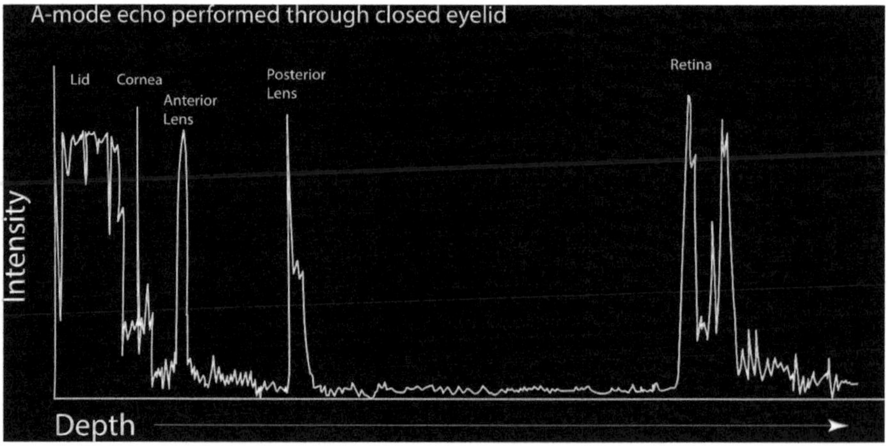

Fig. 15.13 Image output from an 'A mode' ultrasound examination of the eye

as between ribs. Phased array allows a similar field of view but with fewer elements (~130 elements). The elements in this case are activated almost simultaneously, but, by very small careful adjustments in the timing and delays of each element, the collective beam can be made to steer left and right very rapidly. This arrangement is illustrated in Fig. 15.14.

Curvilinear Arrays

Curvilinear arrays have the elements arrayed along an arc to produce a trapezoid field of view.

Motion Mode (M Mode)

Motion (M) mode was the original ultrasound technique which enabled devices to assess and image moving tissues. This technique still has application in cardiac ultrasound to quantify movement and cavity dimensions. A single ultrasound beam is directed into the tissue, and the echoes return from that single line of interrogation. Tissues are moving in that beam, but only the echoes in that single 'pencil lead' beam are collected. The returning echoes have brightness according to intensity and are placed on the screen according to the depth of interface (exactly as per B mode function). This is then repeated at approximately 500 Hz, with each successive collection of data placed next to each other on the x-axis. The x-axis therefore

Fig. 15.14 A phased array transducer probe can be used to improve access through narrow apertures

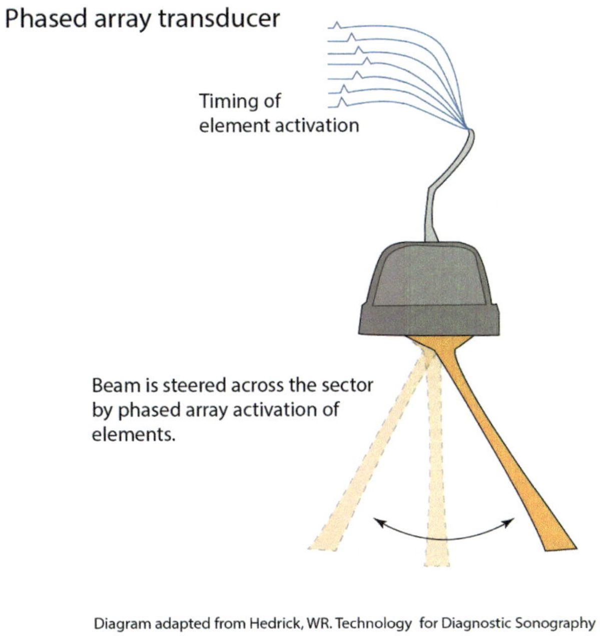

represents time, and the y-axis is depth. The constructed image represents tissue movement and dimensions from one ultrasound beam over time as shown in Fig. 15.15.

Image Artefacts

Artefacts are alterations of the ultrasound image which do not represent an actual image of the area. They are commonly seen in clinical ultrasound examinations. Extra, lost or distorted images or images in the wrong place can be produced by technical imaging errors or result from the interaction of ultrasound waves with biological tissues. Although often considered unhelpful, since they can lead to interpretation errors by obscuring normal anatomy, or be misinterpreted as pathological lesions, some artefacts can be used to aid diagnostic processes. Some examples of image artefacts are displayed in Table 15.3.

Reverberation and Repetition Artefacts

Reverberation artefacts appear as a series of equally spaced lines. This type of artefact results from an ultrasound wave bouncing repeatedly back and forth between two strongly reflective interfaces within the examined tissue. Echoes from these surfaces do not return directly to the transducer for detection; rather, they only

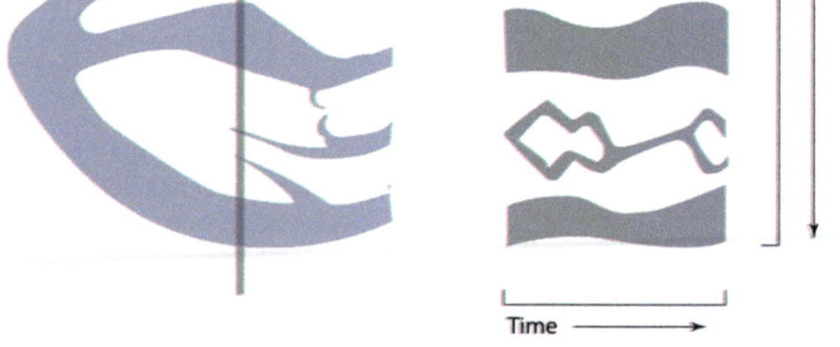

Fig. 15.15 An illustration of how M-mode imaging is constructed

Table 15.3 A classification of image artefacts with examples

Image artefact type	Examples
Extra images	Reverberation artefact
Images in wrong place	Side-lobe artefact, mirror image artefact, propagation speed artefact, refraction
Loss or distortion of images	Acoustic shadowing, acoustic enhancement

return after reverberating between the two reflective surfaces. There is therefore a time delay for these waves, which are consequently interpreted as being returned from extra structures deep to the distal interface. If these reverberations occur between interfaces in a small object, the ultrasound waves are reflected back in close proximity, creating a trail of closely spaced, discrete, very bright, small echoes which appear as a 'greyscale' shadow and can generate a 'comet tail' artefact. When this artefact appears unexpectedly, it may indicate the presence of a needle, metallic pellets, stones or foreign body.

Repetition artefacts can be produced when a pulse returns to the transducer from an (often superficial) highly reflective surface. This echo is partly captured by the probe, but the probe surface itself is reflective, so it returns the echo back into the tissue and the process is repeated. Several equidistant hyperechoic lines, each progressively deeper, are produced. The number of images produced depends on the penetrating power of the beam and the sensitivity of the probe (see Fig. 15.16).

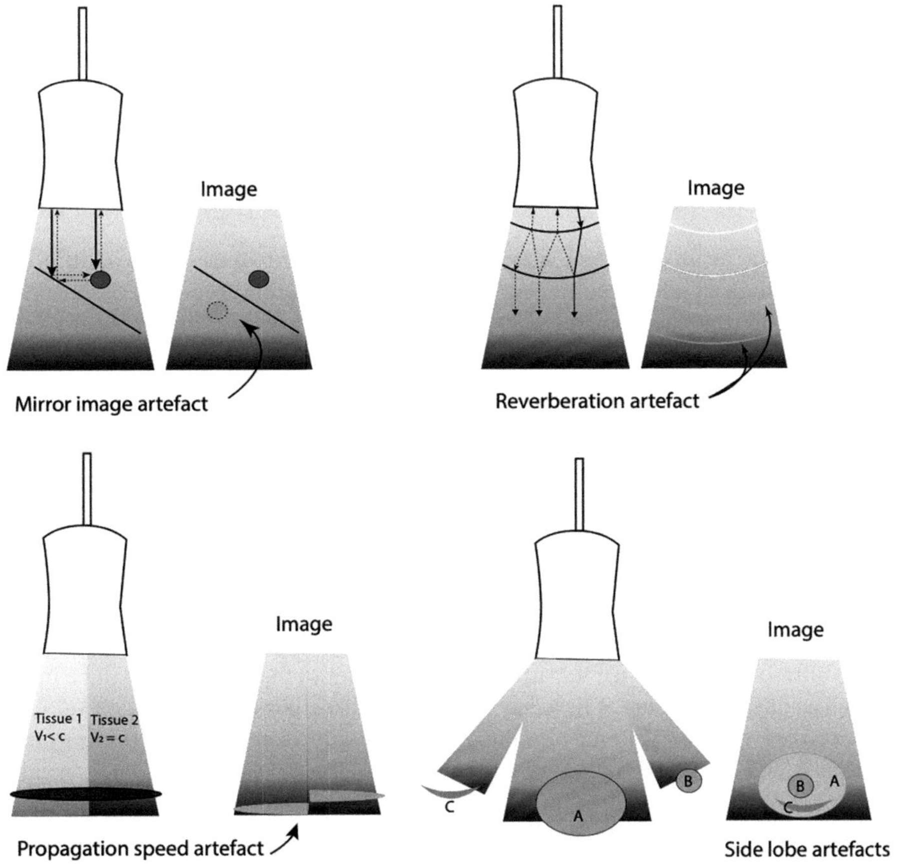

Fig. 15.16 A selection of common ultrasound image artefacts; see text for details

Mirror Image Artefact

This type of artefact is produced from an ultrasound beam that has been reflected from a specular (smooth, mirror-like) surface. The reflected beam is directed laterally and may become incident to objects in the tissue, which in turn then return waves back to the specular surface and up to the transducer. The path of the reflected echoes is physically longer and takes more time to return to the probe. The probe cannot predict refraction events, so it positions this returning signal deeper in the image field, along the original beam axis, at a depth which corresponds with the time delay from the refracted wave (see Fig. 15.16).

Side-Lobe Artefacts

The piezoelectric effect produces a primary ultrasound beam which is generated in the direction of crystal expansion and contraction. Crystals may not however deform perfectly under a given voltage, due to structural imperfections. As a consequence, mechanical displacement in additional axial planes can result with the generation of secondary ultrasound beams. These secondary ultrasound beams are called side-lobe beams, are usually of low intensity and surround the main beam. Despite their low intensity, they may become incident with a highly reflective interface. As with mirror image artefact, the probe assumes that pulses and echoes travel in a straight line from the primary beam. This results in (real) laterally positioned objects being mistakenly placed as if they originated from within the central beam and as such are displayed centrally on the screen image (see Fig. 15.16).

Refraction

An ultrasound beam crossing a tissue interface where the two tissues have differing acoustic velocities may be refracted. The resulting refraction (bending) of the ultrasound beam can cause mispositioning or impair focussing of the beam (see Fig. 15.6).

Velocity/Propagation Error

The acoustic velocity of different types of soft tissue varies (see Table 15.1). However, ultrasound machines use an acoustic velocity of 1540 m s^{-1} when performing depth calculations. If an ultrasound beam traverses tissue that has a slower acoustic velocity than this, echoes from deeper structures are delayed in returning. The time delay is interpreted incorrectly, and the processor places the structure at greater depth than it really is. The converse occurs with tissues of faster acoustic velocity. Similarly, if there is significant variation in tissue composition beneath the same ultrasound beam, then the different return times to the transducer will be interpreted as different depths of tissue as opposed to differences in propagation velocity between the tissues. This may result in discontinuity in the displayed ultrasound image. A propagation error can be commonly observed when performing a sciatic nerve block. When imaging a needle passing under the sciatic nerve, the tip can be seen to separate from the needle and move at an increased depth (see Fig. 15.16).

Acoustic Enhancement (Attenuation Artefact)

If an object attenuates to a different degree than the surrounding tissues, the echoes beneath that object become either hyperechoic or hypoechoic compared to the rest of the tissue.

Sound passing through a poorly attenuating structure undergoes less reflection than that passing through the surrounding tissue. At the deep margin of the poorly attenuating structure, there are therefore more waves present and available to impact the surrounding tissue. Thus, an area of artefactually increased echogenicity is produced right under the structure because more waves are reflected back compared with surrounding tissues at the same depth. It is typically seen with (fluid-filled) cysts, where the structures beneath them produce stronger signals than the surrounding tissues. Conversely, hypoechoic structures produce acoustic shadows beneath them.

Acoustic Shadowing

A strongly reflecting or profoundly attenuating tissue or structure, e.g. deeply calcified tissue, stones or prosthetic tissue, will result in near-total reflection of the propagating sound wave. Consequently, there are very few waves moving forward through the tissue deep to the reflective body, and a 'signal void' is created, resulting in loss of image on the display (appears black).

Doppler

Doppler ultrasound is not an imaging tool, but a method to detect flow, velocity and direction of motion in blood vessels. Doppler transducers typically emit ultrasound with frequencies of between 2 and 10 MHz. Duplex transducers allow simultaneous 2-D imaging and Doppler by pausing real-time imaging for a few milliseconds to allow flow sampling to take place.

Doppler Shift (Effect)

In 1842, Christian Doppler described the phenomenon whereby the observed frequency of a wave changes when the source is moving with respect to the observer (or vice versa). This has become known as the Doppler effect or Doppler shift.

It is important to remember that this is an observer phenomenon. Neither the frequency or wavelength nor the acoustic velocity of emitted waves changes. A simple analogy is to imagine an observer running out through waves in the sea. As the observer moves faster, they encounter the waves with increased frequency, but there is no real change in wave frequency. The shift in the observed frequency with respect to the emitted frequency is proportional to the velocity of the source with respect to the observer.

If a transducer probe is receiving waves from an object moving towards it, the wavelength will appear to shorten; there will be an accompanying increase in frequency, a phenomenon referred to as a positive Doppler shift. Conversely, reflections from a body moving away from the transducer probe will appear to have an increased wavelength and reduced frequency, a negative Doppler shift. This principle is illustrated in Fig. 15.17 .

A positive Doppler shift means that the frequency of received sound waves appears greater than the emitted waves indicating a source moving towards the transducer, and it is usually depicted red in colour flow Doppler mode or above the baseline of a spectral envelope display. A negative Doppler shift is the converse of this and is usually depicted as blue in colour flow Doppler mode.

It is worth noting that the magnitude of the Doppler shift is affected by the angle at which the reflecting source is travelling in relation to the transmitting source. If this is perpendicular, there will be no shift observed since Cosine 90 = 0 (see the Doppler equation in Fig. 15.18).

Somewhat confusingly, the term 'redshift' is often used when describing an increase in the wavelengths (and reduction in frequency) with the Doppler effect.

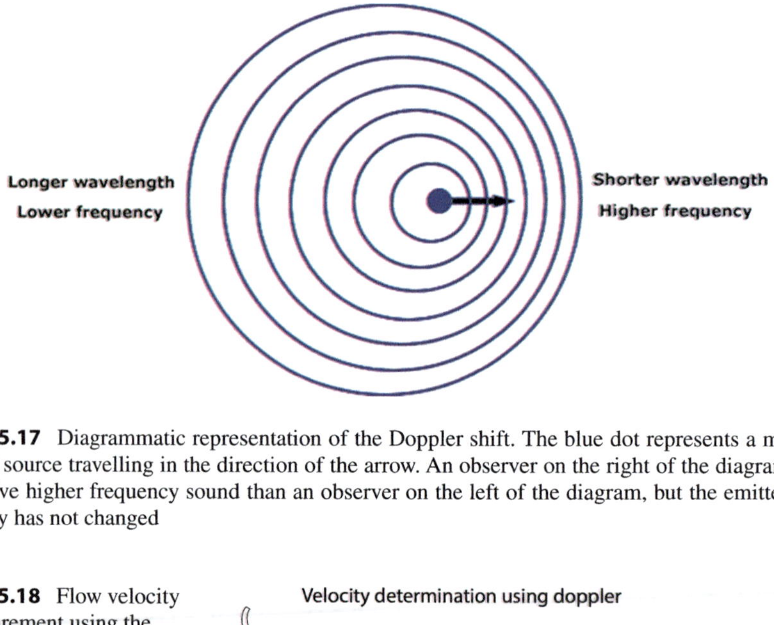

Fig. 15.17 Diagrammatic representation of the Doppler shift. The blue dot represents a moving sound source travelling in the direction of the arrow. An observer on the right of the diagram will perceive higher frequency sound than an observer on the left of the diagram, but the emitted frequency has not changed

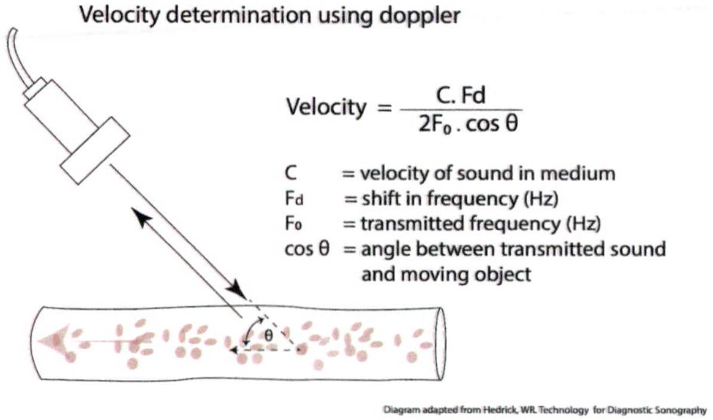

Fig. 15.18 Flow velocity measurement using the Doppler effect. Maximum Doppler shift occurs when $\theta = 0°$ (Cos0 = 1). No shift will be noted when the transmitting source is perpendicular to the motion, since Cos 90 = 0)

The opposite is ‘negative redshift’ or ‘blue shift’. These terms are used because when visible light is subjected to the Doppler effect, red light has longer wavelengths than blue light. This should not, however, be confused with positive and negative Doppler shifts.

Flow Velocity Measurement Using Doppler

Clinically, Doppler techniques can be used to provide measurement of blood flow within vessels. Since the frequency of emitted sound waves from a source does not change, the shift in observed frequency from reflected waves will be proportional to the velocity of the flow (assuming that the probe is static). Additionally, transducer probes need to be inclined at an angle in order to detect the shift in frequency. The more direct-on the transducer is into the flow, the greater the frequency shift and accuracy. Vascular applications usually entail an angle of 30–60°. As angles approach 90°, frequency shift is minimal and accuracy poor. Therefore, a probe perpendicular to blood flow will not be able to measure the flow. The shift in frequency observed with the Doppler effect in clinical applications is typically between 200 and 15,000 Hz in magnitude. This is within the audible range for humans, so can be displayed both visually and audibly on devices.

Spectral Doppler Analysis and Display

Ultrasound waves directed towards a blood vessel will be reflected from blood cells in suspension. Cells are moving at different velocities (and directions) within the axial stream, which creates a variety of frequency shifts (and corresponding calculated velocities) for interpretation. Spectral Doppler techniques use fast Fourier transformations and power spectral analysis to average the frequencies over an epoch (usually 5 ms). Signals therefore contain both frequency and amplitude data, and it is possible to obtain an average frequency shift (F_D) and velocity for the vessel at any given instant.

Graphical displays are presented as a spectral display (hence, spectral Doppler) with frequency shifts plotted against time and brightness representing amplitude of the signal (see Fig. 15.19).

Continuous and Pulsed-Wave Doppler

Continuous-Wave Doppler (CWD)

In this mode, separate piezoelectric crystals are used to simultaneously transmit and receive ultrasound waves, recording velocity along the path of a sound beam. Continuous-wave Doppler is able to record direction and velocity of flow but is not able to localise the origin of velocity elements (a problem referred to as range or depth ambiguity). It can, however, accurately record very high flow velocities, so it is useful for assessing flow across cardiac valves with high flow rates.

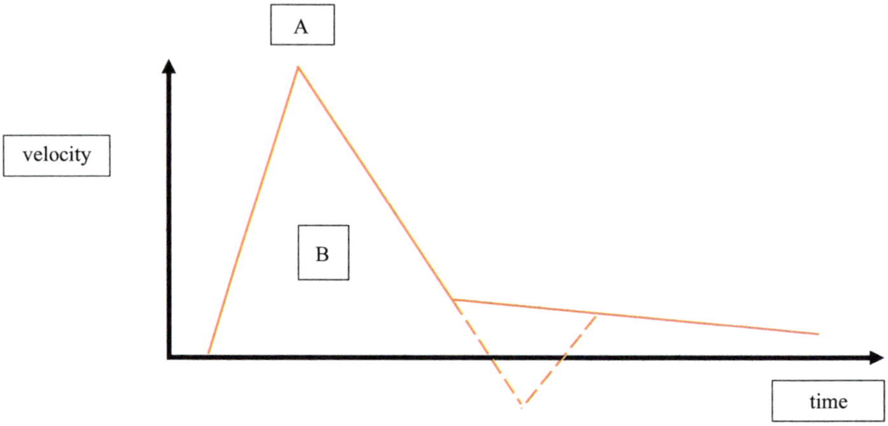

Fig. 15.19 Spectral Doppler display. Flow towards the transducer is represented above the baseline, while flow away from the transducer (broken line) is displayed below the baseline. The peak at point 'A' represents peak velocity. The triangular area B is the spectral window. A narrow range of frequencies gives a sharply defined triangular window

Pulsed-Wave Doppler (PWD)

Pulsed-wave Doppler emits short pulses of sound waves (at the pulse repetition frequency, see above). A user can select a tissue area of interest (a 'sample volume' or 'gate'), and based on the time recorded for returning sound waves, only Doppler shifts observed from the 'sample volume' or 'gate' are calculated.

Small shift changes observed within individual pulses are ignored, but relative phase changes of the pulses are used to determine the frequency shift, since it is the rate of change of phase which is important. Pulsed-wave Doppler is able to localise the origin of velocity elements, but the intermittent sampling methodology results in an error called 'aliasing' (see below), especially when trying to assess deeper, faster moving targets.

Colour Flow Doppler

Colour flow Doppler, colour Doppler imaging or colour Doppler also utilise pulsed-wave interrogation of tissues. As with pulsed-wave Doppler, users select a 'sample volume' or 'gate', and frequency shifts recorded from pulses returning from this area of interest are analysed. They are then colour coded and displayed according to velocity and direction. Each pixel displayed represents a sample volume, and CWD simultaneously analyses multiple sample volumes along a scan line. Velocity and direction of flow are arbitrarily colour coded. Flow away from the transducer is usually blue (negative Doppler effect), and flow that is travelling towards the transducer red (positive Doppler effect). High-velocity flow is often indicated by using paler shades of these colours, while turbulent flow is illustrated with a third colour, often yellow or green. However, there is no standard for colour display when using colour Doppler, and colour settings can even be manually altered by users which may confuse users who subsequent try to interpret images.

Power Doppler

Power Doppler uses the amplitude of a Doppler shift to detect moving matter; as a consequence, it is independent of velocity and direction of flow and therefore remains unaffected by the angle of interrogation. These differences mean that signal aliasing is also avoided (see below). It is a more sensitive technique than colour Doppler, so it allows detection of flow in small vessels with low velocities.

Aliasing and the Nyquist Limit

Aliasing errors occur in signal processing which utilises pulsed signal samples. If the sampling rate (pulse repetition frequency) is too low, direction and velocity of signals are recorded inaccurately and the different reflected signals become 'aliases' of each other when sampled. These errors can be reduced if the pulse repetition frequency is increased.

The Nyquist limit is the maximum measurable shift frequency without inducing an aliasing error and is calculated as half the pulse repetition frequency. Ultrasound machines will display the Nyquist limit as a maximal measurable blood flow velocity or as a value in kHz which represents the maximum measurable Doppler shift. Flow velocities above this level will induce aliasing artefacts on colour or spectral Doppler images. Areas of high blood flow therefore require a high pulse repetition rate.

Transoesophageal Doppler

As illustrated in Fig. 15.20, a transoesophageal Doppler probe can be used to assess aortic blood flow and, by transformation, estimate cardiac output. The descending aorta lies immediately anterior to the oesophagus, so a stationary ultrasound probe in the oesophagus is extremely well positioned to assess blood flow in the descending aorta. The top of the probe is bevelled to provide the necessary angle of sonic interrogation.

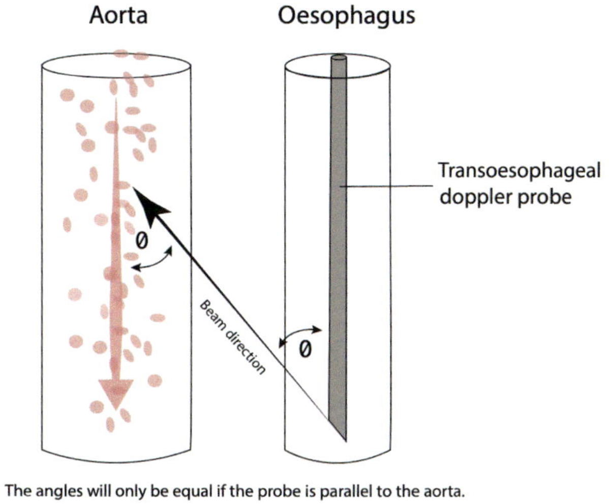

Fig. 15.20 A transoesophageal Doppler probe in place, directing ultrasound towards the aorta

Assumptions and Errors in Transoesophageal Doppler

- The exact 3-dimensional conformational position of the aorta is not usually known, yet assumption of the interrogation angle θ relies on the probe and aorta being parallel. Small errors in θ can make large errors in velocity estimation. For example, if the correct angle is 70°, a 5-degree error leads to a 24% error in velocity estimation.
- If the transducer angle is 90°, frequency shift is minimal and accuracy or measurement extremely poor.
- There is an assumed division of blood flow in the aortic arch of 70% to descending aorta and 30% to brachiocephalic and coronary arteries. Additional transformational algorithms are needed to calculate cross-sectional area of the aorta for cardiac output estimation, hence the need to input patient characteristics when inserting the probe.
- An assumption of negligible diastolic flow is made.
- There is an assumption that all RBCs move at the same speed. This misconception can be countered with Fourier analysis across the vessel diameter.

Further Reading

Basic principles of ultrasound testing. Iowa State University. NT Education Resource Centre Web Site. https://www.nde-ed.org/EducationResources/CommunityCollege/Ultrasonics/Introduction/description.htm. Accessed 25th April, 2020.

Hedrick WR. Technology for diagnostic sonography. St. Louis: Elsevier; 2012.

Powles AE, Martin DJ, Wells IT, Goodwin CR. Physics of ultrasound. Anaesth Intensive Care Med. 2018;19(4):202–5.

Ultrasound artifacts. https://radiopaedia.org/articles/ultrasound-artifacts-3. Accessed 10th May, 2021.

Blood Pressure Monitoring

16

Alan McLintic and Amanda Siu

Non-invasive Blood Pressure Monitoring

Sphygmomanometer

Sphygmomanometer is a non-invasive blood pressure (NIBP) monitor that measures blood pressure (BP) using an inflatable cuff that temporarily occludes blood flow to an artery.

Components

The components of a sphygmomanometer consist of:

- The **pressure monitor** (mercury manometer or aneroid bellows)
- The **'Riva-Rocci' cuff**
  - Note: the width and length of the cuff bladder should be 40% and 80% of the circumference of the patient's upper mid-arm, respectively.

How It Works

The inflation and deflation of the BP cuff produce blood pulsations (Korotkoff sounds), which is detected by auscultation with a stethoscope over the artery. There are five Korotkoff phases:

A. McLintic
Department of Anaesthesia and Pain Medicine, Counties Manukau Health, Auckland, New Zealand

A. Siu (✉)
Department of Anaesthesia and Pain Medicine, Counties Manukau Health, Auckland, New Zealand

University of Auckland, Auckland, New Zealand
e-mail: tsiu001@aucklanduni.ac.nz

C. Birch et al. (eds.), *Physics and Measurement for Anesthesia*,
https://doi.org/10.1007/978-3-031-65060-4_16

I. Sounds appear—this is taken as the systolic BP (SBP).
II. Sounds become quieter.
III. Sounds rise in volume.
IV. Sounds are muffled—8–10 mmHg higher than directly recorded diastolic BP (DBP).
V. Loss of sound—this is taken as DBP (note; sounds may not disappear in hyperdynamic circulation).

Problems and Inaccuracies

Intrinsic Accuracy

- Tends to underestimate SBP and overestimate DBP
- Inter-observer variability may exist
- Does not measure mean arterial pressure (MAP)
  - MAP can be calculated by:

    MAP = DBP + 1/3 (SBP-DBP)

Equipment and Patient Factors

Inaccurate readings may result from equipment factors:

- Leaks or blockages in pneumatic system.
- Cuff misplacement, wrong-size cuff (over-reads if cuff is too narrow).
- Cuff deflated too quickly.
- Manometer tilted or blocked:
  - Unlike an invasive pressure transducer, the position of the manometer relative to the patient makes no difference to the accuracy of the BP reading because the hose connection between cuff and manometer is filled with air, which exerts no mass additive effect on the pressure.

Inaccurate readings may result from patient factors:

- SBP is overestimated in hypotension.
- Arteriosclerosis.
- AF or other arrhythmias.
- Obesity may lead to overestimation of BP.
- Movement, shivering.

Automated Oscillometry

How It Works

An automated oscillometer is an indirect non-invasive automated BP monitor. BP cuff is inflated to occlude blood flow through an artery. As the cuff pressure falls below SBP, the arterial pulsations are transmitted via the cuff to a transducer in the

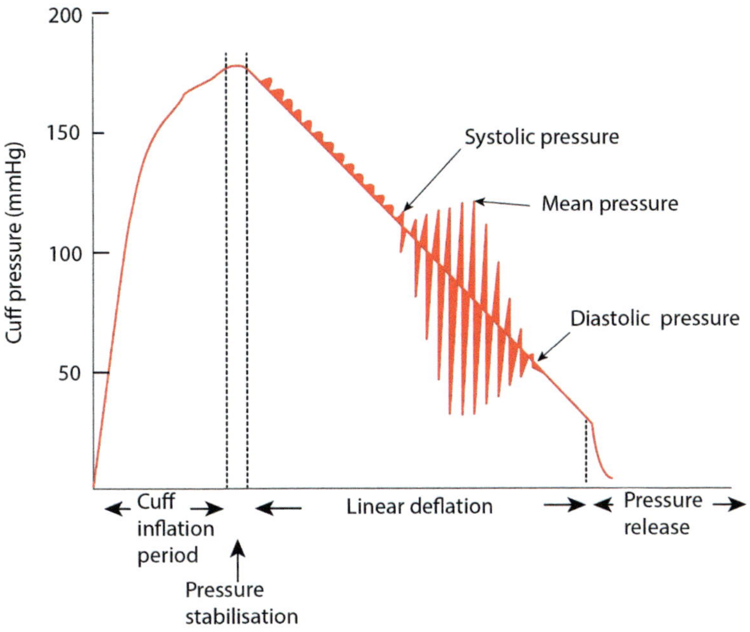

Fig. 16.1 Cuff pressure and oscillations in blood pressure measurement

module, which is controlled by a microprocessor. SBP, DBP and MAP are determined by the oscillations in the cuff detector by the sensor (see Fig. 16.1).

- SBP
  - Sudden increase in amplitude of oscillations
  - Pressure where pulsations are rising and are at 25–50% of maximum
- MAP
  - Lowest pressure at which there is maximum amplitude of oscillation
- DBP
  - Abrupt diminution of amplitude
  - Pressure where pulse amplitude has decreased by 80% of maximum

Note: The methods of determining SBP, MAP and DBP are proprietary empirical algorithms and differ between machines. The above are accepted mainstream explanations. There is no sound theory as to their rationality, but empirical calibration shows these landmarks to be accurate representations of SBP, MAP and DBP.

An example of an automated oscillometry device is the device for indirect non-invasive automated mean arterial pressure (DINMAP).

Problems and Inaccuracies

Intrinsic Accuracy

- SBP and MAP have reasonable correlation with readings from invasive blood pressure monitoring, but DBP is not as well correlated with invasive blood pressure monitoring.

Equipment and Patient Factors

Inaccurate readings may result from equipment factors:

- Leaks or blockages in pneumatic system
- Cuff misplacement
- Over-reading of BP if cuff is too small or narrow
- Under-reading of BP if cuff is oversized

  Inaccurate readings may result from patient factors:

- Hypotension: SBP overestimated
- Hypertension: SBP underestimated
- Arteriosclerosis
- AF or other arrhythmias
- Obesity overestimates pressure
- Movement, shivering

Iatrogenic Injury

- Pain
- Nerve palsy
- Skin haematoma

Automated Methods Using Doppler

Automated blood pressure monitoring using Doppler utilises similar principle to the methods described above. However, the SBP and DBP are established by Doppler interrogation of arterial wall movement. An example of this is the Arteriosonde. The Doppler transducer is incorporated in the cuff and must be positioned over the artery. When the artery is occluded by cuff inflation, no sound is detected. As the cuff is deflated and blood starts to flow, the movement of the arterial wall results in a frequency shift, and a 'murmur-like' sound is generated. This is taken as the SBP. This 'murmur-like' sound disappears when cuff pressure falls below the DBP. This method is said to be more accurate than oscillometry in infants.

Volume Clamp (Penaz) Technique

The Penaz technique is otherwise known as the *vascular unloading* or *volume clamp* technique. It was developed by the Czech physiologist Jan Peñáz in the 1970s. It is a non-invasive method that allows continuous monitoring of blood pressure, cardiac output, PPV and SVV (see cardiac output section).

Arterial Tonometry

Arterial tonometry is a technique based on the linear relationship between pressure and arterial displacement. A tonometer is placed over an artery whereby the artery is partly flattened against the underlying bone. The arterial displacement is read by the sensor and transduced, and the waveform is displayed digitally. As the artery is never completely occluded, this allows continuous measurement of the blood pressure.

Invasive Blood Pressure Monitoring

Invasive blood pressure monitoring is the monitoring of blood pressure directly via the arterial system. The radial artery is commonly used because of its convenient access, ease of placement, collateral ulnar circulation and reasonable approximation to the aortic root MAP.

Components

Cannula and Tubing

The standard adult arterial cannula is a 4 or 6 cm 20G Teflon cannula. It connects to the transducer via low-compliance, wide tubing of minimal length that is practically appropriate.

Pressurised Fluid

Saline is pressurised to 300 mmHg and connected to a continuous slow-flush ('inter-flow') device that allows slow flow of fluid through the transducer, tubing and cannula. This is essential to prevent the cannula from clotting. The flow rate of the fluid is approximately 4 ml h^{-1} at a pressure of 300 mmHg.

It is very important to avoid any air bubbles between the transducer and the patient because the compressibility of air increases the compliance of the system and introduces extra fluid movement. The consequence is reduced natural frequency and increased damping (see below).

Transducer Housing

Typically, the housing will contain the transducer, the interflow device, a stopcock and a fast-flush tab for priming and square-wave testing.

Transducer

The standard arterial pressure transducer is a tiny diaphragm of very low compliance and high natural frequency. The diaphragm surface supports a wire resistor or resistors. Arterial pressure fluctuations are transmitted to the diaphragm causing it to flex and stretch the wire. This increases the wire resistance, which is measured by a Wheatstone bridge. A solid-state alternative to the diaphragm uses a thin piezoelectric element that flexes in response to pressure changes and generates a voltage.

Practical Considerations

Zeroing and Transducer Placement

Blood pressure is 'gauge pressure', which is pressure referenced to the atmospheric pressure. Zeroing is the process whereby the transducer is opened to atmospheric pressure via a stopcock to make the module read that as zero. The standard placement of the transducer is at the level of the right atrium which, in the supine patient, is at the mid-axillary line, fourth intercostal space. For patients in the sitting or beach-chair position, the transducer may be placed at head level to indicate cerebral arterial pressure.

Complications

- Pain on insertion
- Haematoma
- Thrombosis and ischaemia
- Disconnection and haemorrhage
- Flushing, with antegrade or retrograde embolism
- Infection

Definitions and Concepts

Before outlining the physical principles of invasive pressure accuracy, it is important to have a basic understanding of the following concepts.

Static Accuracy

Static accuracy is the accurate measurement of a fixed pressure. Static accuracy requires the following:

- Time stability—accuracy does not change over time
- Linear gain over a range of fixed pressures

From the practical point of view, this means that atmospheric pressure is read as zero, and this baseline does not drift over time. The gain could be checked against a fixed column of mercury, but this is neither practical nor necessary in contemporary modules.

Dynamic Accuracy

Dynamic accuracy is the accurate reproduction of a dynamically varying pressure.

Fundamental Frequency

Fundamental frequency is the slowest component of a repetitive complex waveform. In the context of arterial pressure monitoring, this is the heart rate. This is also termed the first harmonic.

Harmonics

Harmonics are whole-number multiples of the fundamental frequency. For example:

- If the heart rate is 60 bpm, the fundamental frequency is 1 Hz. The 2nd and 10th harmonics are 2 Hz and 10 Hz, respectively.
- If the heart rate is 120 bpm, the fundamental frequency is 2 Hz. The 4th and 6th harmonics are 8 Hz and 12 Hz, respectively.

Fourier Analysis

Fourier analysis is the process of analysing a complex sine wave into its component frequencies, namely the fundamental frequency and a series of harmonics. Fourier analysis is not part of the normal invasive arterial pressure processing, but a grasp of the concept helps to understand an arterial pressure waveform as a repetitive sine wave comprised of multiple frequencies (see Fourier analysis).

Natural Frequency (F_N)

It is the frequency at which a system oscillates naturally when disturbed. Tap the transducer tubing, and you will see the pressure oscillate briefly at its natural frequency. Damping reduces the F_N a little, so sometimes it is referred to as the *damped natural frequency* (F_D). For simplicity, F_N will be used in the text.

Resonance

A system may also oscillate because an oscillating force (the arterial pressure wave) is driving it. As the frequency at which it is being driven approaches the natural frequency, the transducer system gains increasing energy from the driving force and the output oscillations become amplified relative to the driving oscillations. This is termed *resonance*. Transducer resonance leads to over-reading, waveform distortions and superimposed pressure spikes. Amplification is maximum at the natural frequency, so this is often termed the *resonant frequency*. The distinction is unimportant for the rest of the section, so the term natural frequency will be used. When the driving frequency exceeds the natural frequency, the transducer is unable to keep

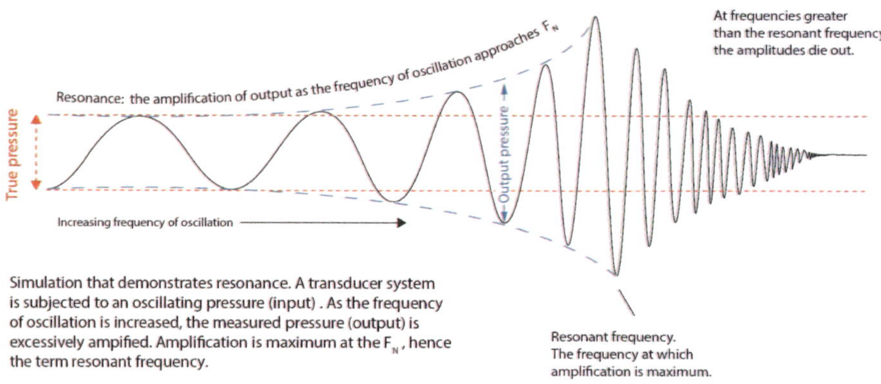

Fig. 16.2 Diagram representing the concept of resonance

up, the driving frequency and transducer will go out of phase and amplitudes die out (see Fig. 16.2).

The heart rate (fundamental frequency) is not high enough to cause transducer resonance, but some of the high-frequency harmonics, such as those of the systolic upslope and dicrotic notch, do have that potential.

Frequency Response/Bandwidth

The frequency response, or bandwidth, is the range of frequencies that are reproduced with minimal amplification relative to the true arterial pressures. Ideally, the ratio of transducer output to input would be near to 1.0 for most frequencies, and this is termed a flat frequency response. In clinical practice, an acceptable frequency response is achieved with a ratio up to 1.4. This sounds quite lax, but remember that we are mostly only interested in SBP and MAP.

Physical Principles of Dynamic Accuracy: Natural Frequency and Damping

Natural Frequency (F_N)

The arterial pressure waveform is a complex waveform comprised of multiple different frequency components. Some of those components are high-frequency driving forces that will resonate the transducer if their frequency is close to the system F_N. Examples are the systolic upslope and the dicrotic notch. To prevent this, the F_N of the system must be designed to be as high as possible, well above the frequency of those biological signals (see Fig. 16.3).

Rule of Thumb Regarding F_N

- At least ten times the fundamental frequency.
- At least ¼ of the heart rate (bpm).
- At least 40 Hz:

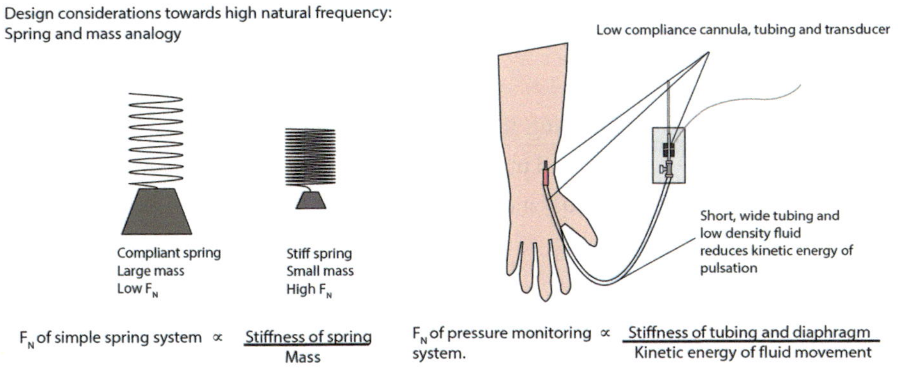

Fig. 16.3 Design features in an arterial pressure monitoring system that influence damping

- The Edwards TruWave IAP system has an F_N of 200 Hz for the transducer alone and 40 Hz for the whole system.

Design Features Leading to High F_N

- Non-compliant cannula, tubing and diaphragm:
  - Air bubbles increase the compliance of the system and must be eradicated.
- Short, wide tubing:
  - The kinetic energy of fluid motion in the tubing is the equivalent of the mass of the spring. Short, wide tubing means that there is less fluid moving and at lower velocity, hence lower kinetic energy.
- Low-density fluid reduces kinetic energy of the pulse wave.

Damping

Damping is the tendency for a system to resist oscillation through frictional forces. Damping reduces the amplitude of oscillation. Damping can be good or bad. Some inbuilt damping helps to oppose resonance, but we must try to avoid extra imposed clinical damping from air bubbles, clots and kinks. Our transducer systems come out of the packet underdamped. The following sections explain why that is and why it does not matter.

Design Features That Influence Damping

Damping is caused by fluid friction in the transducer system. Design features that reduce damping are:

- Short, wide tubing
- Low-compliance cannula, tubing and transducer
- Low-viscosity fluid such as saline
- Low-density fluid? You will read that damping is reduced when fluid density is high. This is because high-density fluids are less compressible and, therefore, produce less fluid movement. This is relevant in other science contexts (e.g. if the

fluid is a gas), but saline is virtually incompressible and is perfectly suited for our purpose.

$$\text{Damping} \propto \frac{\text{Tubing length.Compliance.Fluid viscosity}}{\text{Tubing diameter. Fluid density}}$$

Thus, the design features that increased F_N are also minimising damping!

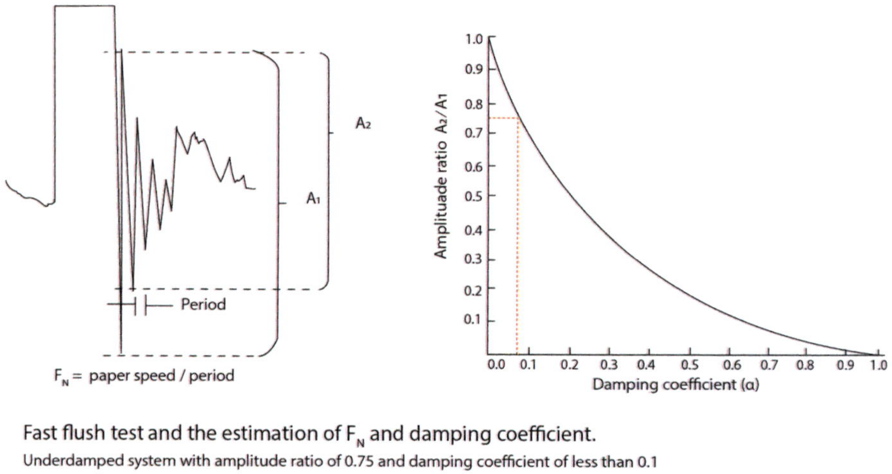

Fig. 16.4 The fast-flush test and the estimation of F_N and damping coefficient

Table 16.1 Degree of damping and their effect on oscillation amplitude

Degree of damping	Damping coefficient (α)	Notes
No damping	0.0	Oscillations do not die away at all in this hypothetical situation. See Fig. 16.5
Underdamped	0.3[a]	The damping in our systems is about 0.2–0.3. In this situation, successive oscillations diminish in amplitude by more than 60% each time. See Fig. 16.5
Optimal damping	0.64	Rapid diminution of oscillation with an amplitude ratio of only 7% of the previous oscillation. See Fig. 16.5
Critically damped	1.0	The minimal amount of damping where there are no oscillations after the square wave. A system damped to this degree would produce little or no useful information. See Fig. 16.5

[a]There are a range of coefficients that could be described as underdamped. This approximates to our systems when they are taken out of the packet

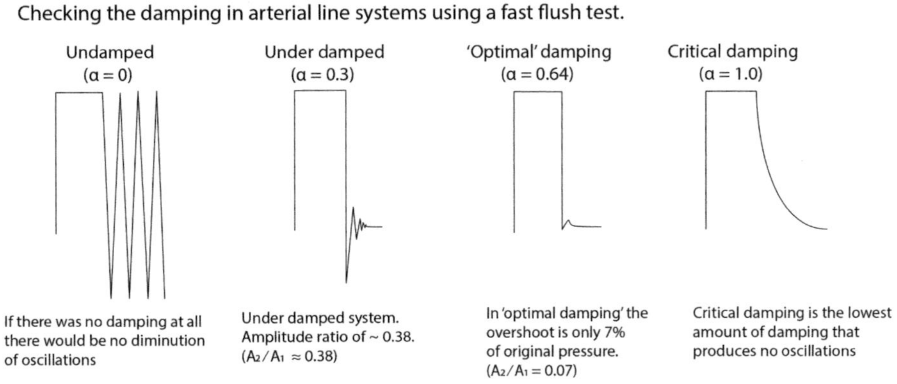

Fig. 16.5 Fast-flush test in different damping conditions in an arterial line system

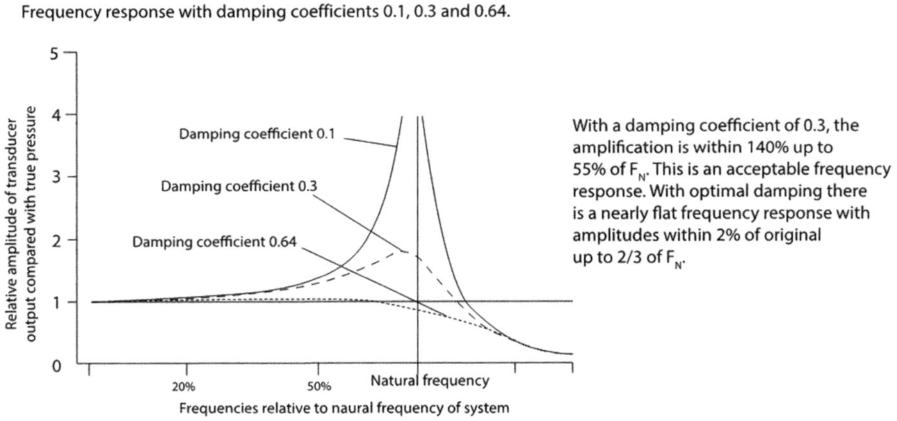

Damping Coefficient

The degree of damping is described by the damping coefficient (α). The damping coefficient is based on how rapidly oscillations die out after a sudden square wave pressure is applied in a fast-flush test shown in Fig. 16.4. The degree of damping and their effect on oscillation amplitude are shown in Table 16.1.

How Much Damping Do We Need? The Relationship Between Natural Frequency and Damping

Summary

Our transducer systems are designed to have high F_N, and this means that they have minimal damping. But don't we want some damping to oppose resonance? The answer is that we do not need to worry too much, as long as the F_N is well above the frequency of our biological components. It is the high F_N that we will mainly rely on to prevent resonance.

Working Illustration

A working illustration is shown in Fig. 16.6. Consider a typical underdamped system with damping coefficient of $\alpha = 0.3$. Experimentally, it is known that a damping coefficient of 0.3 produces an acceptable frequency response up to 55% of the F_N. As mentioned earlier, 'acceptable' in clinical practice means that the transducer pressure output-to-input ratio is no more than 1.4. Our important high-frequency components therefore need to be within that 55% of the F_N.

Fig. 16.6 The frequency response with damping coefficients 0.1, 0.3 and 0.64Thus, if $\alpha = 0.3$ and F_N is 15 Hz, there will be an acceptable frequency response up to 55% of 15 Hz, which is 8 Hz (rounded down). This is the 8th harmonic if the HR is 60 bpm but only the 4th harmonic if the HR is 120 bpm.

The general standard is that there should be an acceptable frequency response up to the 10th harmonic for a normal range of heart rates, although, for most purposes, 6–8 harmonics are adequate. It is clear that the 4th harmonic is not adequate.

The F_N must, therefore, be much higher to cope with underdamped systems. Most systems have F_N of around 40 Hz. With a damping coefficient of 0.3, this would provide an acceptable frequency response up to 55% of 40 Hz, which is 22 Hz. This is the 22nd harmonic at a heart rate of 60 bpm and the 11th harmonic at a heart rate of 120 bpm.

Optimal Damping

The flattest frequency response is obtained when the system has a damping coefficient of around 0.64. This is termed optimal damping and will produce a flat frequency response to 66% of F_N. A flat frequency response means the output amplitudes are within 2% of the input. Optimal damping is of interest, but, as described above, the systems we use are underdamped, at least to start with. It becomes more important to have damping coefficients around 0.64 in systems of lower F_N (see Fig. 16.7).

Phase Lag

Dynamic accuracy depends on not only the accurate reproduction of the amplitude of harmonics but also the harmonics that are in phase with each other. The inertia of

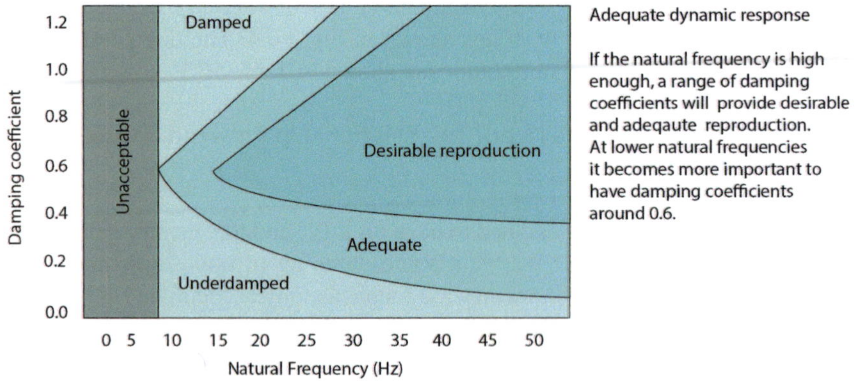

Fig. 16.7 Different damping conditions with damping coefficient and natural frequency

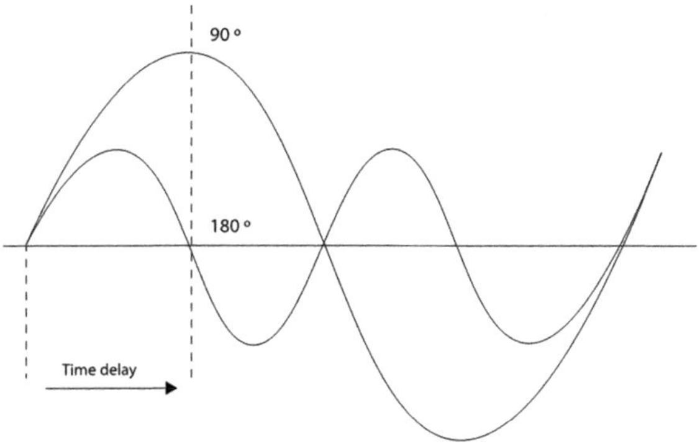

If the same time delay is applied to both components the 5 Hz waveform is delayed by 90° and the 10 Hz wave is delayed by 180°. The phase delay is in proportion to the frequency of the wave. This is best achieved at optimal damping ($\alpha = 0.64$)

Fig. 16.8 Phase lag

the pressure monitoring system means that there is a time delay between arterial pressure wave and the monitor signal. This does not matter if all components of the waveform are delayed by the same time interval. Because time intervals of sine waves are described in terms of phase, the technical term for this is that the *phase lag must be in proportion to the frequency of the wave*. This is best achieved with a damping coefficient of around 0.64, optimal damping (see Fig. 16.8).

Invasive Pressure Accuracy: In a Nutshell

Static Accuracy

- Fixed pressures, such as the zero baseline, must be reproduced accurately and must not drift with time.

Dynamic Accuracy

- Accurate reproduction of a complex sinusoidal pressure waveform.
- High-frequency components near the natural frequency of the system may cause resonance.
- The transducer system is designed to have a very high F_N, well above the frequency of the biological signals.
- This results in an underdamped system, and we lose some of the helpful aspect of damping, which is to oppose resonance.
- This will not be a problem if the F_N is well above the frequency of the biological components.

Further Reading

Davis PD, Kenny GN. Basic physics and measurement in anaesthesia. Butterworth-Heinemann; 2015.

Teplick R. Basic principles and limitations of hemodynamic monitoring. In: Foundations of anesthesia. Mosby; 2006. p. 173–88.

Vibration. Wikipedia. 2020. Available at https://en.wikipedia.org/wiki/Vibration#Damped_and_undamped_natural_frequencies. Accessed 8 May 2020.

Pulmonary Artery Catheter, Cardiac Output and Indices of Fluid Balance

17

Alan McLintic and Amanda Siu

Central Venous Pressure

A normal central venous pressure (CVP) trace is demonstrated in Fig. 17.1. The CVP waveform can change in pathology; some examples are listed in Table 17.1.

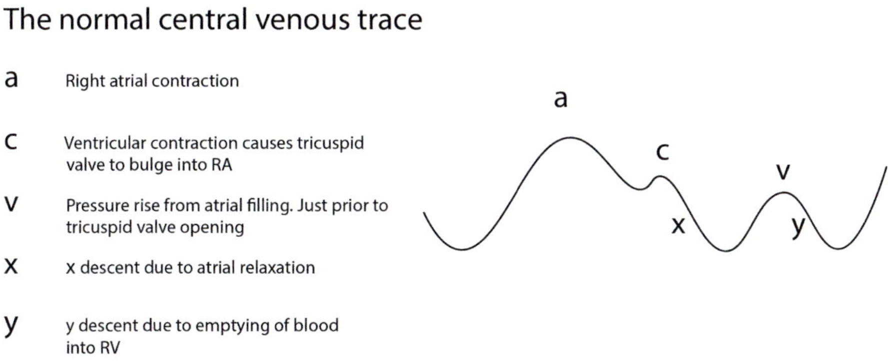

Fig. 17.1 The central venous pressure trace

A. McLintic
Department of Anaesthesia and Pain Medicine, Counties Manukau Health, Auckland, New Zealand

A. Siu (✉)
Department of Anaesthesia and Pain Medicine, Counties Manukau Health, Auckland, New Zealand

University of Auckland, Auckland, New Zealand
e-mail: tsiu001@aucklanduni.ac.nz

C. Birch et al. (eds.), *Physics and Measurement for Anesthesia*,
https://doi.org/10.1007/978-3-031-65060-4_17

Table 17.1 The central venous pressure waveform in pathology

CVP waveforms in pathology	
Cannon waves	Atrioventricular dissociation (e.g. complete heart block) causes large rapidly rising 'a' waves
Large 'a' waves	Tricuspid stenosis
Absent 'a' waves	Atrial fibrillation
Large 'c–v' waves	Tricuspid incompetence
Rapid 'y' descent	Constrictive pericarditis
Slow 'x' or 'y' descent	Tricuspid stenosis

Potential Complications of CVP Line Insertion

- Haemorrhage and haematoma
- Infection
- Pneumothorax, haemothorax
- Damage to surrounding structures including carotid artery, nerve plexus, trachea, tamponade, thoracic duct, etc.
- Arrhythmia
- Embolus of air, Teflon or thrombus

CVP as an Indicator of LV Filling

- There is a long history in medicine of using the CVP as a guide to optimise left ventricular filling and stroke volume, and to guide fluid challenges. This is now seen as inherently flawed for the following reasons:
  - The relationship between CVP and LV end-diastolic volume (LVEDV) is uncertain in the critically ill because of changes in venous tone, pulmonary vascular resistance, intrathoracic pressures and RV and LV compliance plus valve dysfunction and other mechanical changes.
  - The only purpose of giving fluid is to improve stroke volume, and this will only occur on the ascending part of the Frank-Starling curve. It is now clear that neither CVP nor pulmonary capillary wedge pressure (PCWP) is a reliable indicator of a patient's position on the Frank-Starling curve and therefore is a poor indicator of fluid responsiveness (see Fig. 17.2).

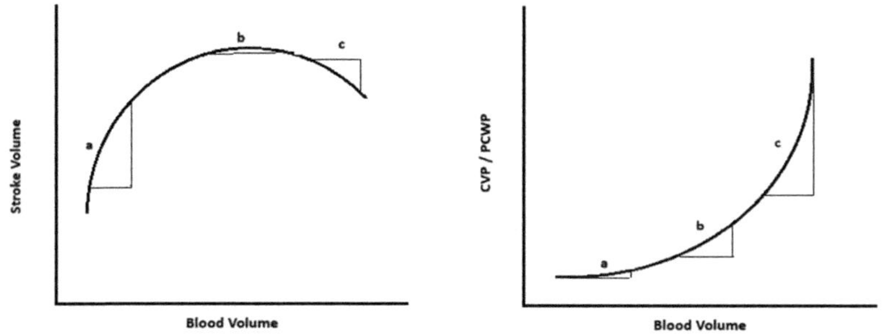

Fig. 17.2 The use of CVP and PCWP as indicators for fluid responsiveness

Pulmonary Artery (Swan-Ganz) Catheter

Components

A typical PA catheter is 50 cm in length and has three lumens and the following construction:

- The proximal lumen that opens 30 cm from the tip
- The distal lumen that opens at the tip
- An air-filled lumen to allow inflation of a small balloon situated just proximal to the opening of the distal lumen. The balloon is inflated by injecting 1–1.5 ml air from a syringe at a lockable connection at the hub.
- A thermistor is situated 4 cm back from the tip and has electrical connection at the hub.

Modifications of This Basic Design May Include

- An additional lumen for infusions.
- Ability to perform mixed venous oximetry via fibre-optic transmission (e.g. Edwards CCOmbo volumetrics catheter).
- A thermal element that emits a heat signal in the right ventricle. This allows continual cardiac output measurement by a heat dilution technique (e.g. Edwards Continuous CO catheter).

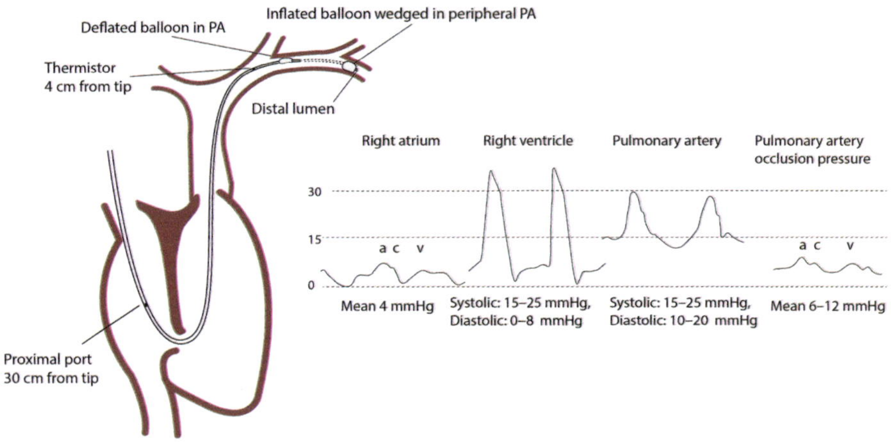

Fig. 17.3 Pressure trace of the pulmonary arterial catheter as it advances through the right atrium, right ventricle and pulmonary artery and finally wedged in the peripheral pulmonary artery

Insertion

The PA catheter is inserted through a major central vein, commonly the right internal jugular vein. The catheter is progressed through the heart and tracked by observing the distal lumen pressure trace (see Fig. 17.3). When the right atrium (RA) trace is observed, the balloon is inflated, and the catheter is advanced. The flow of blood encourages passage into the right ventricle (RV) and then to the left main pulmonary artery (MPA). The catheter can then be advanced further until the balloon becomes wedged in a small distal pulmonary artery. At this point, the distal lumen is registering pulmonary capillary back pressure from the left atrium (LA) that is indicative of left ventricular end-diastolic pressure (LVEDP) and left ventricular end-diastolic volume (LVEDV). The pressure obtained from the wedged catheter is colloquially termed the pulmonary capillary wedge pressure (PCWP) or more correctly the pulmonary artery occlusion pressure (PAOP). The catheter must not be left in the wedged state for more than 30 s or pulmonary infarct may occur. Once the balloon is deflated, the catheter should spring back into the MPA on its own accord and can be left in that position for subsequent pressure and cardiac output measurements.

Potential Complications

Potential Complications of CVP Line Insertion

- Haemorrhage and haematoma
- Infection
- Pneumothorax, haemothorax
- Damage to surrounding structures including carotid artery, nerve plexus, trachea, tamponade, thoracic duct, etc.

- Arrhythmia
- Embolus of air, Teflon or thrombus

Arrhythmia

Ventricular ectopics or short runs of VT are particularly common when the PAC passes through the tricuspid valve into the RV.

Catheter Knot

In situations of high right-heart pressures, it may be impossible to float the catheter into the PA, and, if this is not recognised, it is easy to develop coils of catheter in the RV with the danger of a knot forming.

Pulmonary Artery Rupture

If the uninflated catheter wedges on its own accord and is unrecognised, subsequent inflation of the balloon may rupture the pulmonary artery causing haemorrhage and haemoptysis.

Practical Considerations and Inaccuracies

1. Catheter tip must lie in West zone 3

   For the PAOP to equal LVEDP, there must be an uninterrupted pressure conduit from pulmonary artery through to pulmonary veins. This can only happen if the catheter tip lies in West zone 3 where the $P_{PA} > P_{PV} > P_{alv}$. Indications that the tip is in West zone 3 include:
   - Tip points downwards on erect CXR or below RA on lateral CXR.
   - 'a' and 'v' waves can be seen on the PAOP trace.
   - Should be able to aspirate blood from the wedged catheter.
   - The $PA_{diastolic}$ > PAOP.
2. Artefact
   - The PA catheter has lower natural frequency (25–35 Hz) than an arterial line and is therefore more subject to resonance.
   - In a hyperdynamic circulation, the catheter 'whips' around, causing artefact and distorting the trace.
3. Mean PAOP underestimates LVEDP in normal physiology
   - The part of the PAOP trace that most closely represents LVEDP is the peak of the 'a' wave, but it is not feasible to attempt to isolate and track the 'a' wave in the clinical setting, so it is the mean PAOP that is used to direct therapy. The mean PAOP underestimates the LVEDP by a small amount (see Fig. 17.4).
4. Effect of IPPV and PEEP
   - Increased intra-thoracic pressure has an additive effect on PAOP resulting in overestimation of LVEDP.

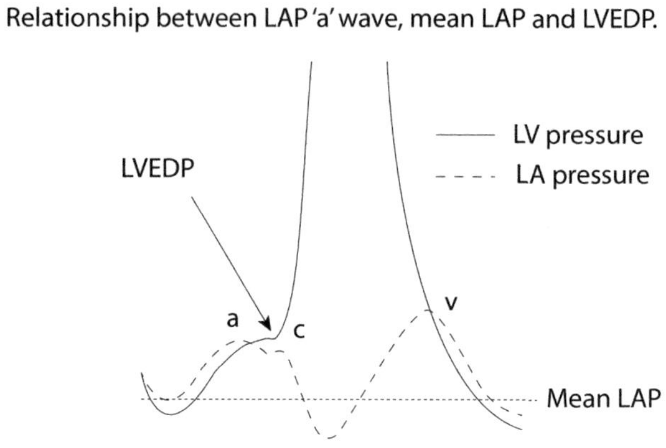

Fig. 17.4 Relationship between left atrial pressure 'a' wave, mean left atrial pressure and left ventricular end-diastolic pressure

5. Conditions changing the LAP and LVEDP relationship
   - The LAP and therefore the PAOP may overestimate LVEDP in:
     - Mitral stenosis or regurgitation.
     - Tachycardia. This is due to inadequate time for diastolic filling.
   - The LAP and therefore the PAOP may underestimate LVEDP in:
     - Aortic regurgitation. AR jet can cause premature closure of the mitral valve. The LV pressure then continues to rise after closure.
6. LVEDP and LVEDV relationship
   - Non-compliant left ventricles require higher than normal filling pressures.

Mixed Venous Oxygen Saturation

Overview

Central mixed venous Hb saturation ($ScvO_2$) reflects the balance between oxygen delivery and consumption. Therefore, in case of arterial Hb saturation, Hb concentration and oxygen consumption remain stable, and $ScvO_2$ can be used as an indirect indicator of cardiac output:

$$ScvO_2 = SaO_2 - \frac{\dot{V}O_2}{\dot{D}O_2} \quad \text{or} \quad ScvO_2 = 1 - \text{Extraction ratio}$$

Technology

Measurements are made by fibre-optic oximetry incorporated in the central venous lines or pulmonary artery catheters. These are reflection oximeters. Light emitted from LEDs at the transducer end travels up one fibre-optic channel and is reflected off RBCs back down a second fibre-optic channel to the detector.

Interpretation

- Normal value of $ScvO_2$ ~70%
- Causes of decreased $ScvO_2$:
  - Reduced oxygen delivery (decreased cardiac output, decreased SaO_2)
  - Increased oxygen consumption
- Causes of increased $ScvO_2$:
  - Reduced metabolic demand
  - Inability to use delivered oxygen (e.g. sepsis)
  - Elevated cardiac output
  - Shunting

Indication for Use

- Indicates adequacy of tissue oxygenation
- Indication of cardiac output and adequacy of cardiac output
- Surveillance/early warning parameter
- Guide for adjusting therapy

Caveats

- $ScvO_2$ does not reflect the adequacy of *regional* oxygenation. An organ can be ischaemic, while another has luxury perfusion.
- Indicates cardiac output only if the other parameters are stable.
- Surveillance triggers are not reliably defined.
- Evidence for benefit is lacking.

Cardiac Output: Fick Principle

The amount of a substance taken up by an organ is the product of the flow through the organ and its arterio-venous content difference. When the Fick principle is used to calculate cardiac output, the organ is the lungs (or strictly the whole body) and the 'uptake' is oxygen consumption.

- Arterial O_2 content = 20 ml dl^{-1}
- Mix venous O_2 content = 15 ml dl^{-1}
- Oxygen consumption = 250 ml min^{-1}. Oxygen consumption can be derived from differences between inspired and expired minute volumes and oxygen concentrations using a bedside metabolic computer:

$$CO = \frac{250 \text{ml} \min^{-1}}{20 - 15 \text{ml} \text{dl}^{-1}} \times 100 = 5 \text{L} \min^{-1}$$

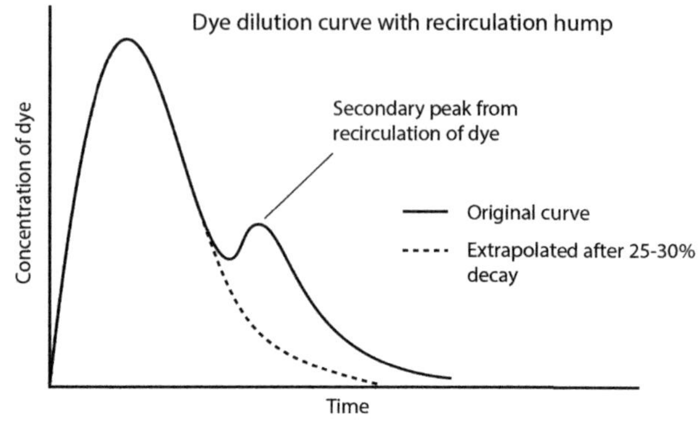

Fig. 17.5 Dye dilution curve

Cardiac Output: Indicator Dilution

Dye Dilution

Overview

The measurement of cardiac output by dye dilution is a modification of the Fick principle but is more meaningfully described as a conservation of mass technique: if a known mass of dye is added to a volume and you measure the concentration after dilution, you can work out the volume. The basic principle is to give a bolus of dye into a central vein and measure the rate of dilution by the blood flow of the heart. This is the dye dilution curve as shown in Fig. 17.5. The greater the rate of dilution, the greater the cardiac output.

How It Works

The most used dye is indocyanine green. Others include Evans blue, methylene blue and bromsulphalein. The dye concentration is typically measured by a densitometer using light absorption principles, with sampling taking place continuously at the radial artery. Non-invasive detectors are also available with similar design to a pulse oximeter probe.

Dye Dilution Curve

- The area under the curve (AUC) is inversely proportional to the cardiac output:

$$\text{Cardiac output} \propto \frac{\text{Mass of dye}}{\text{AUC}}$$

- Repeated measurements cause a gradual rise in baseline from zero.
- Recirculation of dye causes a recirculation hump. If this was included in the calculation, the cardiac output estimate would be falsely low. To correct for this, the curve is allowed to decay for 25–30%, and the rest of the curve is extrapolated.

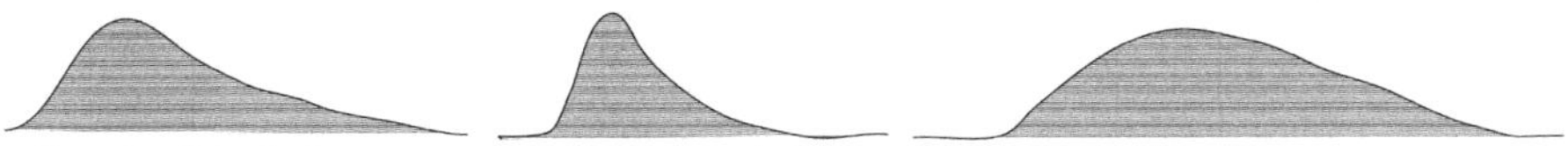

Fig. 17.6 Thermodilution curve in different cardiac output states

Thermodilution

Overview

The measurement of cardiac output by thermodilution is a modification of the Fick principle but is more meaningfully described as a conservation of mass technique. Ten millilitres of room-temperature 5% dextrose is injected as rapidly as possible into the RA via the proximal port of the PA catheter. The temperature of the injectate is measured by a thermistor attached to the injection port. The blood temperature (T_B) is measured in the MPA by the thermistor 4 cm proximal to the PA catheter tip. The rate of dilution of the coldness is proportional to the cardiac output.

Dilution Curve and Calculation

- The AUC is inversely proportional to the cardiac output (see Fig. 17.6):

$$\text{Cardiac output} \propto \frac{\text{Mass of coldness}}{\text{AUC}}$$

$$\text{Cardiac output} = \frac{\text{Volume}_{\text{inj}} \times \left(T_{\text{blood}} - T_{\text{injectate}}\right) \times K}{\text{AUC}}$$

- The computation constant (K) depends on volume, specific heat and density of injectate and catheter size.
- The original Stewart-Hamilton equation relates to dye dilution. The modified Stewart-Hamilton equation is for thermodilution and expands on the above with formal integration notation for AUC in the denominator:

$$\text{Cardiac output} = \frac{\text{Volume}_{\text{inj}} \times \left(T_{\text{body}} - T_{\text{injectate}}\right) \times K}{\int_0^{\infty} \Delta T_{\text{B}}(t)\,\mathrm{d}t}$$

Practical Aspects

- Typically, the average three measurements that are within 10% of each other are taken.
- Iced injectates improve signal-to-noise ratio and reduce variability but may cause reflex bradycardia. Iced injectate can also increase contractility and cardiac output as a consequence of reduced temperature in the coronary circulation.
- Thermodilution has the advantage of no recirculation hump although there can be some elevation of baseline in serial measurements with cold injectates.
- Temperature in the RV varies with respiration. This is because there is a temperature difference between IVC and SVC blood and their proportions in the venous

return vary with respiration. This variation makes it difficult to determine when the curve reaches baseline. It is usual therefore to extrapolate the exponential curve after it has decayed by 25–30% of peak.

- Some devices such as PiCCO and LiDCO (see below) record the dilution curve from a peripheral artery rather than the PA. Even if the total cardiac output does not pass the sampling site, the change in indicator concentration is the same in every arterial branch. Thus, the AUC will be the same in any part of the circulation.

Situations When Results May Be Invalid

- Tricuspid incompetence leads to underestimation
- Right-to-left shunt
- Concomitant rapid infusion into SVC
- Haemodialysis
- RA port lying within the introducer sheath

Edwards Continuous CO Catheter

This PA catheter has a thermal coil that emits pulses of heat every 30–60 s into the RV. The dilution of the heated blood is measured by a thermistor in the MPA. Background changes in temperature are compensated for by analysing cooling of random heat pulses. This causes a delay through averaging.

Advantages of this system include:

- Convenience, less handling, less disconnection, less infection risk
- Continuous estimation of cardiac output
- No need for repeated boluses of fluid which contribute to fluid load

Cardiac Output: Pulse Contour Analysis (PCA)

Cardiac output can be derived by analysing the arterial pressure waveform. Pulse contour analysis will be used as a general term for this process, but the algorithms differ between manufacturers, and they use different terms such as pulse pressure analysis (Edwards FloTrac) and pulse power analysis (LiDCOplus).

Invasiveness and Calibration Requirement

PCA methods vary in their invasiveness and their need for prior calibration by dilution. For example:

- Arterial line PCA + prior cardiac output calibration by thermodilution
  - (PiCCO, Edwards VolumeView)
- Arterial line PCA + prior cardiac output by lithium dilution
  - (LiDCOplus)

- Arterial line PCA with no prior calibration
  - (FloTrac, PiCCO ProAQT, LiDCOrapid)
- Non-invasive PCA using Penaz technique
  - (ClearSight, LiDCO CNAP)

Technique with Calibrated Devices

The technique with calibrated devices is to first perform thermodilution or lithium dilution cardiac output measurement while the arterial pressure waveform is analysed. Indicator injection is via a central line, and measurement of the dilution curve is via a femoral or radial arterial line. The arterial pulse contour is analysed in the context of the measured cardiac output, and, from then on, pulse contour analysis provides a continual estimation of cardiac output.

How Is Cardiac Output Derived from Pulse Contour Analysis?

The points of interest and algorithms differ between manufacturers. In general, the algorithms use the heart rate, an estimation of stroke volume or pump performance and an index of large vessel impedance or compliance to derive cardiac output.

Indication of Stroke Volume and Pump Performance

The classic parameters used to indicate stroke volume and pump performance include:

- Gradient of systolic upslope (d*p*/d*t*) related to contractility
- AUC of systolic ejection portion proportional to stroke volume
- Pulse pressure

Pulse contour analysis and variables of interest in estimating stroke volume are shown in Fig. 17.7 (left). However, there are several proprietary algorithms analysing different parameters.

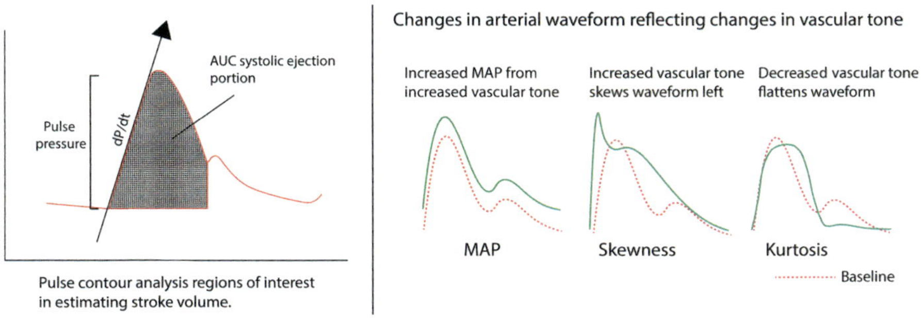

Fig. 17.7 Pulse contour analysis and variables of interest in estimating stroke volume (left), and changes in arterial waveform with changes in vascular tone (right)

Indicators of Large Vessel Impedance or Compliance

There is a correlation between patient's biometric data such as age, gender, height, weight and MAP with respect to aortic compliance. Correction factors can be derived from these variables. Arterial waveform contours can also indicate large vessel compliance. Changes in parameters such as MAP, kurtosis (how peaked or flat the contour is) and skewness (lack of symmetry) are used during dynamic monitoring to adjust for compliance changes (see Fig. 17.7 (right)).

Calculation of Cardiac Output

The algorithms differ between devices, but all of them have the same overall pattern as above. A simple algorithm described by the Edwards ClearSight device is:

$$\text{Stroke volume} = \frac{\text{AUC systolic ejection portion}}{\text{Vascular impedance}}$$

- Vascular impedance is estimated from patient biometrics.
- The SV is then multiplied by heart rate to give cardiac output.

Intrathoracic Blood Volume (ITBV) and Extravascular Lung Water (EVLW)

Calibrated PCA devices, including PiCCO and Edwards VolumeView, provide estimates of ITBV and EVLW or variants of them. These are highly derived indices deduced from parameters of the thermodilution curve including pulmonary circulation volumes and transit times. The ITBV is an indication of LV preload, while the EVLW is an index of capillary permeability and interstitial oedema.

LiDCOplus

The LiDCOplus follows the basic principles of the calibrated devices described above. The measurement of lithium dilution is taken via a lithium-sensitive electrode, which is a 'flow-through' attachment to an arterial line. The passage of lithium across a lithium-selective membrane creates a voltage. It is pulse power that is analysed rather than a pulse contour. This technique cannot be used in patients taking lithium and is contraindicated in the first trimester of pregnancy. Measurements may also be upset by benzylisoquinolinium muscle relaxants.

Stroke Volume Variation (SVV) and Pulse Pressure Variation (PPV)

All contemporary pulse contour type devices provide either PPV or SVV or both, as guides to volume responsiveness.

Changes in Arterial Pressure During Spontaneous Breathing

In normal subjects breathing spontaneously, the blood pressure decreases on inspiration by about 5 mmHg. Pulsus paradoxus is the exaggeration of this phenomenon in cardiac tamponade and other states. The normal arterial pressure swing during inspiration is due to the following interrelated factors:

- Negative intra-thoracic pressure increases right ventricular return.
- Improved filling and dilatation of RA reduce compliance of LA and reduce LA filling.
- Reduced LA filling reduces LV preload and LV stroke volume (SV).

Changes in Arterial Pressure During IPPV

During positive-pressure ventilation, the cyclic variation in pressure is amplified and reversed; the arterial pressure rises during inspiration and falls in the expiratory phase. This is called reverse pulsus paradoxus. This pressure swing is the result of positive-pressure ventilation leading to increased intra-thoracic pressure (ITP). Increased ITP leads to decreased venous return to RA with decreased RV filling, decreased RV stroke volume, decreased pulmonary blood flow and decreased LV stroke volume. The increased alveolar pressure creates West zone I and II conditions, which leads to increased RV afterload. Increased alveolar pressure squeezes capillary blood towards the left heart and increases LV preload. Positive pleural pressure reduces thoracic blood volume and therefore reduces LV afterload. The net effect is that, while the LV stroke volume increases in inspiration, the RV stroke volume is at the same time decreasing. Because the pulmonary transit time of blood is about 2 s, the effect of the RV insufficiency is not felt in the LV until 2–3 beats later, which will be in the expiratory phase. Thus, during expiration, the LV preload is reduced causing a drop in LV stroke volume and arterial pressure. This effect is exaggerated in hypovolaemia (see Fig. 17.8).

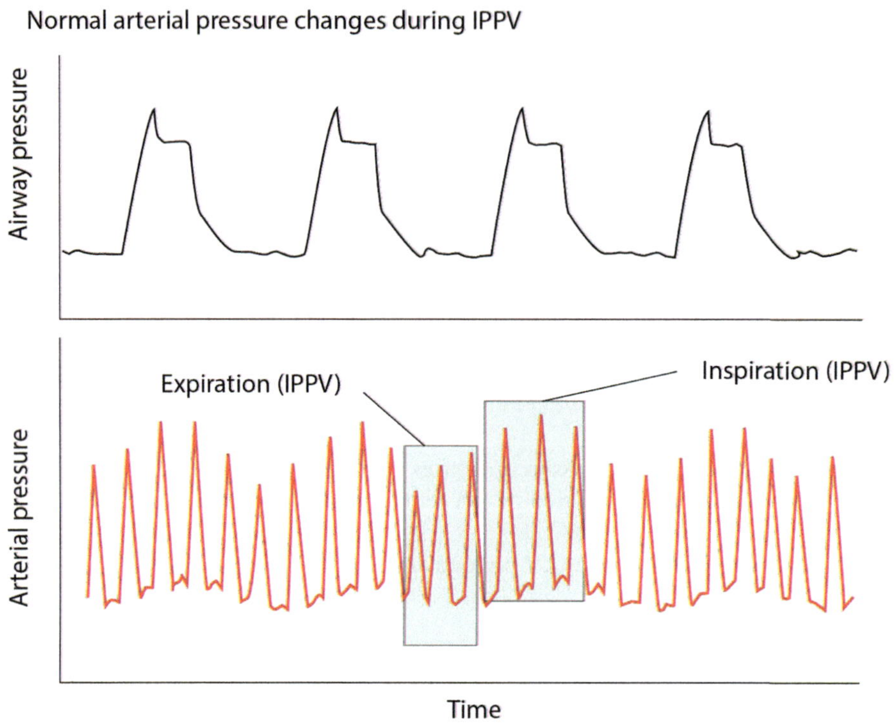

Fig. 17.8 Pulse pressure variation with respiration cycle

Pulse Pressure and Stroke Volume Variation

The pulse pressure is the difference between the systolic pressure (SBP) and the preceding diastolic pressure.

The PPV has been shown to be directly proportional to SV and inversely related to arterial compliance.

Calculation of PPV

$$\text{PPV}(\%) = \left(\frac{\text{PP}_{\text{max}} - \text{PP}_{\text{min}}}{(\text{Average PP})} \right) \times 100 = \left(\frac{\text{PP}_{\text{max}} - \text{PP}_{\text{min}}}{(\text{PP}_{\text{max}} + \text{PP}_{\text{min}})/2} \right) \times 100$$

Inferences

The inspiratory effects on RV insufficiency are made worse in conditions of hypovolaemia resulting in large swings in stroke volume and arterial pressure. In these conditions, the LV operates on the steep part of the Frank-Starling curve and is particularly sensitive to volume changes. Large swings in pressure therefore suggest not only that the patient is inadequately filled, but that they may respond to volume loading. There are minor differences between devices, but a PPV or SVV of <13% suggests that the patient is unlikely to be fluid responsive.

Volume Clamp 'Penaz' Technique

The *Penaz* technique is otherwise known as the *vascular unloading* or *volume clamp* technique. It was developed by the Czech physiologist Jan Peňáz in the 1970s. It is a non-invasive method that allows continuous tracking of blood pressure, cardiac output, PPV and SVV. Examples of the Penaz technique include Edwards ClearSight and LiDCO CNAP.

Components

The components of a volume clamp device consist of an inflatable finger pressure cuff, infrared light source with a detector incorporated within the pressure cuff and a module that allows rapid servo feedback between light detector signal and the cuff.

Working Principle

The infrared system continuously measures the arterial diameter within the finger as a surrogate for arterial volume. This is fed back rapidly to the cuff, which gradually inflates until the arterial wall is 'unstretched'. This means that the internal arterial pressure is balanced, not by the arterial wall tension, but by the external pressure from the cuff. The volume in the artery at this point is termed the unloaded volume, hence one of the names for this technique. From then on, the cuff pressure varies, increasing in systole and decreasing in diastole, to clamp the arterial volume at the unloaded volume, hence the other name, the volume clamp technique. The continuously changing cuff pressure corresponds to arterial pressure. The arterial pressure waveform is continuously displayed and undergoes pulse contour analysis to produce CO, SVV and PPV as described above.

Practical Considerations

- The ClearSight has the facility for two finger cuffs so that fingers can be alternated.
- The ClearSight has a heart reference sensor that must be levelled at the heart to compensate for hydrostatic pressure differences between heart and finger.
- Performance may be adversely affected in conditions of shock, vasoconstrictor therapy and mechanical obstruction to hand or arm.

Further Reading

Marik PE, Monnet X, Teboul JL. Hemodynamic parameters to guide fluid therapy. Ann Inensive Care. 2011;1(1):1–9.
Marik PE, Baram M, Vahid B. Does central venous pressure predict fluid responsiveness?*: a systematic review of the literature and the tale of seven mares. Chest. 2008;134(1):172–8.
McGee WT, Headley JM, Frazier JA, Lichtenthal PR. Quick guide to cardiopulmonary care. Edwards Lifesciences; 2014.
Teplick R. Basic principles and limitations of hemodynamic monitoring. In: Foundations of anesthesia. Mosby; 2006. p. 173–88.

Electrocardiography 18

Alan McLintic and Amanda Siu

What Are the Measurements on an ECG? See Table 18.1.

Table 18.1 ECG conventions

ECG conventions	
Paper speed/sweep speed	25 mm/s
Time interval one small square	0.04 s = 1mm
Time interval one large square	0.2 s = 5 mm
Voltage calibration	10 mm = 1 mV

A. McLintic
Department of Anaesthesia and Pain Medicine, Counties Manukau Health, Auckland, New Zealand

A. Siu (✉)
Department of Anaesthesia and Pain Medicine, Counties Manukau Health, Auckland, New Zealand

University of Auckland, Auckland, New Zealand
e-mail: tsiu001@aucklanduni.ac.nz

C. Birch et al. (eds.), *Physics and Measurement for Anesthesia*,
https://doi.org/10.1007/978-3-031-65060-4_18

What Does the Vertical ECG Deflection Represent?

It is an electrical vector which is the net magnitude and direction of depolarisation as sensed by a particular electrode.

- By convention, depolarisation towards an electrode will be displayed with positive deflection.
- The magnitude of deflection is in the order of 1–2 mv, the signal being attenuated by lung air, muscle and other tissues from the original 90 mV myocardial potential.

What Is Einthoven's Triangle?

The Einthoven's triangle as depicted in Fig. 18.1 is an inverted equilateral triangle with the heart at the centre that uses three extremities as recording points. The recording points are chosen so that the majority of deflections were positive.

The 12-Lead ECG System

The 12-lead ECG system as demonstrated by Fig. 18.2 consists of standard limb lead, augmented leads and unipolar chest leads.

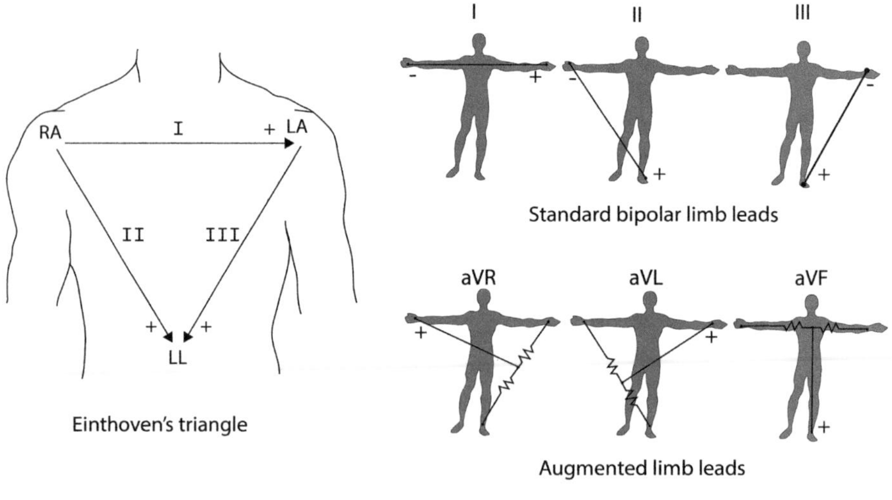

Fig. 18.1 Einthoven's triangle

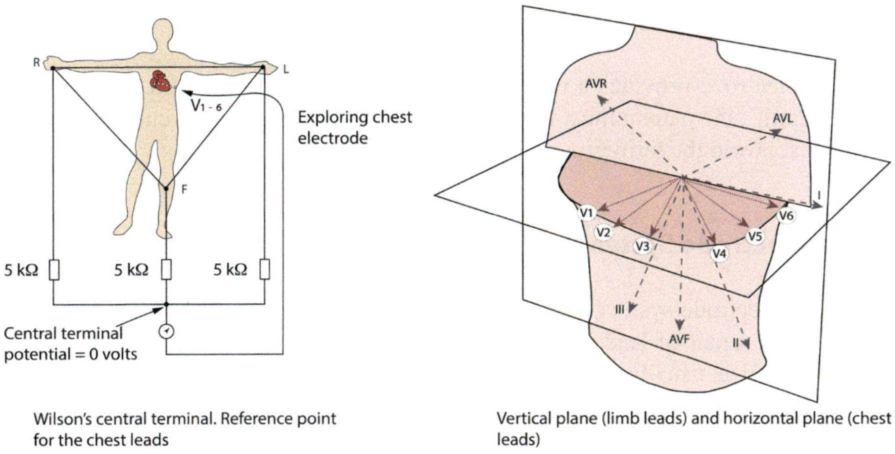

Fig. 18.2 The 12-lead ECG system

Standard Limb Leads

Standard limb leads are bipolar leads that record differences in potentials between pairs of electrodes in the Einthoven's triangle. One of the pairs is designated +ve. If the overall vector is towards that electrode, the deflection is positive:

- Lead I: RA – LA (+)
- Lead II: RA – LL (+)
- Lead III: LA – LL (+)

Augmented Leads

Augmented leads are unipolar leads whereby one Einthoven electrode is compared against the average of the other two:

- aVR: RA – 0.5 (LA + LL)
- aVL: LA – 0.5 (RA + LL)
- aVF: LL – 0.5 (RA + LA)

Unipolar Chest Leads

When the three electrodes are joined together, the potentials cancel each other out, and the net electrical potential is zero. This is called Wilson's central terminal, and it provides a reference zero against which six exploring precordial chest electrodes can be measured. Depolarisation towards an exploring electrode is given a positive deflection.

What Is the Purpose of the Right Leg (RL) Electrode?

The RL electrode provides a reference for background potentials. It is absolutely not an 'earth'; the patient must never be connected to earth. To prevent ambiguity, I would also avoid the term ground.

Three-Electrode System

The three-electrode system consists of RA, LA and LL pairs as per standard limb leads. When a pair of lead is being used, the third electrode is the reference electrode. Lead II is usually used as the reference electrode, as the axis is parallel to normal vector axis and P waves show up well. However, the three-electrode system has limited ability to detect anterior ischaemia.

Five-Electrode System

The five-electrode system as shown in Fig. 18.3 consists of RA, LA, LL, RL and one chest lead. This system allows recording of six standard limb leads and precordial unipolar lead. It has an improved sensitivity for the detection of myocardial ischaemia.

Modified 3-Lead Systems

Of all the 12 ECG leads, V5 is the lead with the highest sensitivity (75%) to detect myocardial ischaemia. The configuration of the normal 3-lead system can be

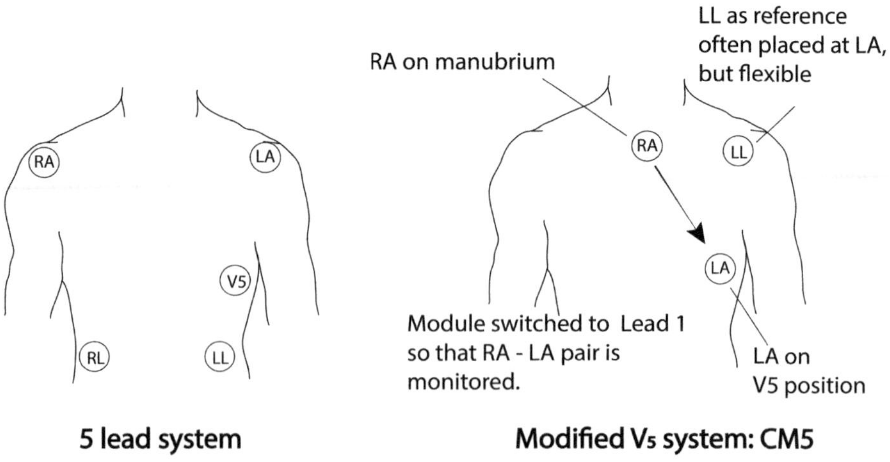

Fig. 18.3 The 5-lead ECG system (left) and the modified V5 system (right)

modified to approximate V5 to increase sensitivity. There are at least five configurations. The most common is the CM5 configuration as shown in Fig. 18.3, as follows:

- RA is placed over the manubrium.
- LA is placed at precordial V5 position.
- LL can go anywhere but is usually placed at the normal left arm position.
- Switch monitor to lead 1.

Electrocardiogram Axis

Frontal (Vertical) Axis

The limb leads depict the direction of the ventricular depolarisation in the vertical (frontal) plane. Frontal axis can be approximated using the hexaxial reference system. The normal axis is −30° to +105°. The rightward limit of normal varies between texts. An axis >+90° is likely to indicate abnormality outside infanthood. Calculation of the precise vertical axis based on Einthoven triangle is inherently flawed because the placement of electrodes is not, in reality, equilateral (see Table 18.2 and Fig. 18.4).

Rule of Thumb Calculation

The ECG axis can be assessed using leads I–III (see Fig. 18.5).

−30° (normal limit):	Lead I positive and lead II equiphasic
<−30 (left axis deviation):	Lead I positive and lead II and III negative
+90° (normal limit):	Lead I equiphasic and lead II and III positive
>+90° (right axis deviation):	Lead I negative and lead II and III positive

Table 18.2 Polarity and axis of standard limb leads and augmented limb leads

Lead	Limbs	Polarity	Axis if vector directed towards +ve electrode	Axis if vector perpendicular to +ve electrode
Standard limb leads				
I	RA-LA	LA +ve	0°	±90°
II	RA-LL	LL +ve	+60°	−30° or +150°
III	LA-LL	LL +ve	+120°	+30° or −150°
Augmented limb leads				
AVR	RA − 0.5 (LA + LL)	RA +ve	−150°	−60° or +120°
AVL	LA − 0.5 (RA + LL)	LA +ve	−30°	+60° or −120°
AVF	LA − 0.5 (RA + LA)	LL +ve	+90°	0° or 180°

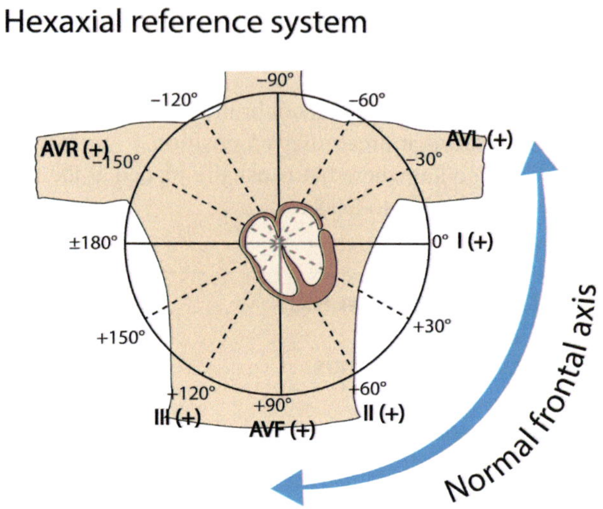

Fig. 18.4 Hexaxial reference system

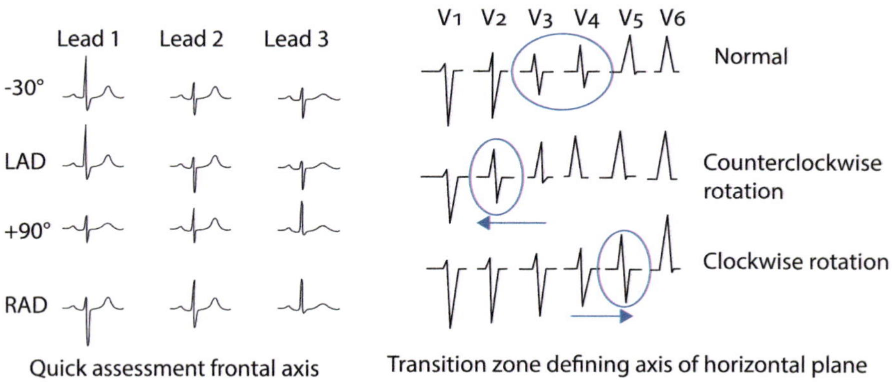

Fig. 18.5 ECG axis

Physiological Variations in Frontal Axis

Age

At birth, the QRS axis is right of the normal adult, with mean 75° and range from 60° to 160°. The right-sided dominant pattern usually reverts by 3 years of age but may persist into the 8–12-year group. Axis moves more leftward with ageing.

Body Habitus

Thin people have more vertical (rightward) axis. Obese people tend to have more leftward axis.

Horizontal Plane Axis

The cardiac axis in the horizontal plane is described in terms of the transition from a dominant S wave (rS pattern) in the right chest leads to a dominant R wave (Rs pattern) in the left chest leads. The horizontal vector is imagined as rotation clockwise or counterclockwise as you look up on the heart from below.

- Counterclockwise rotation: rS has changed to Rs by V3.
- Clockwise rotation: rS pattern remains at V4 or further leftward.
- Normal: transition between V3 and V4 so there is as dominant S wave in V3 and dominant R wave in V4.

Implications

In general, clockwise rotation is associated with worse cardiac and non-cardiac outcomes including mortality. Counterclockwise rotation has less associated morbidity although certain conditions are specifically associated with dominant R waves in the right chest leads. These include:

- RV hypertrophy
- HOCM
- True posterior MI
- Left septal fascicular block
- RBBB
- WPW

The Normal Electrocardiogram

Figure 18.6 demonstrates the ECG waves (P wave, QRS wave, T wave and U wave) and the intervals (PR interval, ST interval, QT interval and RR interval)

P Wave

What Is the P Wave?

P wave represents atrial depolarisation. The early part of the P wave is RA depolarisation; the mid-portion is RA, LA and inter-atrial septum depolarisation; and the late portion of the P wave is LA depolarisation.

Normal Axis

A normal axis may be anterior, leftward or inferior. P waves are always upright in I and II and V3–V6. They are always inverted in AVR and often biphasic in V1.

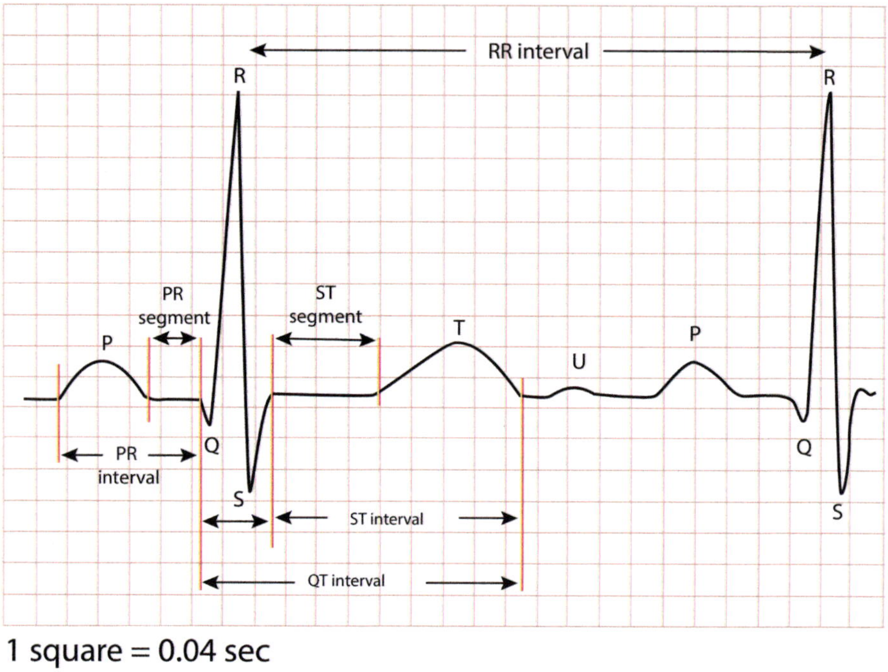

Fig. 18.6 ECG waves and intervals

Normal Dimensions

Normal P waves are <3 mm in height and <0.12 s in duration.

Why Does Left Atrial Hypertrophy Give a Bifid P Wave But Right Atrial Hypertrophy Give a Peaked P Wave?

Mitral stenosis causes LA hypertrophy. This increases LA voltages and prolongs depolarisation of the mid- to late portion of the P wave causing a bifid waveform. However, P pulmonale is RA hypertrophy. This increases RA voltages and prolongs depolarisation of the early to mid-portion of the P wave. Summation with the LA potentials results in a peaked waveform. This is demonstrated in Fig. 18.7.

PR Interval

The PR interval is the interval between the onset of atrial depolarisation and the onset of ventricular depolarisation. It is measured from the onset of P wave to the beginning of Q, or the R wave if there is no Q wave. The PR interval represents depolarisation of the atria, AV node, His bundle, bundle branches and Purkinje fibres. It does not include SA node activity.

Dimensions

A normal duration for the PR interval is 0.12–0.2 s.

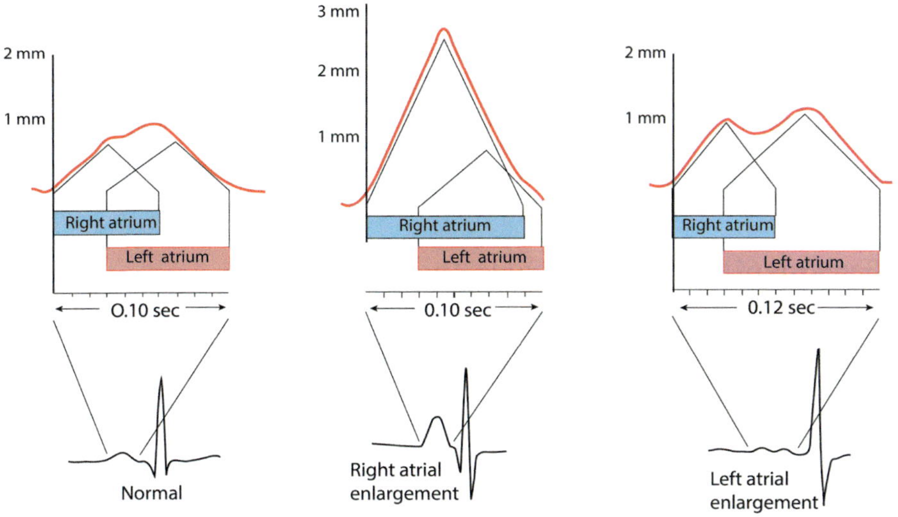

Fig. 18.7 P wave in the normal ECG (left), right atrial enlargement (middle), left atrial enlargement (right)

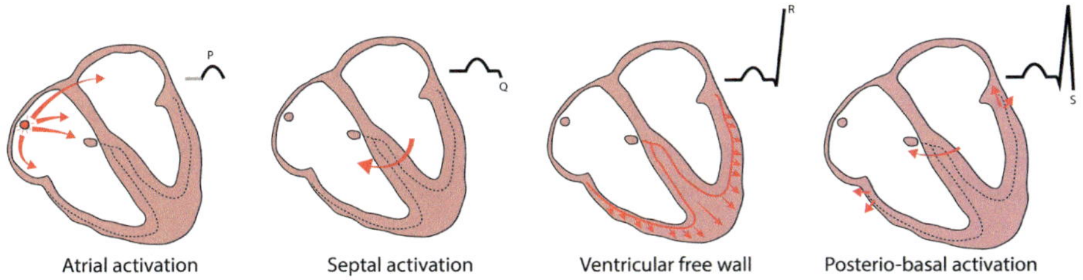

Fig. 18.8 Sequence of action potential through the heart

Physiological Variation

PR interval increases with age and decreases with tachycardia.

PR Segment

The PR segment starts from the end of the P wave to the onset of ventricular depolarisation. It is used as baseline for ST segment measurement.

QRS Complex

There are three phases of ventricular activation (see Fig. 18.8):

- Septal wall: small, anterior, left to right vector

- Free wall vector: simultaneous activation of both ventricles from endocardium to epicardium
- Terminal vector: basal septum and posterior-basal region of LV activated last plus a few Purkinje fibres; shown in a small posteriorly directed vector

Dimensions of QRS

A normal duration for the QRS complex is <0.12 s.

Diagnosis of LVH from Amplitude R and S Waves

- Sum of S in V1 or V2 and R in V5 or V6 >35 mm.
- R wave in AVL >11 mm.
- ST-T wave abnormalities lend supporting evidence.
- There are many other proposed ECG parameters, but each has diminishing sensitivity and specificity.

Q Waves

The Q wave is a negative deflection occurring when the vector of the initial QRS activation is directed away from the exploring electrode. Sometimes, it is termed *septal Q* waves. It is most commonly seen in leads I, II, III, AVL, AVF and left precordial leads and more common in those <40 years of age. *Q* waves are more common if there is counterclockwise rotation because more of the left chest leads will see septal activation as directed away from them. Septal activation is registered by anterior chest leads (V1, V2) as a small R wave (see Fig. 18.8).

Normal Dimensions

The normal duration of a *Q* wave is <0.03 s and <25% of the height of the following *R* wave as long as the *R* wave is ≥5 mm. The depth of the *Q* wave in limb leads is <4 mm except in lead III where it can be 5 mm.

Pathological Q Waves

Pathological *Q* waves may indicate infarcted, electrically silent tissue as a result of a change in the vector of ventricular activation away from the exploring electrode.

ST Segment

The ST segment represents a state of full ventricular polarisation between depolarisation and start of repolarisation.

Measurement

The ST segment is measured from the end of the QRS to the beginning of the T wave. The junction between the end of QRS and beginning of ST is called the J point. The J point is identified as the beginning of a change of slope of the rising S wave. It is often difficult or impossible to determine. The end of the ST segment is the point at which the slope starts to rise at the T wave. This is also often difficult to determine. The ST baseline is usually taken as the PR segment.

Physiological ST Changes

- ST elevation in the chest leads is very common (90%) in normal subjects. V2 and V3 may have up to 3 mm elevation, particularly in thin young males.
- ST depression is abnormal in any chest leads and is rarely normal in limb leads.

Diagnostic Criteria for Ischaemic ST Segment Shifts

Upsloping ST segment depression is much less specific for myocardial ischaemia than horizontal or downsloping ST depression. Upsloping ST depression therefore requires greater magnitude of depression at greater distance from the J point. The further from the J point that ST depression is detected, the greater the specificity for ischaemia. Diagnostic criteria for ischaemic ST segment shifts include:

- Horizontal ST depression: 0.1 mm ST depression at 0.6–0.8 s after the J point.
- Upsloping ST depression: 0.2 mm ST depression at 0.8 s after the J point.
- ST elevation usually requires 2 mm ST elevation and is less specific in the right chest leads, especially in the presence of Q wave.

The Dräger Zeus anaesthetic machine default measurement is 80 ms after J point with baseline taken at 28 ms before the beginning of QRS. These settings can be manually adjusted.

Mechanism for ST Shift in Ischaemia

The mechanism for ST shift in ischaemia remains controversial, but, in summary, a potential difference develops between the ischaemic tissue and healthy tissue and a current of injury flows between that is detected as ST segment shift. The diastolic hypothesis is as follows:

- Loss of intracellular potassium results in decrease in intracellular resting membrane potential from −90 mV to −70 mV.
- The balancing positive potential on surface is proportionately reduced.
- The injured surface is now relatively negative in respect to healthy cells.
- A current of injury flows from healthy to injured cells in diastole.
- Electrodes oriented towards the injured zone register a depressed baseline during diastole (before the QRS). The amplifier, however, compensates by returning the baseline to control levels.
- When healthy cells are activated in systole, their external surface becomes more negative, the current of injury is reduced and baseline returns to normal. Thus,

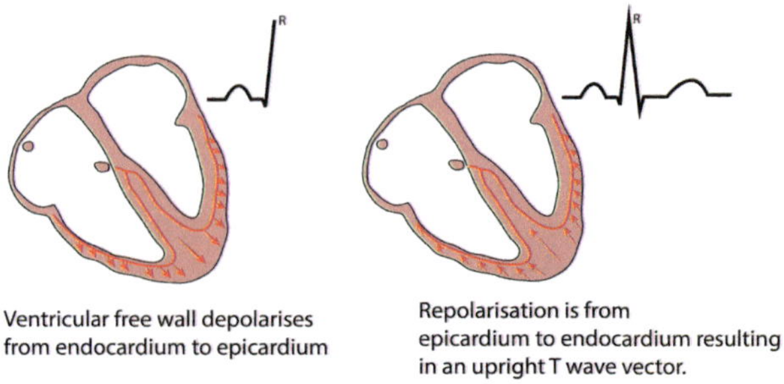

Fig. 18.9 Ventricular free wall depolarisation and repolarisation

the ST segment returns to normal in systole but is seen as ST elevation because of the amplifier's diastolic compensation.

The direction of ST shift depends on the direction of the current of injury in relation to the recording electrode. It thus depends on the position of the electrode, the location of the ischaemia and whether the ischaemia is endocardial, epicardial or transmural.

T Wave

The T wave represents ventricular repolarisation (see Fig. 18.9). The T wave has an upright vector. This is because the recovery of polarity is in general direction of ventricular depolarisation, but the reversing polarity is counterbalanced by an epicardium to endocardium direction. Paradoxically, the first cells to be depolarised are the last to be repolarised.

Normal Dimensions

A normal T wave is <6 mm amplitude in limb leads and up to 12 mm in right precordial leads. T wave can be very tall in young slim males. Normal T waves are usually asymmetrical, having a shallower upstroke.

Persistent Juvenile Pattern

Persistent T wave inversion in V1 occurs in 50% of women. Persistent T wave inversion in V2 occurs in 10% of normal women. However, persistent T wave inversion in V3 is rarely normal.

QT Interval

The QT interval represents the duration of ventricular electrical systole depolarisation and repolarisation. It is measured from the beginning of QRS to the end of the T wave. The upper limit of normal QT interval is 0.44 s. The QT interval varies inversely with heart rate, and there are several ways of correcting for this, for example, the Bazett's formula:

$$QTc = QT\,\text{interval} / \sqrt{RR}.$$

What Is the Problem with Long QT?

Long QT syndromes are caused by either an increase in depolarisation currents or a decrease in repolarisation currents. The arrhythmogenic mechanisms are complex and varied but arise from alteration in conduction velocities, shortening of the refractory period or action potential prolongation (after-depolarisation).

U Wave

U wave is a small deflection immediately following the T wave. It is usually <25% of the T wave amplitude with maximum amplitude of 1–2 mm. The amplitude of the U wave is in the same direction as T wave. The size of the U wave increases as heart rate falls. U waves are prominent in hypokalaemia, LVH and digoxin use. There are several theories of the aetiology of the U wave:

- Delayed repolarisation of Purkinje fibres
- Delayed repolarisation of papillary muscles
- Prolonged repolarisation of mid-myocardial 'M cells'
- After-potentials resulting from mechanical forces in the ventricular wall

Filtering and ST Monitoring

Why Filter the Signal?

Filtering is required to reduce environmental artefact.

- High-frequency filter: reduces artefact from EMG, electromagnetic interference, 50 Hz electrical interference.
- Low-frequency filter: stabilises baseline by reducing artefact from respiratory movement, positional changes and poor electrode contact.

Most contemporary monitors have two or three different filtering bandwidths depending on the requirement. Specifications and names differ between machines, but the following are typical:

Diagnostic Mode (0.05–100 Hz)

Upper limit allows high-fidelity reproduction and analysis of QRS morphology and tachyarrhythmias. Lower limit allows accurate reproduction of low-frequency features including ST segment and P wave.

Monitoring Mode (0.5–40 Hz)

Upper and lower limits are reduced to stringently eliminate high- and low-frequency interference. The ECG looks 'clean', but the new lower limit can produce ST segment distortion including false or excessive depression. Broadly, this is because the ST segment has a frequency of around that lower limit, 0.05 Hz. Waveforms at the extremes of a filtering bandwidth are prone to distortion.

ST Analysis Mode (0.05–40 Hz)

The lower limit is reduced to provide accurate reproduction of the ST segment, while the high-frequency filter remains.

Artefact

Electrode Contact Problems

General Contact Problems

Motion and changes in skin impedance may cause artefact and baseline wander. This can be minimised by shaving hair and cleaning with alcohol.

Electrode Potentials

The interface between lead and skin involves metal, gel and skin electrolytes. The interactions can generate electrical potentials, which will be registered as interference or baseline drift. This can be reduced by minimising the differences between interfaces by using an electrode of silver coated with silver chloride which, in turn, is in contact with penetrating chloride gel solution. Despite this, after defibrillation, the potential can be so large that the ECG signal is lost altogether.

Powerline interference

Powerline interference is seen as 50 Hz AC voltage on an ECG trace. This is easily seen as 50 spikes per five large squares. This can be minimised by shielding the leads in conductive, earthed material that draws away stray current.

Capacitance

The movement of electrons on a nearby appliance such as a theatre light induces movement on the electrode or lead.

Inductance

Magnetic fields induced by transformers or coiled wires induce currents in ECG leads, producing 50 Hz interference.

EMG

EMG is high frequency and random. It can be minimised by:

- Placing electrodes over bony prominences rather than over muscle.
- The use of a common mode rejection (CMR) amplifier. The ECG amplifier is a differential amplifier in that it measures only the difference between two electrodes. Any signals that are applied to both electrodes are eliminated. Common mode rejection thus helps to eliminate interference that is applied more generally to the patient such as 50 Hz mains interference and EMG.

Electrocautery

Electrocautery results in very-high-frequency artefact. This can be minimised by the use of separate power source from the ECG, by placing reference electrode close to ground pad and by the use of high-frequency filter.

Others Sources of Artefacts

- Static charge
- Infusion pumps, blood warmers
- Physical contact with plastic tubing

Further Reading

Dickinson DF. The normal ECG in childhood and adolescence. Heart. 2005;91(12):1626–30.

Hemmings HC, Hopkins PM. Foundations of anesthesia: basic sciences for clinical practice. Elsevier Health Sciences; 2006.

Patel S, Kwak L, Agarwal SK, Tereshchenko LG, Coresh J, Soliman EZ, Matsushita K. Counterclockwise and clockwise rotation of QRS transitional zone: prospective correlates of change and time-varying associations with cardiovascular outcomes. J Am Heart Assoc. 2017;6(11):e006281.

Riera ARP, Ferreira C, Ferreira Filho C, Ferreira M, Meneghini A, Uchida AH, Schapachnik E, Dubner S, Zhang L. The enigmatic sixth wave of the electrocardiogram: the U wave. Cardiol J. 2008;15(5):408–21.

Tse G, Chan YWF, Keung W, Yan BP. Electrophysiological mechanisms of long and short QT syndromes. IJC Heart Vasc. 2017;14:8–13.

Vincent GM, Abildskov JA, Burgess MJ. Mechanisms of ischemic ST-segment displacement. Evaluation by direct current recordings. Circulation. 1977;56(4):559–66.

Zimmerman, F. Clinical electrocardiography: review & study guide; 2004.

Spiromety and Flow Sensors 19

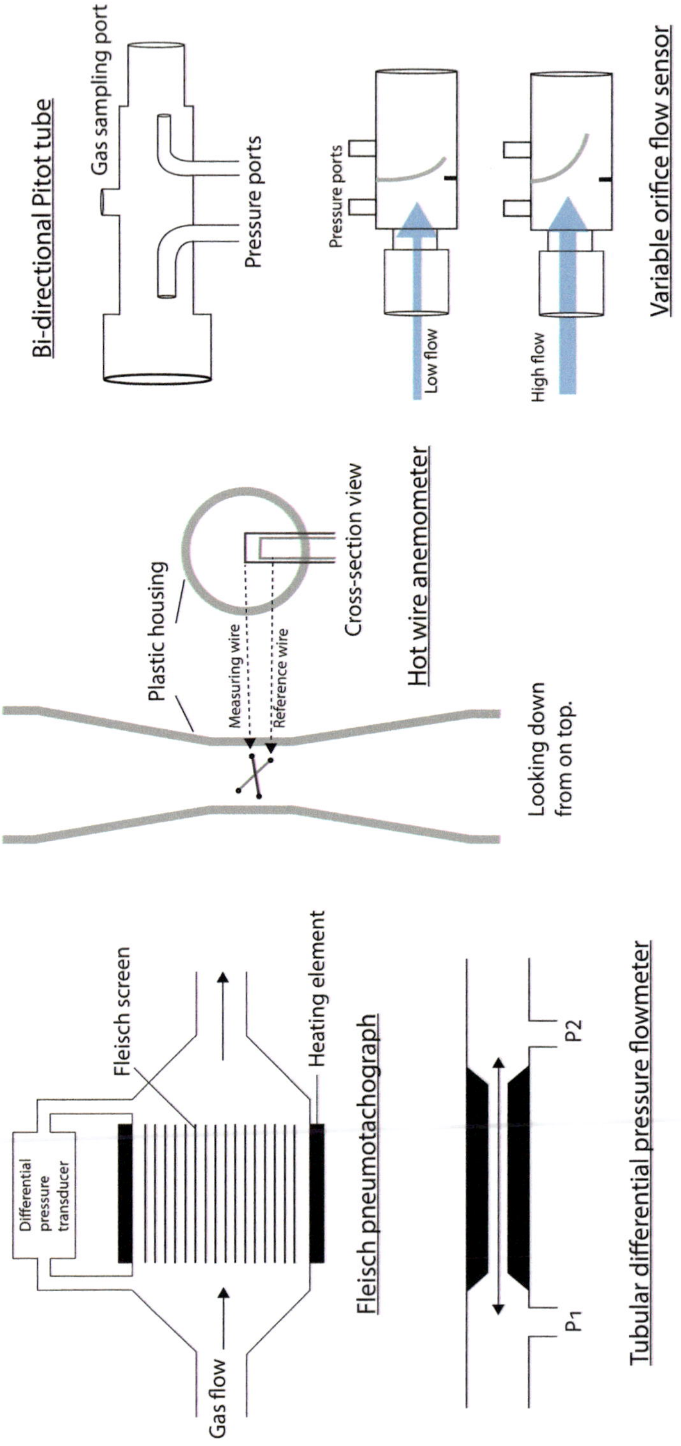

Fig. 19.1 Schematics of various flow sensors used in anaesthesia equipment

Pitot Tubes

The pressure exerted by a gas in a blind-ending tube is related to the gas velocity, as well as the density, viscosity and specific heat capacity of the gas mixture. It is a common method for monitoring flows in GE anaesthetic machines (GE/Datex D Lite spirometry sensor) (Fig. 19.1):

- Two tubes face in opposite directions within the gas flow.
- At the other end of each tube is a pressure transducer. One tube is subject to the flow and measures the *stagnation pressure*, while the other is used for reference (*static pressure*). The roles reverse as flow changes direction. The difference in pressure is related to flow rate.
- Gas mixtures are sampled to add correction factors for the physical properties of different gas mixtures.

Differential Pressure Methods

Fleisch and Lilly Pneumotachographs

Context

This is a common flow sensor in PFT labs and in clinic spirometers. A Fleisch pneumotachograph is the flow sensor in contemporary Vitalograph spirometers (Fig 19.1).

Principle

If flow is laminar, the pressure drop across a known resistance is proportional to flow:

$$\text{Flow} = {}^{\Delta P}\!/_{R}$$

- Resistance
  - In the Fleisch pneumotachograph, the resistance is provided by the bundle of capillary tubes. The arrangement of tubes ensures that flow is laminar.
  - In the Lilly pneumotachograph, the resistance is a series of gauze screens.
- Pressure transducers on either side of the resistance.
- Resistive element is heated to prevent condensation.
- Calibrated for a specific gas, because laminar flow is viscosity dependent.

Simple Tubular Differential Flow Sensors

- Smaller tubular differential pressure sensors of other designs are used in anaesthetic machines either alone or in combination with Pitot tubes and other methods (Fig. 19.1).

Variable Orifice Flow Sensor

A flow sensor of this type is used in the Datex-Ohmeda Aestiva and GE Aisys ventilators:

- A hinged plastic flap sits in the gas flow.
- As flow increases, the flap opens more and alters the pressure drop across the orifice.
- This system improves sensitivity at low flows compared with a fixed resistance or orifice.
- The differential pressure measurements are compared with an empirical algorithm calibrated for flow.

Turbine Flow Sensors

The gas flow rotates a vane, and the rate of rotation is related to flow. This is a very common method of measuring flow in clinical spirometry including small handheld devices. The MicroLab Spirometer, Spiropalm and Discovery-2™ are examples:

- A vane is mounted in the path of the gas.
- The rate of rotation is detected using optical or electromagnetic methods.
- Microprocessing and integration with time allow multiple different functions of volume and flow to be assessed. See below (Fig. 19.2).

Ultrasonic Flow Sensors

Transit Time

Sound waves are passed at an angle across the gas flow stream. Sound travels faster downstream than upstream. Sound transit times are measured.

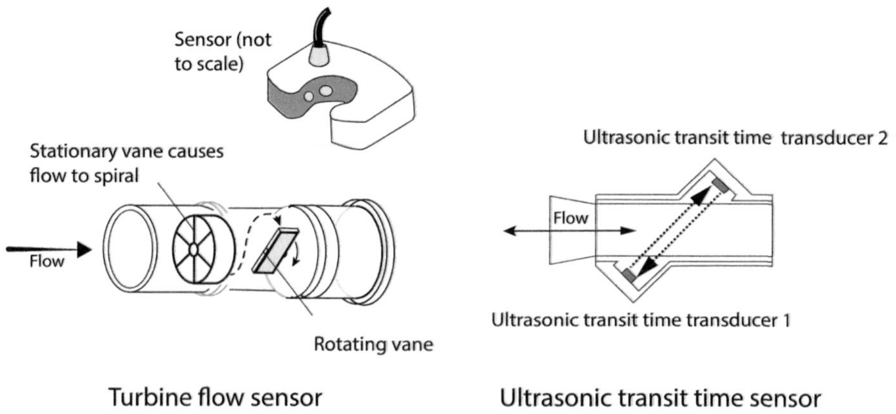

Fig. 19.2 Schematics of turbine and ultrasonic flow sensors

There are numerous variants of this technology. The Easy®One Air is a handheld version for clinic spirometry.

Respiratory: Spirometry

Overview

A spirometer is a device that measures the volume of inspired and expired air. The residual volume, FRC and TLC are therefore not measured.

- Most spirometry is flow-sensing spirometry: flow is measured and integrated over time to provide volumes required for V_T, MV and PV loops.
- The volume displacement methods are of academic interest in contemporary anaesthesia.

Spirometry	
Flow-sensing spirometers	Most spirometers are flow-sensing spirometers (see above)
Volume displacement methods	Turbines: *Wright respirometer*
	Bellows: *Vitalograph*
	Water seal: *Benedict-Roth spirometer*
Monitors of thoracic movement	Strain gauges
	Inductive plethysmography
	Impedance pneumography

Flow-Sensing Spirometry

Context

This is by far the most common method in clinics and in ventilation monitoring. Flow is measured and converted to volume.

Method

Flow is measured using one of the above flow sensors. Microprocessing integrates flow with time to produce volume (see previous section):

- Some spirometers register temperature as well and can correct ATPS measurements to the equivalent at BTPS.

Volume Displacement Methods

These methods measure the volume rather than a surrogate such as flow. They are not in common use in contemporary anaesthetic practice.

Turbine Spirometers (e.g. Wright Respirometer)

Context

The Wright respirometer was one of the original methods to measure V_T and MV in circuits. Turbine methods are still common, but they are usually designed to measure flow and integrated with time to give volume.

Method

The Wright (volume) respirometer contains a single vane connected to a series of gears. Gas flowing through the vane causes it to rotate and drive a pointer that registers volume. A second pointer registers the cumulative volume of multiple breaths and so can indicate MV. It is unidirectional only.

Contemporary turbine spirometers are bidirectional and monitor the vane's rotation optically or electromagnetically.

Bellows-Type Spirometers ('Vitalograph')

Context

The classic was the Vitalograph that produced a characteristic volume/time curve on a paper chart. Vitalograph has supplanted this technology with an electronic version that has no bellows.

Method

The subject blew through a mouthpiece that inflated a collapsible bellows. As the bellows inflated, it moved a marker vertically over a paper chart. At the beginning of exhalation, a motor automatically started and moved the chart sideways. Thus, the chart was recording volume on the vertical axis and time on the *x*-axis to produce an expiratory volume/time curve (Fig. 19.3).

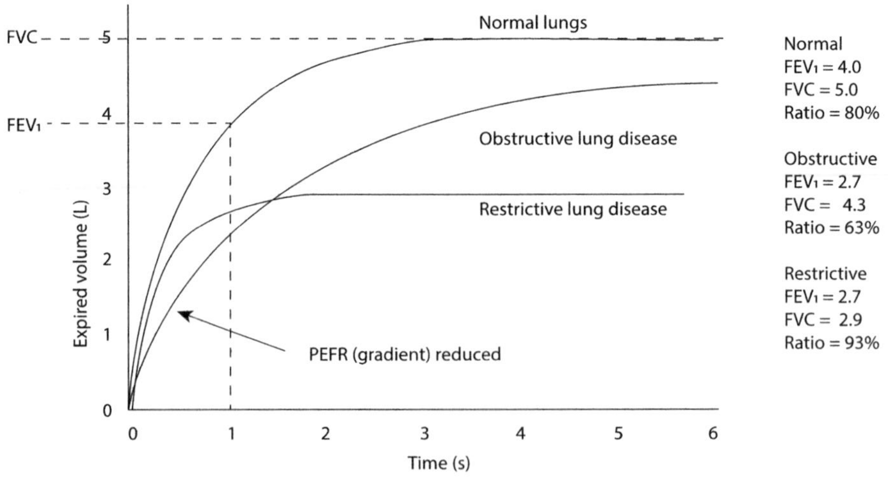

Fig. 19.3 Examples of expiratory volume-time traces

Water-Seal Spirometers (e.g. Benedict-Roth)

Context

The Benedict-Roth spirometer was the classic spirometry method for over 100 years, and, although water-filled bells play no part in contemporary pulmonary function testing, the characteristic trace is still a staple in textbooks and exams. The trace is now obtained through electronic spirometry (see trace below: Fig. 19.4).

Method

An upturned bell is submerged in a water tank. Patient breathes in and out through a mouthpiece that communicates via a tube to the underside of the bell. Breathing thus moves the bell up and down, and this drives a chart marker in the vertical axis. At the same time, the chart rotates so that time is registered on the x-axis. As this is a multi-breath process, there must be a CO_2 absorber in circuit as well as a basal oxygen supply. Volumes measured are at ATPS and must be corrected to BTPS.

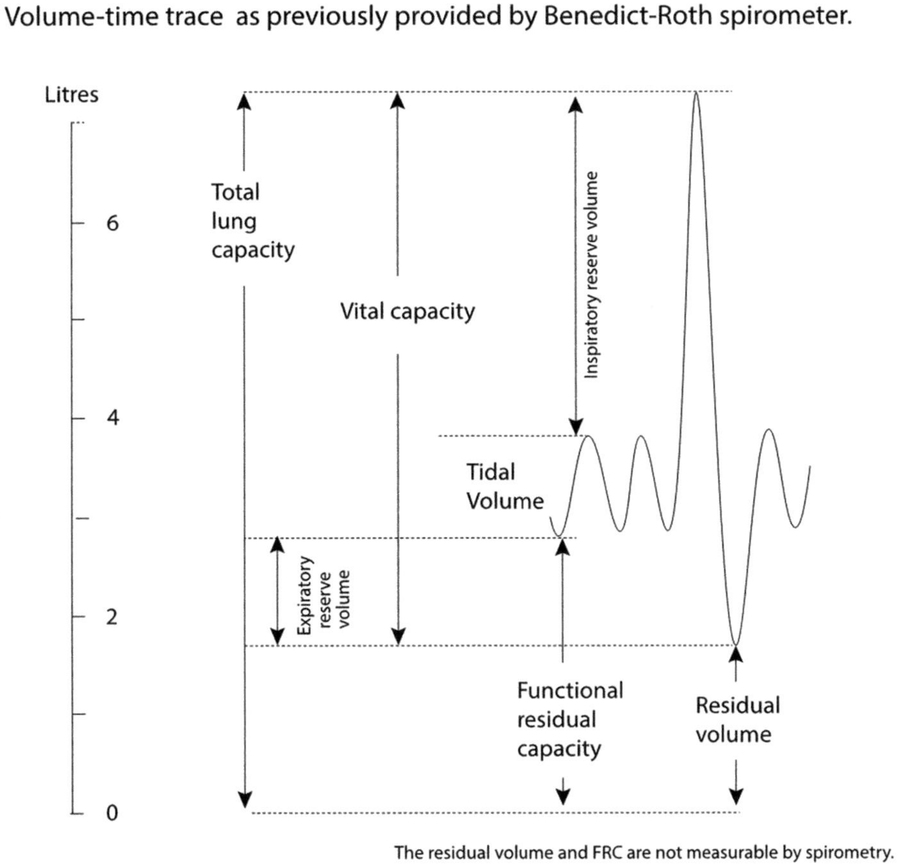

Fig. 19.4 Lung volumes and capacities characterised by spirometers

Monitors of Thoracic Movement and Effort

These methods enable monitoring of breathing in unintubated patients including neonates. They require prior calibration with spirometry if volumes are to be monitored accurately.

Strain Gauges

Belts are placed around both the thorax and the abdomen. Each belt contains a piezoelectric strain gauge that emits a voltage in response to a change in length.

Inductive Plethysmography

Belts are placed around both the thorax and the abdomen. Within each belt, a current flows through an electrical coil and generates an electromagnetic field that opposes the current flow. This is termed a back EMF. During respiration, the cross-sectional area of the thorax and abdomen changes and alters the tightness of the coils. This alters the back EMF and the current flow, and the effect is calibrated for V_T.

Impedance Pneumography

A high-frequency current is passed across the thorax. The impedance to current flow varies with the volume of air in the thorax.

Spirometry Traces

Volume-Time Trace Showing Classical Subdivisions of Lung Volume

This trace used to be produced using the Benedict-Roth spirometer but is now recorded using flow-sensing spirometry.

Expiratory Volume-Time Trace

This is a very common printout in both clinic spirometry and formal pulmonary function tests. It was previously produced by the bellows-type vitalograph.

Other Measurements

- PEFR: tangent at the beginning of expiration

- Maximum mid-expiratory flow rate: average gradient between 25% and 75% of FVC. Removes effort-dependent first 25% of FVC. More reproducible.
- FEV_6: FEV in 6 s. Easier and more precise than FVC.

Flow-Volume Loops

Most clinic spirometry will provide expiratory and sometimes inspiratory flow-volume loops. The following depicts normal plus five disease states. Remember that the residual volume cannot be measured with spirometry, so total lung capacity is not measured with this test (Fig. 19.5).

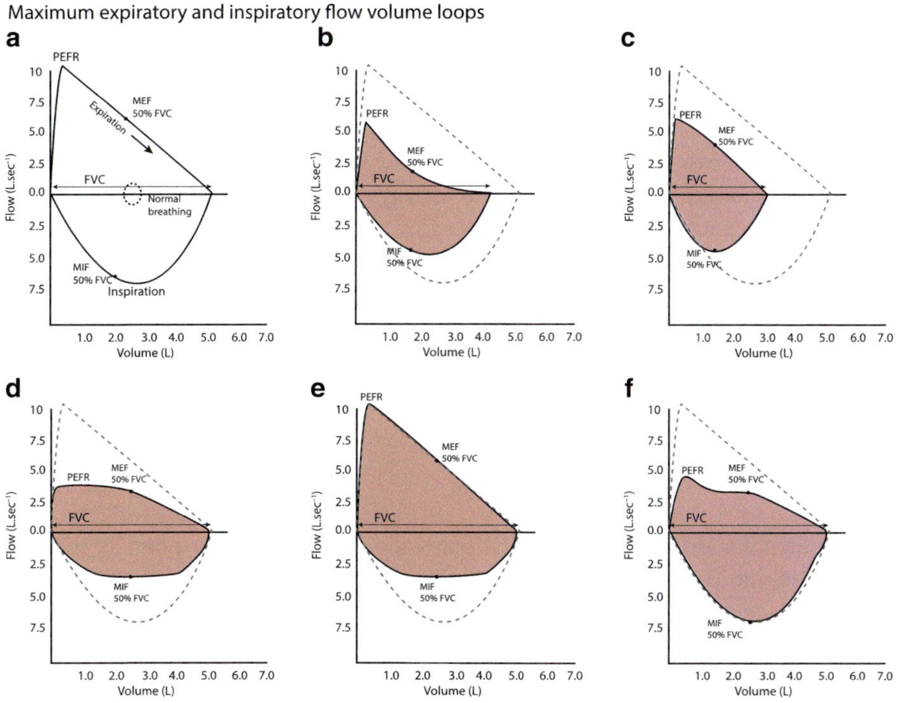

Fig. 19.5 Examples of flow/volume loops in disease states(**a**) Normal: Maximum expiratory flow rate at 50% FVC (MEF 50% FVC) is usually a little lower than the equivalent in inspiration because of dynamic compression of the airways in expiration. (**b**) Severe obstructive lung disease: The PEFR is markedly reduced as is the MEF 50% FVC. FVC is reduced, and the expiratory trace is scalloped. This is because of delayed emptying of lung units with long time constants. RV and TLC may be increased but cannot be depicted with spirometry. (**c**) Restrictive lung disease: The PEFR is reduced, but flow rates may be increased for a given lung volume because elastic recoil is increased. This gives the expiratory curve a convex appearance. FVC is reduced. RV and TLC may be reduced but are not depicted with spirometry. (**d**) Fixed obstruction of the upper airway (e.g. goitre, laryngeal cancer): Limited flow in both inspiration and expiration. MEF 50% FVC may equal MIF 50% FVC. (**e**) Variable extrathoracic obstruction (e.g. laryngospasm or other vocal cord dysfunction): Patient may have stridor. Markedly reduced flows on inspiration. MEF 50% FVC > MIF 50% FVC. (**e**) Variable intrathoracic obstruction (e.g. tracheomalacia): During forced inspiration, the trachea is held open by negative intrapleural pressure. During expiration, the trachea collapses

Partial Flow-Volume Curves

These are initiated from lower lung volumes. The calibre of the airways and bronchomotor tone are dependent on the immediately preceding breathing pattern. A full inspiration minimises lung recoil and bronchomotor tone with opposite effects on flow during the forced expiration. Initiation from lower lung volumes maintains bronchomotor tone better and allows the influence of drugs on tone to be better assessed.

Effort Independence

Why Does Flow Rate Become Independent of Effort?

Dynamic compression of the airways:

- During quiet exhalation, gases are driven down the airways by a positive alveolar pressure caused by lung recoil. The airways are held open by the distending forces of negative intrapleural pressure.
- During forced expiratory efforts above a certain level, the larger positive pressures applied externally to the alveoli are also compressing the downstream airways, preventing an increase in airflow. This system is an example of a *Starling resistor* where the system resistance is dependent on the external pressure collapsing the system.

Equal Pressure Point (EPP) Theory

As the alveolar driving pressure dissipates along the airway, a point is reached where the intrabronchial pressure equals the extrabronchial pressure. This is the EPP:

- Intrabronchial pressure falls from alveolus to mouth on expiration.
- The alveolar pressure is the sum of that produced from lung recoil and positive intrapleural pressure from forced expiration.
- The EPP occurs where there has been dissipation of pressure along the airway of the magnitude of that caused by lung recoil. The pressure drop along the airway to the EPP is equal to the lung recoil pressure.

EPPs and Lung Volume

- During forced expiration at high lung volumes (>50% VC), the lung recoil component is large and the EPPs lie fairly far downstream in the large segmental and lobar airways. The structural rigidity of these airways prevents collapse and flow limitation.
- As lung volume falls, the lung recoil component of the intrabronchial pressure also falls and the EPPs move upstream to smaller, more compressible airways.

Respiratory: Measurement of Functional Residual Capacity

20

Alan McLintic and Nic Randall

Body Plethysmograph

Basic Principle

Body plethysmograph measures lung volumes by the application of Boyle's law. Functional Residual Capacity (FRC) is an important respiratory concept, it has implications in mechanics, lung function and is practically utilised for pre-oxygentation during the induction and extubation phase of anaesthesia.

Boyle's Law

Boyle's law states that if temperature is constant, the absolute pressure of a mass of gas varies inversely with its volume:

$$P \propto \frac{1}{V}$$

For the measurement of FRC lung air is sealed off with a shutter at FRC (end expiration), and the subject pants. During panting, the lung air volume moves up and down Boyle's curve. The pressure volume relationship remains constant during that exercise, and, by measuring the changing pressures, it is possible to derive the starting volume, FRC (Fig. 20.1).

Apparatus and Process

- The subject sits inside an airtight box and breathes through a mouthpiece; a nose clip is applied. The mouthpiece is connected to a pressure transducer; a shutter

A. McLintic · N. Randall (✉)
Department of Intensive Care, Counties Manukau Health, Auckland, New Zealand
e-mail: nic.randall@middlemore.co.nz

C. Birch et al. (eds.), *Physics and Measurement for Anesthesia*,
https://doi.org/10.1007/978-3-031-65060-4_20

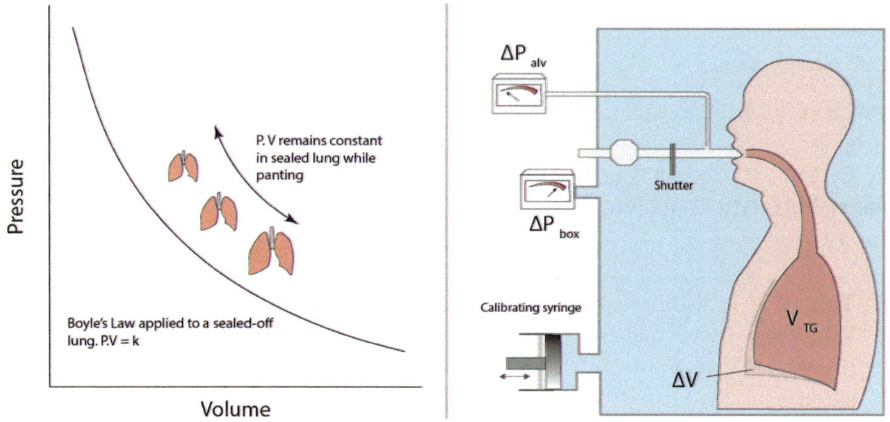

Fig. 20.1 Measurement of functional residual capacity requires the application of Boyle's law and a sealed box in which the subject sits

Pressure in alveoli at FRC is barometric pressure ~ 101 kPa

When panting against a closed shutter there is no air flow, so the alveolar pressure is equal to the mouth pressure.

$$P_{bar} \cdot V_{FRC} = P_{alv} \cdot (V_{FRC} + \Delta V)$$

FRC is the volume we are looking for.

During panting, the lung volume is changing by ΔV and the thoracic volume change is also compressing the box air by ΔV. This is causing a change in box pressure. The prior calibration allows us to deduce ΔV from $\Delta P_{box\ air}$

Fig. 20.2 FRC is derived by the application and solving of Boyle's law

lies between the subject and the outside of the box. Box pressure (relative to ambient pressure) is measured by a separate transducer.

- Prior to the test, the box air volume/pressure relationship is determined using a large automated calibrating syringe or an automated 'lung' that is placed in the box. These devices alter the box air volume while the resultant box pressure is measured, establishing the PV relationship.
- During testing, a subject is asked to pant gently after a normal exhalation—this will occur around or slightly above FRC. The shutter is closed; the subject is asked to continue to pant gently against the shutter. While this is occurring, mouth pressure and box pressure are being monitored. The lung is now going up and down the Boyle curve by a small amount.

Solving the Equation

This is an automated process, the following explains the derivation of FRC. Although gas in the chest is unknown, from Boyle's law, chest PV must equal box PV (Fig. 20.2).

On the left of the equation is the product of pressure and volume (at FRC) and on the right is the product during an inspiratory pant. The equation can now be solved for V_1 which is FRC:

- The pressure in the alveoli at FRC is barometric pressure (P_{bar}).
- When the shutter is down, there is no airflow between mouth and alveoli so the pressure measured at the mouth is assumed to be equivalent to alveolar pressure (P_{alv}).
- The change in lung volume during panting is the same as the change in thoracic volume, which compresses the box air by the same amount. This compression causes the box pressure to swing proportionately; the box pressure change is converted to ΔV from the calibration.

Notes

- The box described above is constant volume variable pressure. This is the most commonly used technique, however another version has the opening in the box connected to a spirometer. Box air is shunted in and out during thoracic expansion and contraction and is measured by a spirometer (giving volume). This version is called the constant pressure, variable volume box.
- The volume that is measured is the lung volume when the shutter comes down. The shutter timing mechanism is such that the lung is usually slightly above FRC at closure, so the volume measured is often termed thoracic gas volume (V_{TG}) rather than FRC. V_{TG} can be corrected to FRC.
- The technique relies on $P_{mouth} = P_{alv}$ during the shutter manoeuvre. In severe airflow obstruction, it is possible that the pressure change in alveolus is not fully transmitted to the mouth, and this can lead to inaccuracies.
- The body plethysmograph measures everything within the visceral pleura including trapped gas. This is an advantage over the helium dilution techniques (below) in which only ventilated areas are measured.
- Another advantage of this is that the test can be repeated as many times as is necessary. This is not possible with helium dilution techniques as you must wait until all the helium is flushed out of the lungs.

In a Nutshell

- The body plethysmograph is a method of measuring lung volumes by the application of Boyle's law.

- The subject sits in an airtight box and breathes through a tube connected to a mouth pressure manometer and a shutter. The pressure-volume product at FRC is equal to the pressure-volume during an inspiratory pant:
  - Pressure at FRC is barometric pressure.
  - The alveolar pressure during an inspiratory pant is the same as the mouth pressure with the shutter down.
  - The change in lung volume is reflected in the change in the box air volume and the box air pressure.
  - The change in box pressure can be read as volume change because of prior pressure-volume calibration.

Inert Gas Dilution

Basic Principles

- The subject breathes from a closed-circuit system containing a known volume (V_1) and concentration (C_1) of an inert tracer gas such as helium, argon or neon.
- They breathe until the concentration in the system reaches a plateau. This takes approximately 3 min but may take over 10 min in airway disease.
- The lung and system gas concentrations are now in equilibrium and can be measured (C_2).
- Now the mass balance equation can be used to determine FRC (V_2) (Fig. 20.3):

$$C_1.V_1 = C_2\left(V_1 + V_2\right)$$

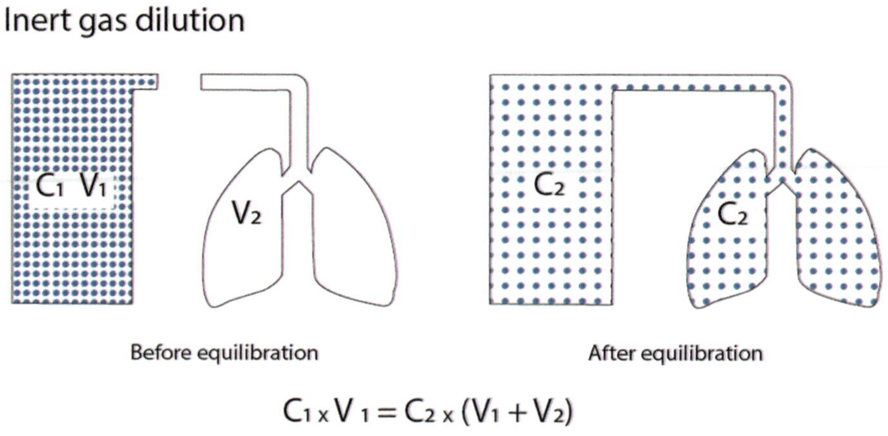

Fig. 20.3 Inert gas (helium) dilution technique uses the mass balance equation to determine the FRC

Practical

- 20% Helium in air is commonly used.
- For FRC to be measured, the patient must start breathing at FRC.
- The system includes a CO_2 absorber and basal oxygen supply.
- Dilution methods only measure ventilated areas.
- Areas of air trapping are not measured.
- Helium is measured by thermal conductivity (see gas analysis).

Nitrogen Washout

This technique is not used in contemporary practice and was described in 1940 by Darling. It is a dilution technique in which the tracer gas is the subject's own lung nitrogen.

Basic Principles

- The subject begins breathing 100% oxygen from FRC; this washes out the nitrogen (known concentration 79%) until all lung N_2 has been eliminated.
- Takes at least 7–8 min.
- Expired gas can be collected into a Douglas bag via a non-rebreathing valve, or tidal volume and N_2 concentration are measured on a breath-by-breath basis.
- From the collected gas, volume of N_2 can be calculated ($V \times C$).
- As with inert gas dilution, this technique cannot measure regions of trapped air.
- The mass balance equation is used to solve for FRC:

$$V_{\text{FRC}} \cdot \equiv C_1 = \left(V_{\text{FRC}} . C_2\right) + \left(V_{\text{Douglas bag gas}} . C_3\right)$$

- $C_1 = N_2$ concentration in lung at start
- $C_2 = N_2$ concentration in lung after washout (negligible)
- $C_3 = N_2$ concentration in gas collected in Douglas bag

Further Reading

Anon. Measurement of lung volumes and capacities; n.d.—https://derangedphysiology.com/

Darling RC, et al. Studies on the intrapulmonary mixture of gases. Nitrogen elimination from blood and body tissues during high oxygen breathing. J Clin Investig. 1940;19(4):591–7.

Respiratory: Closing Volume and Anatomical Dead Space

21

Alan McLintic and Nic Randall

Familiarisation of the different volumes and capacities obtained from a spirometry trace is essential to the complete understanding of the concepts described in this chapter. Readers are encouraged to seek out this material.

Closing Volume

Closing capacity (CC) is the volume remaining in the lungs when small airways begin to close during expiration. Closing volume (CV) can be calculated from the closing capacity minus the residual volume (RV).

Closure of small airways during expiration is a normal phenomenon; it occurs first in the basal, dependant regions of the lungs because of a gravity-dependent increase in intrapleural pressure and the lack of parenchymal support occurring in distal airways. In health, airway closure does not occur during normal tidal breathing as the functional residual capacity (FRC) is usually greater than closing capacity keeping the lungs open.

With ageing and in diseased states, CC can exceed FRC, increasing the work of breathing and reducing PaO_2. Prone and supine positions contribute markedly to the degree to which the closing capacity will impact FRC and are a significant cause of atelectasis and mild intraoperative hypoxia. The measurement of closing volume is not a routine pulmonary function test but can be performed using the following techniques.

A. McLintic · N. Randall (✉)
Department of Intensive Care, Counties Manukau Health, Auckland, New Zealand
e-mail: nic.randall@middlemore.co.nz

C. Birch et al. (eds.), *Physics and Measurement for Anesthesia*,
https://doi.org/10.1007/978-3-031-65060-4_21

Single-Breath Nitrogen Washout

The subject breathes out to residual volume (RV) and then takes a maximal vital capacity breath of 100% oxygen; this is followed by exhalation through a mouthpiece from VC to RV (maximal expiration); nitrogen concentration is recorded at the mouth using a nitrogen meter. Figure 21.1a shows a typical trace obtained, and an explanation of this follows.

During the inspiration phase, the apex of the lung receives less of the inspired oxygen than the base. This occurs due to the base being more compressed than the apex, which is already relatively well distended; therefore, at the end of inspiration, the upper alveoli have a greater concentration of N_2 than the lower.

During expiration, the alveoli empty evenly until airway closure begins; small airway closure happens in the dependant areas (lower alveoli) first and is represented in Fig. 21.1a by the sudden increase in N_2 concentration. This occurs because the basal areas having the highest oxygen concentration and the lowest nitrogen concentration. The CV is the expired volume from inflection point to the end of expiration.

Xenon or Argon Bolus Technique

This technique has a subtle but important difference from that described above. The tracer used is a bolus of xenon or argon. Due to the regional distribution observed in the lung during inspiration, the bolus of xenon (or argon) goes preferentially to the upper alveoli. This is because it is injected at the very start of the inspiratory phase, compared to the oxygen tracer (above) which is delivered throughout inspiration.

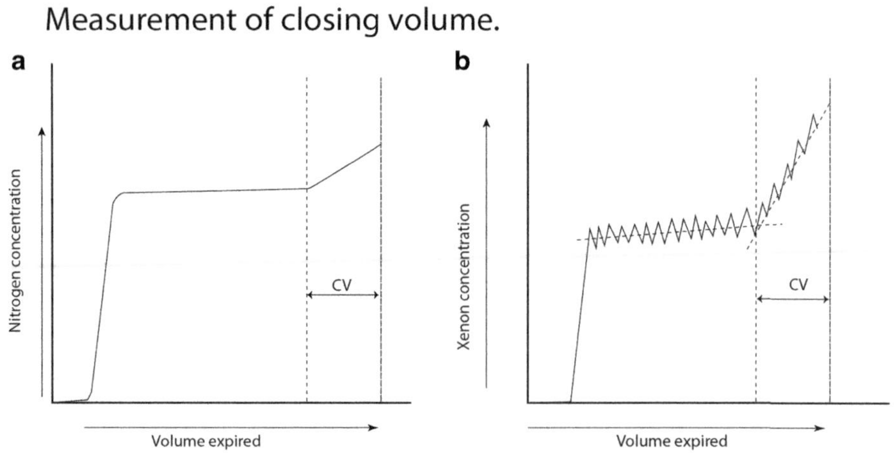

Fig. 21.1 Measurement of closing volume (CV) using single-breath nitrogen washout (left, **a**) and argon or xenon tracer technique (right, **b**)

Now during expiration, the alveoli empty evenly until airway closure begins. This happens in the dependant (lower) areas first. It is signalled by a sudden increase in tracer concentration as the xenon- or argon-rich upper airways begin to contribute more to expiration (Fig 21.1b).

Vascular oscillations are superimposed because of the amplification required with low gas concentrations.

Anatomical Dead Space

Historical Note: Fowler's Method

In 1948, Ward S. Fowler (University of Pennsylvania) published a paper on the measurement of anatomical dead space.[1] *He used nitrogen as the tracer gas and, in examining the robustness of his findings, compared the results of a vital capacity (VC) breath with that of normal 'quiet' expiration. He concluded that taking a VC breath increased dead space by about 100 ml compared with quiet exhalation. Fowler described what is commonly referred to as phase I, II and III, but there was no mention of the phase IV inflection point; he did not measure closing volume.*

Anatomical Dead Space Measurement (Fowler's Method)

The subject takes a vital capacity breath of 100% oxygen and then exhales using the same apparatus as previously described (single-breath nitrogen washout). Both the expired nitrogen concentration (nitrogen gas analyser) and the expired volume (spirometer) are measured. A typical trace is shown in Fig. 21.2.

Notes

CO_2 can be used as the tracer instead of nitrogen.

Fowler initially calculated the anatomical dead space from his experimental results using the Bohr equation. He then found that the method described above was an accurate and easier substitute. Most texts describe the procedure using a VC breath but, unlike the closing volume measurement where a VC breath from RV is essential; it is not here.

[1] Fowler, Ward S. "Lung function studies. II. The respiratory dead space." American Journal of Physiology-Legacy Content 154.3 (1948):405–416.

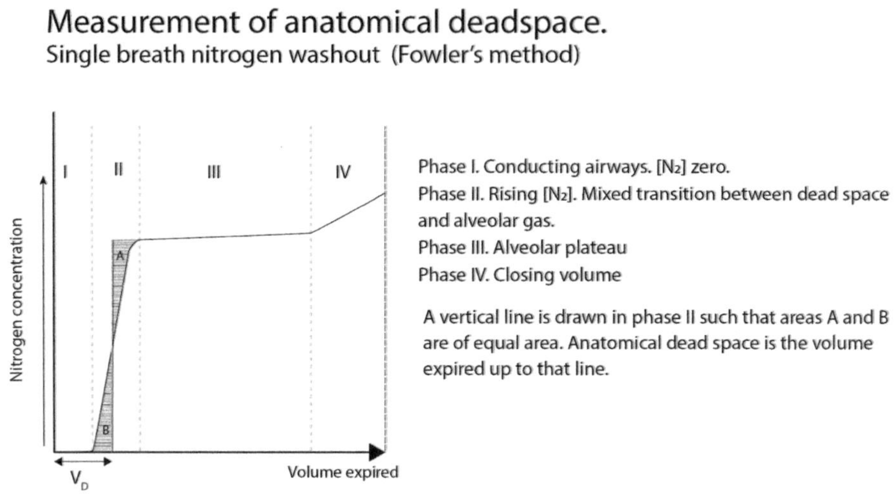

Fig. 21.2 Nitrogen washout trace showing the phases of expiration and demonstrating the approach to calculate anatomical dead space (V_D)

Fowler did not measure CV; therefore, the term Fowler's method should be reserved for V_D measurement only, but examiners may not expect such a strict demarcation in an exam answer!

Respiratory: Measurement of Airway Resistance

22

Alan McLintic and Craig Birch

See Table 22.1.

Table 22.1 Methods of measuring airway resistance (AJ McLintic)

Measurement of airway resistance	
Body plethysmograph	
Non-standard	Interrupter technique
	Subtraction technique
	Forced oscillation
Indirect assessment of airway resistance	
Peak expiratory flow rate	See spirometry chapter
Flow-volume loops	See spirometry chapter
Expiratory volume-time curves	See spirometry chapter
Assessment of airway resistance in the anaesthetic machine	
Ventilation patterns	PV loop bulge
	$P_{peak} - P_{plateau}$ /flow
Capnography	Upsloping capnograph plateau

A. McLintic · C. Birch (✉)
Department of Anaesthesia, Counties Manukau Health, Auckland, New Zealand

C. Birch et al. (eds.), *Physics and Measurement for Anesthesia*,
https://doi.org/10.1007/978-3-031-65060-4_22

Introduction

Whatever the method being used, the required measurements have to include the pressure difference between the mouth and the alveolus during airflow measurement:

$$R_{AW}\left(\mathrm{cmH_2O / L.\ sec^{-1}}\right) = \frac{\text{Mouth pressure} - \text{Alveolar pressure}}{\text{Flow rate}}$$

The flow rate and mouth pressure are easy enough to measure, but determining alveolar pressure during flow measurement is not straightforward.

Measurement of Airway Resistance Using the Body Plethysmograph

Context

This is the standard method for measuring airway resistance when patients are sent for formal pulmonary function tests.

Method: Two Steps

1. The patient sits in the sealed body plethysmograph as described (see Chap. 20 on functional residual capacity) and breathes through a flow meter. The flows ($\dot{V}$) are measured, as well as simultaneous measurement of box pressure (P_{box}). The box pressure swings because the thoracic volume is changing during the breathing.
2. Calibration: A shutter comes down, and the patient is asked to pant gently against the shutter. The mouth pressure (which is equivalent to alveolar pressure with the shutter closed (P_{alv})) is measured along with the box pressure (P_{box}). Thus, changes in box pressure have been calibrated in terms of changes in alveolar pressure

Processing

We now have two relationships: (i) the relationship between flow rates and box pressure changes ($P_{box}/\dot{V}$) and (ii) the relationship between box pressure changes and alveolar pressure changes (P_{alv}/P_{box}). The microprocessor can simply combine these two relationships to produce the alveolar pressure changes during flow rates and, as mouth pressure was barometric pressure (zero) during flow rates, we have the airway resistance:

$$\frac{P_{box}}{\dot{V}} \times \frac{P_{alv}}{P_{box}} = \frac{P_{alv}}{\dot{V}} = R_{AW}$$

Notes

- Airway resistance decreases at higher lung volumes and increases at lower lung volumes. To correct for this, the R_{AW} can be multiplied by FRC to give the specific airway resistance (sR_{AW}).
- Normal values:
  - R_{AW} 0.5–2.0 $cmH_2O/L \quad s^{-1}$
  - sR_{AW} 2.0–4.0 $cmH_2O/L \quad s^{-1}$
- Dräger pressure units are in hectopascals. 1 hPa = 1.02 cmH_2O.

Non-standard Methods of Measuring Airway Resistance

Context

These are not standard methods in day-to-day practice, so the following explanations are brief sketches only.

Forced Oscillation

A low-amplitude high-frequency oscillating airflow is superimposed on the subject's normal tidal breathing. The relationship between the oscillating imposed pressure and the oscillation of the induced airflow is a function of the total mechanical impedance of the respiratory system. This comprises impedance of volume expansion (compliance), impedance of flow (resistance) and impedance to acceleration (inertance). By adjusting the oscillation frequency, the compliance and inertance components cancel each other out leaving that due to airflow.

Subtraction Techniques

Flows are recorded, while intrapleural pressure is measured with an oesophageal monometer. The intrapleural pressure is a function of the pressure required to overcome airway resistance and that required to overcome lung elastance. In subtraction techniques, the lung compliance is determined in a separate investigation and subtracted from intrapleural pressure to leave the resistance component.

Interrupter Techniques

During flow measurement, a shutter briefly interrupts airway pressure measurements. The mouth pressure at these cessations of flow is assumed to be the same as the alveolar pressure. Resistance is calculated using the flow measurement just before the shutter comes down, and the pressure difference is seen in mouth (measured before the interruption) and alveoli (measured at the end of the interruption).

Assessment of Airway Resistance in the Anaesthetic Machine

Overview

Contemporary anaesthetic machines can provide an estimate of airway resistance.

Airway pressures are measured within the body of the anaesthetic machine by a piezoresistive transducer; the pressure stretches a material on a diaphragm and alters its resistance. Flow measurements are made by hot-wire anemometry at the entry and exit points of circle hose attachments (see chapter on flow measurement).

Volume-Controlled Ventilation Pressure-Time Trace

Volume-Controlled Ventilation

A tidal volume is preset, and the ventilator drives gas down the airways at constant flow until that volume is delivered.

Pressure-Time Trace

The pressure required to do this is a function of the volume delivered, the total respiratory compliance and the total airway resistance during inflation. The peak pressure (P_{peak}) is the pressure required to overcome lung/chest wall elastance plus that required to overcome airway resistance.

As soon as flow stops, the airway resistance component is lost and the pressure falls to plateau pressure ($P_{plateau}$). Because the expiratory valve is not yet open, this pressure is the same throughout the airways all the way down to the alveoli. Thus, the magnitude of ($P_{peak} - P_{plateau}$) is the driving pressure required during flow, and dividing it by the flow rate gives the airway resistance (Fig. 22.1).

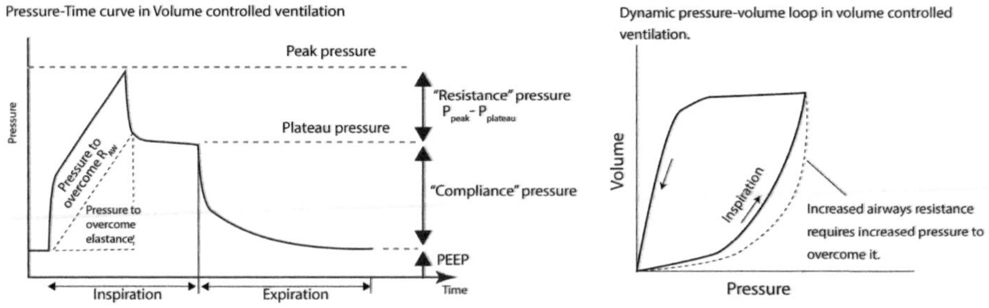

Fig. 22.1 Pressure-time curve in volume-controlled ventilation, and dynamic pressure-volume loop (AJ McLintic)

Notes

- It is important to remember that these estimates do not separate the resistance of the patients' airways from that of tubing, airway and circuits. The estimates are therefore of total respiratory resistance.
- Airway resistance measured during volume-controlled ventilation fairly reflects total respiratory R_{AW}, but it cannot do this during pressure-controlled ventilation without significant microprocessing, as there is a decelerating flow pattern during inflation.
- As noted above, the pressure transducers are within the anaesthetic machine and that is fine for the measurement of R_{AW} during IPPV. However, if we want to measure R_{AW} during spontaneous respiration, we require the alveolar pressure. Thus, the R_{AW} displayed during spontaneous ventilation only reflects the resistance of the ventilator channels and circle, not that of the patients' airways.

Dynamic Pressure-Volume (PV) Loops During IPPV

The gradient of the PV loop during IPPV reflects total thoracic compliance. The extra pressure required to overcome airway resistance is manifest as a bulge to the right during inflation. The greater the airway resistance, the greater the bulge.

Capnography

The classic capnography sign of increased airway resistance is a steeply upsloping plateau phase (phase III). This is because of uneven emptying of lung units, some having considerably prolonged time constants.

Further Reading

Lumb AB, Thomas CR. Nunn and Lumb's applied respiratory physiology. 9th ed. Elsevier; 2020.

Urbankowski T, Przybyłowski T. Methods of airway resistance assessment. Adv Respir Med. 2016;84(2)

Respiratory: Pressure-Volume Loops 23

Alan McLintic and Nic Randall

Work of Breathing - Important Definitions

$$\text{Work}(\text{J}) = \text{Force}(\text{N}) \times \text{Distance}(\text{m})$$

Work is done when a force moves an object; SI unit is the joule (J).

One joule of work is done when a force of one newton moves an object one metre in the direction of the force.

Power is the rate at which work is being done; SI unit is the watt ($1 \text{ W} = 1 \text{ J s}^{-1}$).

How Is Work Expressed in Respiratory Mechanics?

In respiratory mechanics, we are more concerned with pressure and the changes that occur in volume (usually the lung), rather than force and distance—so work of breathing is expressed as follows:

$$\text{Force} = \text{Pressure} \times \text{Area}$$

$$\text{Distance} = \text{Volume} / \text{Area}$$

Therefore,

$$\text{Work} = \text{Pressure} \times \text{''}\ \text{Volume}$$

A. McLintic · N. Randall (✉)
Department of Intensive Care Medicine, Counties Manukau Health, Auckland, New Zealand
e-mail: nic.randall@middlemore.co.nz

C. Birch et al. (eds.), *Physics and Measurement for Anesthesia*,
https://doi.org/10.1007/978-3-031-65060-4_23

Lung Pressure-Volume Loops

Forces to Be Overcome in Inspiration

Inspiration is an energy-requiring process with energy being required to overcome the following:

Elastic Forces

The lung has an intrinsic elastic recoil with a tendency to collapse inwards. Energy used in expanding the lung (by breathing or with the use of mechanical ventilation) is stored as elastic potential energy; this energy is utilised and released as heat during expiration, normally a passive activity. This natural inward (elastic) force is balanced, at the functional residual capacity (FRC), by the tendency of the chest wall cage to 'spring' outwards. Functional residual capacity is approximately 30 mL/kg for adults, is directly related to height and is approximately 10% less in females. Whilst the lung has relatively low concentrations of elastin, it mimics the physical properties of an elastic body due to the action of surfactant on surface tension within the alveoli. Surfactant plays a pivotal role in alveoli stability and preventing collapse.

Resistive Forces

There are also 'non-elastic' forces that act to oppose inspiration; these include frictional resistance to airflow (80%) and the force required to overcome frictional forces between tissues (20%) as they move past each other. This energy is not able to be stored and is lost immediately as heat. Due to the variable size and branching nature of the bronchial tree, airflow within the lung is a complex combination of laminar, transitional and turbulent flow.

Inertia

A small amount of extra work is also required to initiate airflow acceleration. Given that the mass of air being accelerated is very small in comparison to the other resistive forces, this energy is usually ignored.

Energy and Efficiency

Efficiency

- Around 10% of the energy produced by the muscles of respiration during breathing goes towards inflating the lung; the rest (90%) is lost as heat during the respiratory cycle.
- Normal resting work of breathing is around 300–350 mJ/L, with an oxygen cost of 0.25–0.50 mL O_2 per 1000 mL of ventilation (approximately 1–2% of basal metabolic rate).
- Approximately 50% is used to expand the elastic tissues, and the rest to overcome airway resistance.

- Energy used to overcome elastic forces is stored as (elastic) potential energy for expiration, but that used in overcoming resistive forces is converted to heat.

Power (Watt, W)

- Power is work per unit time. Power of breathing is approximately 2.5 J/min (resting).
- The power requirement varies with the type of flow:
- Laminar flow is more likely in quiet resting breathing.
- Turbulent flow requires higher driving pressures than laminar; therefore, oxygen consumption increases in situations where turbulence is more likely, such as hyperventilation, asthma and exercise. Energy required for breathing can be over 50% of the total energy expenditure during periods of severe illness and vigorous exercise.
- Work and power are linearly related to metabolic oxygen consumption (VO_2) and can increase in well-trained athletes up to 6000 mL/min, requiring minute ventilations of around 30 L/min.

PV Loop During a Spontaneous Tidal Breath

Figure 23.1 shows a schematic diagram that illustrates the work required to inflate the lung for a tidal volume from FRC; it is a useful way of demonstrating the various elements of the work of breathing. These convenient representations are not normally based on human experiments, but provide a useful visual method to describe forces and the transfer of energy that occurs.

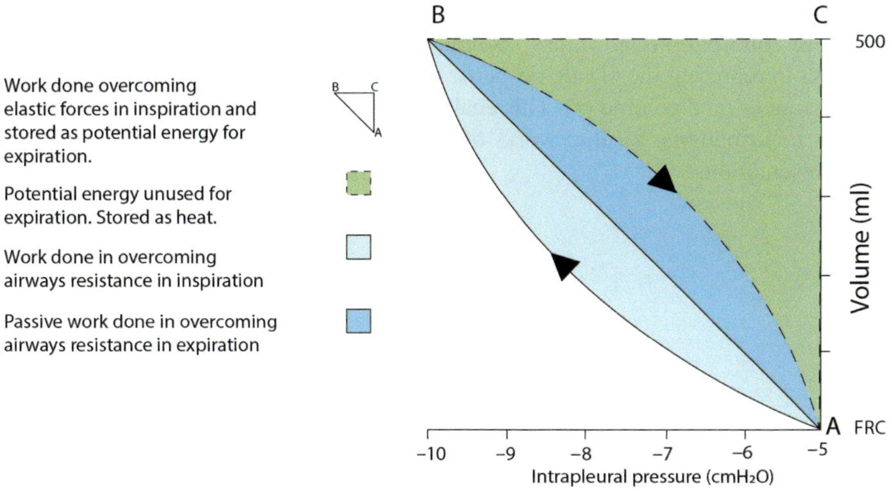

Fig. 23.1 Schematic diagram illustrating the division of work in one spontaneous breath

The triangle (ABC) is a representation of the work required to overcome the elastic properties of the lungs, and inflate them from FRC to a tidal volume, during spontaneous breathing. Intrapleural pressure is negative with the energy being provided by the patient.

A similar diagram could be drawn using positive pleural pressure (mechanical ventilation); in this case, the diagram would be a flipped (mirror) image, and required energy for inflation is supplied by the ventilator; expiration remains a passive process.

How Could This PV Loop Be Measured?

The patient would breathe slowly in and out through a spirometer during tidal volume breaths, and the intrapleural pressure changes are measured using an oesophageal manometer or pleural catheter.

Limitations of this Diagram

- The diagram does not illustrate the passive work that the elastic outward force of the chest wall has made in stretching the lung up to FRC.
- The diagonal compliance line over V_T is depicted as a straight line. In reality, it is a little curved.
- The intrapleural pressure is not uniform throughout the lung. Gravitational forces cause variation from apex to base.
- The elastic contribution that the chest wall makes to inflation diminishes over the tidal breath. A more physiologically correct graph would have the *y*-axis bowing to the right as volume increases to depict the extra work being required as chest wall contribution diminishes.

  These contributions are more accurately described in Fig. 23.2. The diagram seeks to represent the elastic properties of the lung and the chest wall, alongside pressure (x) and volume (y). This enables more complex calculations of the various contributions to the work of breathing and a more complex visual representation.

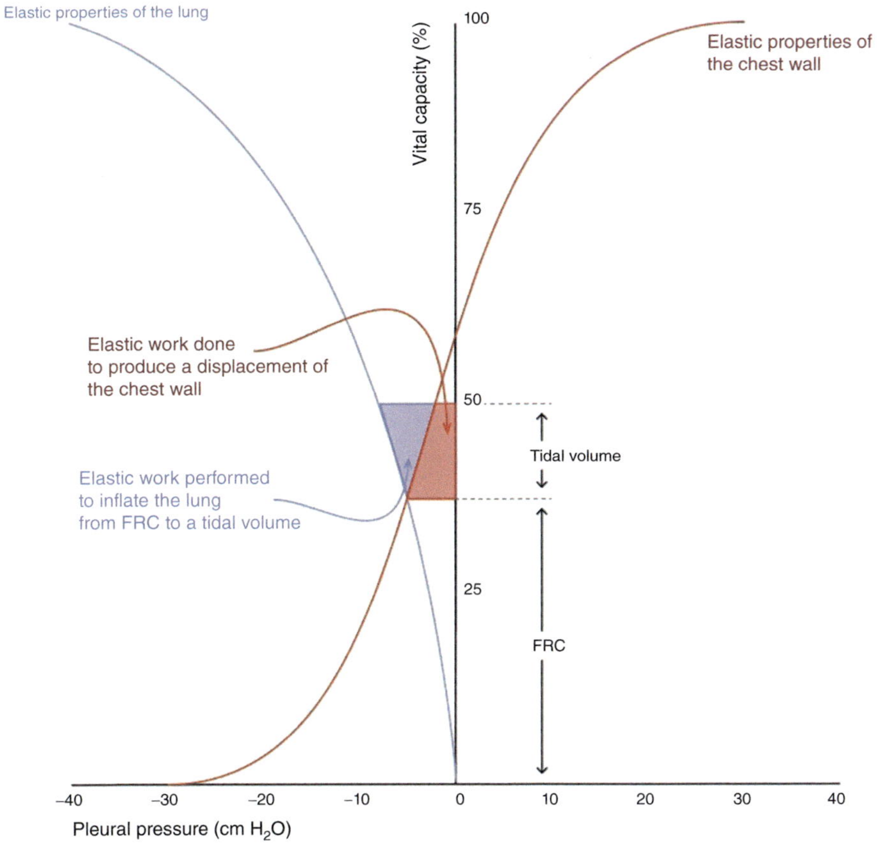

Fig. 23.2 Representation of the various contributions to the work of breathing

PV Loops in Disease

See Fig. 23.3.

Notes

Patients with lung disease often breathe with different tidal volumes (V_T) to those with normal lungs.

To minimise the work of breathing, patients with restrictive lung disease will maintain minute volume (MV) by breathing with smaller V_T but at faster rates.

Patients with obstructive lung disease will minimise work by breathing slower but with larger V_T, thereby maintaining MV.

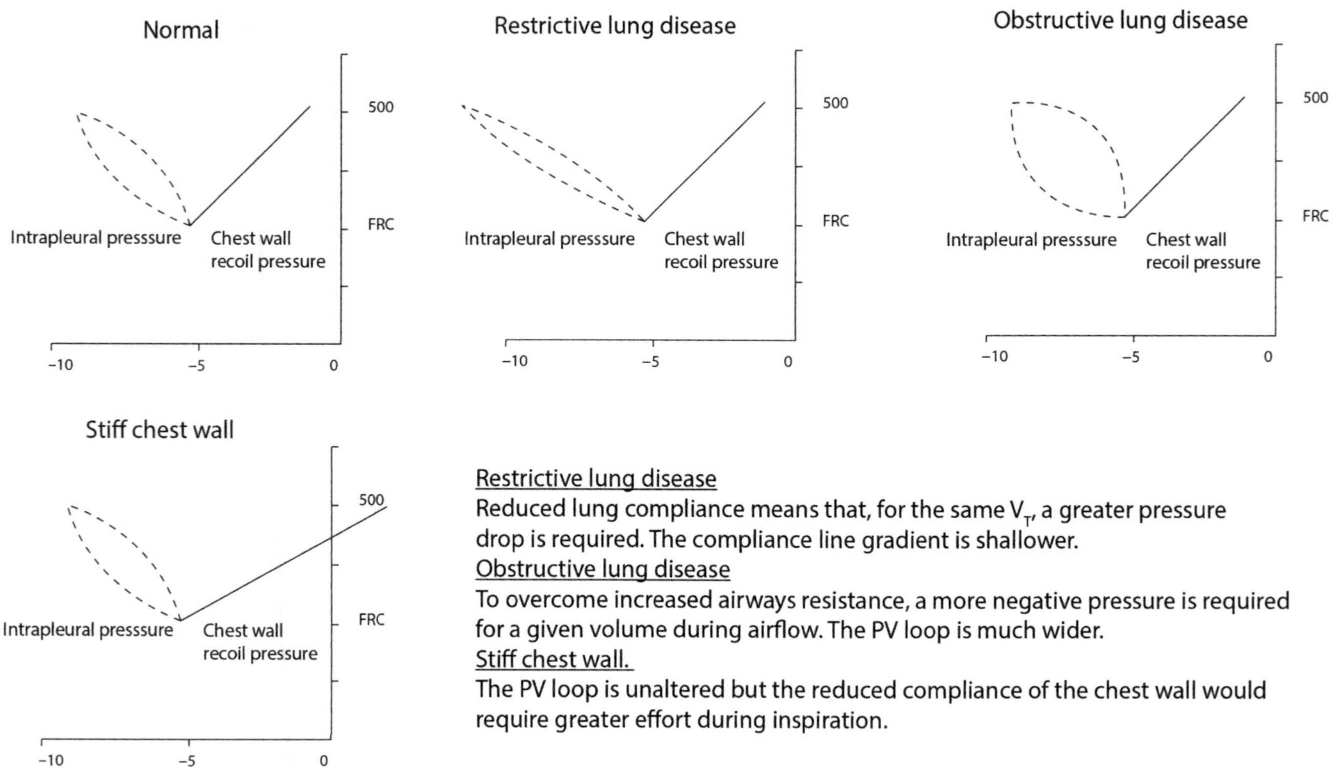

Fig. 23.3 Pressure (cmH_20) versus volume (mLs) loops in various disease states

Pressure-Volume Loops from the Anaesthetic Machine

The pressure-volume loops described above are largely academic illustrations of lung mechanics extrapolated from animal and computer simulation models. The PV loops seen displayed on anaesthetic machines are real-time representations of a particular patient's mechanical interaction, but have different inferences and interpretations because of where the pressures are being measured and depending on whether the patient is breathing spontaneously or mechanically.

Flow and volume measurements are made by hot-wire anemometry (see measurement of flow) at the entry and exit points of circle attachments. The airway pressures are measured within the tubing of the anaesthetic machine—this is of critical importance in understanding the meaning of the PV loops displayed.

Pressure-Volume Loops in Volume-Controlled Ventilation

Pressure is measured by the ventilator during volume-controlled ventilation (VCV); this comprises the pressure required to overcome the elastance of the equipment, the lung and chest wall, as well as resistance to airflow in the tubing, endotracheal tube (ETT) and patients' airways.

This work is displayed by the pressure-volume loop (PV loop) (shape of the area of the displayed PV loop therefore reflects the work done by the ventilator in overcoming all those impedances).

Notes (Figs. 23.4 and 23.5)

- The gradient of the PV loop in VCV reflects total thoracic compliance (lung + chest wall) plus a little from non-rigid equipment tubing.
- These are dynamic PV loops, so the gradient becomes less true to compliance with faster respiratory rates and in disease states.
- Inferences about respiratory resistances can only be made if flow is constant. This is the case in VCV but not in pressure-controlled ventilation (PCV) in which there is a decelerating flow rate. PV loops in PCV are therefore less informative about airway resistance. If there is no airflow at end inspiration and end expiration, the gradient should reflect total thoracic compliance.
- The PV loop in IPPV runs anticlockwise. In spontaneous breathing, it runs clockwise.
- Assessment and interpretation of PV loops can provide important information about the clinical state of the patient—for example, a characteristic PV loop can be seen when there is increased airway resistance due to bronchospasm, secretions or a narrow or kinked tube.

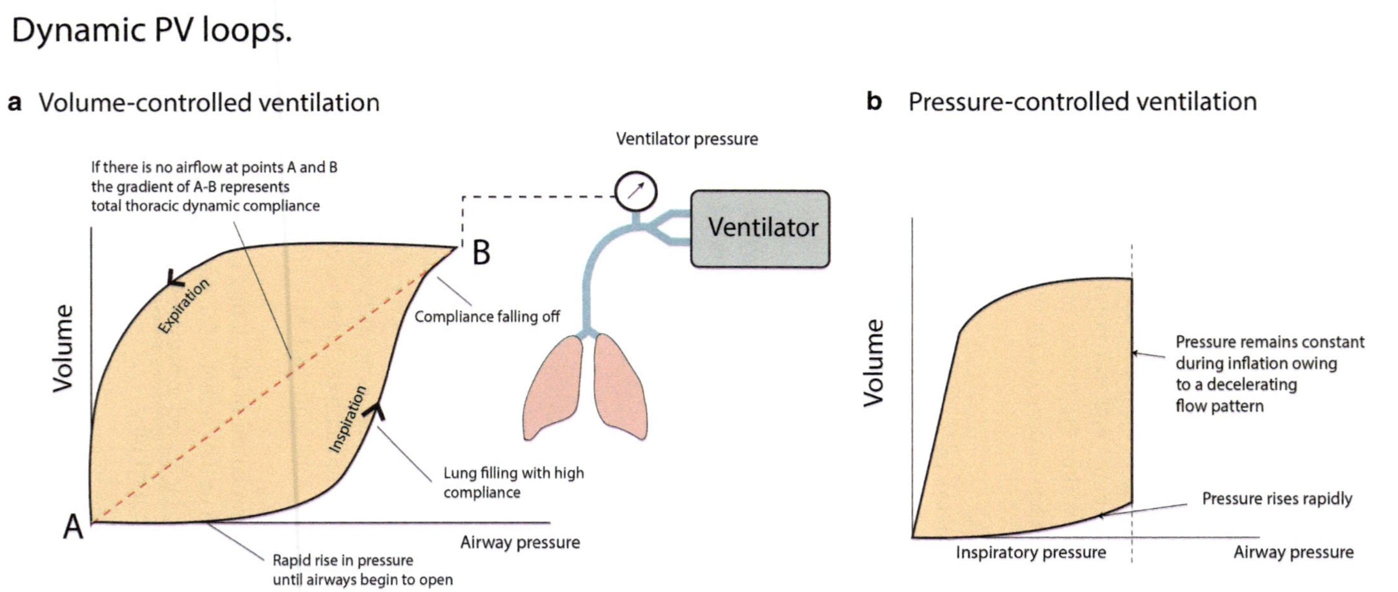

Fig. 23.4 Schematic representation of dynamic pressure versus volume during volume control (**a**) and pressure control (**b**) mechanical ventilation as maybe seen on an anaesthetic display

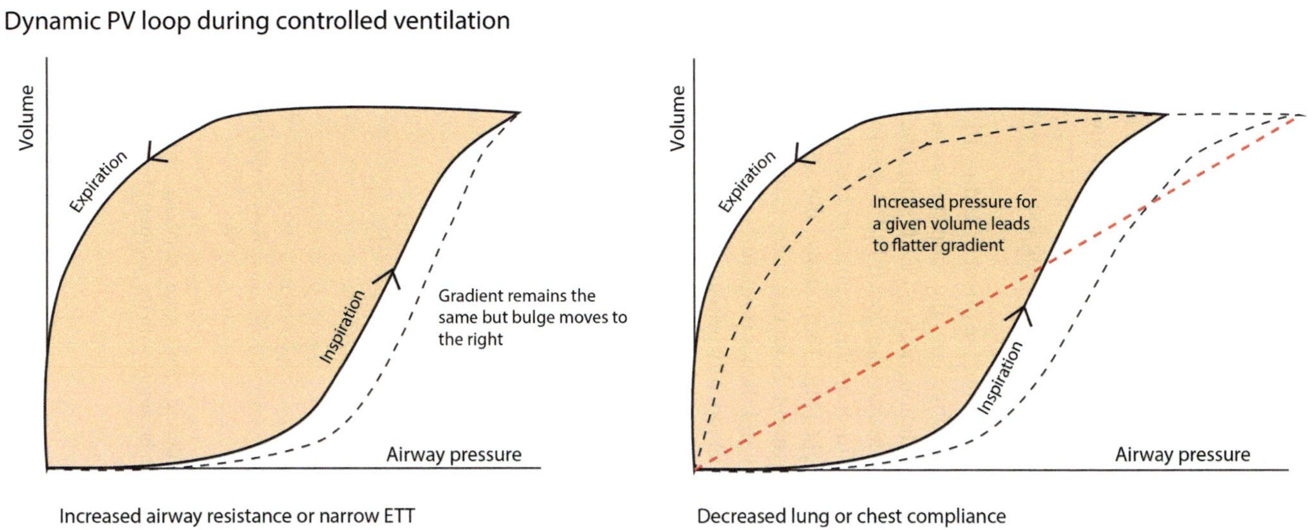

Fig. 23.5 Representation of increased airway resistance as seen with bronchospasm, secretions or a narrow endotracheal tube

Anaesthetic Machine Pressure-Volume Loops During Spontaneous Breathing

Can PV loops during spontaneous breathing inform us about the work of breathing, patient airway resistance or thoracic compliance?

The answer is no, because the pressure is being measured on the wrong side of those impedances. To register those impedances, the pressure would have to be measured in the alveoli (resistance) or intrapleural space (lung compliance).

Because the pressure is measured within the ventilator, the PV loops simply represent the work done in overcoming the resistance of the ventilator tubing. Ventilator manufacturers take pride in making the area within the PV loop as small as possible.

The left figure (Fig. 23.6) shows the effect of adding PEEP to a dynamic PV loop in spontaneous breathing. Notice how the loop moves in the opposite direction to that seen in controlled ventilation; adding PEEP shifts the curve to the right. Actual work done maybe slightly lower with added PEEP due to a reduction in atelectasis and a more favourable position on the respiratory compliance curve.

The diagram on the right (Fig. 23.6) shows the effect of pressure support in a spontaneously breathing patient. Note that there is a negative pressure at the initiation of breathing (trigger) and then a positive curve is seen with the pressure support. This diagram nicely shows why pressure support reduces the work of breathing as much of the work is performed by the ventilator, after the initial patient trigger.

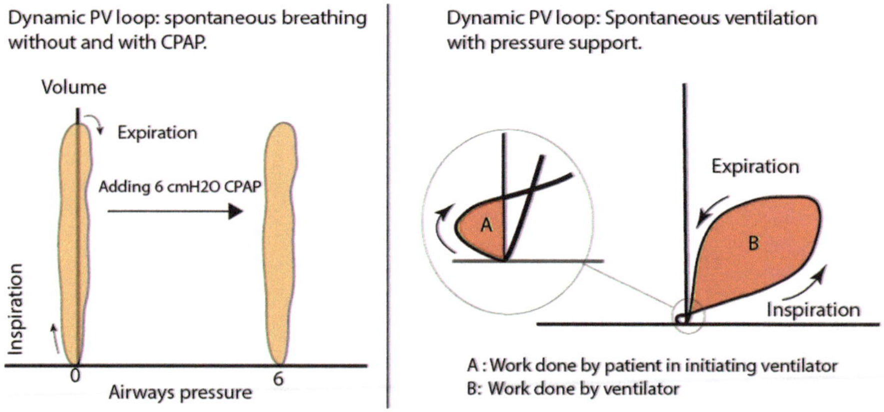

Fig. 23.6 Dynamic PV loops during spontaneous breathing, with and without added PEEP (left). Work done during spontaneous breathing with the addition of pressure support (right)

Compliance

24

Alan McLintic and Nic Randall

Static Lung Compliance

Lung compliance is change in volume for a given change in pressure. Static and dynamic compliance can be measured and represent different measurement techniques, they are frequently confused and the terms (incorrectly) interchanged.

Static lung compliance is measured during a condition of no airflow (breath-holding); it is the change in lung volume per unit pressure difference between the intrapleural space and the alveoli ($P_{pl} - P_{alv}$):

- The normal value for static lung compliance is 150–200 ml cmH_2O^{-1}.

Method

- Volumes are measured using either a spirometer or the body plethysmograph, and the intrapleural pressures are measured with an oesophageal monometer. In conditions of no airflow, the alveolar pressure will be equivalent to mouth pressure, which is barometric pressure.
- The subject inspires to vital capacity and holds their breath until the pressure settles.
- The subject then breathes out in increments, each time holding their breath for 1–2 s, while the pressure settles and is recorded. This procedure is repeated several times to obtain a sufficient data to construct a curve from TLC to FRC (Fig. 24.1). For a mechanically ventilated patient, static compliance can be still calculated, the technique uses the ventilator to slowly deliver the stepwise volume change to a paralysed patient whilst recording the pressure.

A. McLintic · N. Randall (✉)
Department of Intensive Care, Counties Manukau Health, Auckland, New Zealand
e-mail: nic.randall@middlemore.co.nz

C. Birch et al. (eds.), *Physics and Measurement for Anesthesia*,
https://doi.org/10.1007/978-3-031-65060-4_24

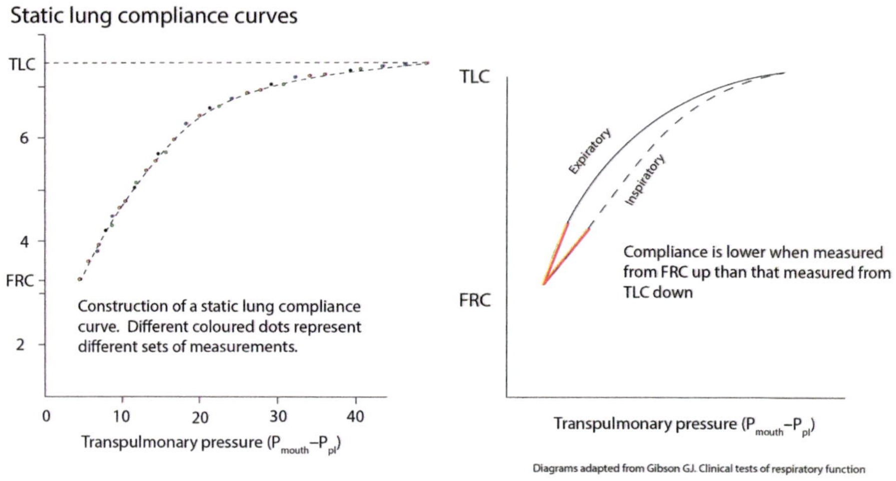

Fig. 24.1 Construction of static lung compliance curve for the subject breathing out incrementally from total lung capacity. Transpulmonary pressure is obtained from the difference between alveolar (barometric) and pleural (oesophageal) pressure

Notes

- The usual summary of lung compliance is obtained by fitting a straight line to the curve from FRC up to 500 or 1000 ml and finding its gradient.
- If measurements are made starting from FRC, the recoil pressures for a given volume are a little larger than when the curve is constructed from TLC down.
- Pulmonary compliance is less on the way up than on the way down; this is known as hysteresis and reflects the greater degree of distension/recruitment of lung units occurring when starting from TLC.
- This curve can be extended below FRC, where it takes on a sigmoid shape. This is most obvious if the curve is constructed from lower lung volumes back up to FRC.
- Lung compliance varies with the size of the lungs, even between normal individuals, and is possibly related to quantitative differences in numbers of alveoli. Specific lung compliance accounts for this by expressing compliance as a percentage of predicted FRC or TLC.

Dynamic Lung Compliance

Dynamic lung compliance is lung compliance measured during quiet breathing. Volumes are measured via a spirometer, and intrapleural pressure is measured using an oesophageal manometer. Theoretically, end expiration and end inspiration are points of zero flow; the gradient of a line drawn between them represents lung compliance; however, a difference exists between the static and dynamic gradients due to regional variation in ventilation and lung time constants.

Notes

- In the normal patient, the dynamic compliance is less than the static curve constructed in expiration but close to the static curve constructed in inspiration.
- In disease, dynamic compliance measurement may be markedly less than the static, due to the Pendelluft effect, whereby air continues to be redistributed in slow lung units even though flow has ceased or reversed at the mouth. This effect is seen in more markedly ventilated patients and reflects a heterogeneous disease pattern in the lungs.
- The static–dynamic differences increase as respiratory rates increase as there is less time for uniform distribution of gas to occur.

Dynamic and static lung compliance

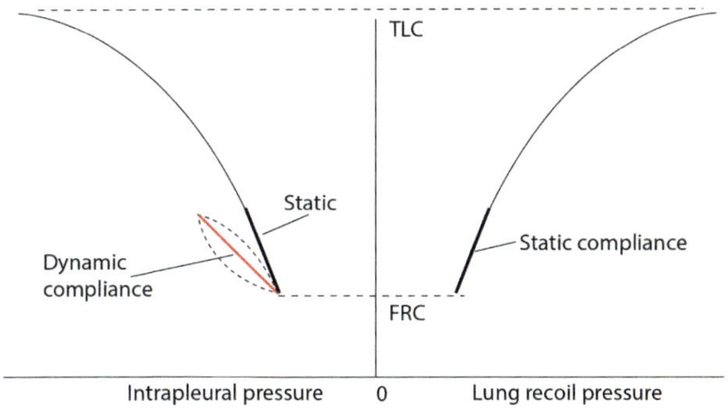

Diagrams adapted from Gibson GJ. Clinical tests of respiratory function

Compliance Measured in the Anaesthetic Machine

An estimation of total thoracic (lung + CW) compliance during ventilation is usually available in contemporary anaesthetic machines. It is important to understand that this is an estimation as oesophageal monitoring is not routinely available and hence the transpleural pressure measurement requires a number of assumptions.

Dynamic Compliance from PV Loops

As described above, a gradient drawn between the end-expiratory and end-inspiratory points of the PV loop in controlled ventilation represents total thoracic dynamic compliance. It is this dynamic compliance that is most commonly displayed in ventilators, but can only be calculated for mechanical (positive pressure) ventilation. Pressure and volume are measured at the start of inspiration and the end, and compliance is calculated. This may be displayed as a number or as part of a compliance V time graph. The pressure-volume loop during spontaneous ventilation is not able to provide any information on lung compliance, as it is impossible to calculate the intrapleural (oesophageal) pressure measurement.

Static Compliance from the Pressure-Time Trace

An estimation of total thoracic static compliance can be made from the pressure-time trace in volume-controlled ventilation (VCV), using an inspiratory pause. In VCV, tidal volume is preset, and the ventilator drives gas down the airways at constant flow until the preset volume is delivered. The pressure required to deliver the tidal volume is measured within the ventilator and is a function of the volume delivered, the total respiratory compliance and the total airway resistance encountered during inflation.

When flow stops, the airway resistance component is lost, and the pressure will fall to plateau pressure (zero flow, $P_{plateau}$); this is only achieved if enough time is allowed for redistribution to occur. When a true plateau pressure is obtained, pressure is same throughout the transmitting airways, from trachea to alveoli; this pressure can be recorded at the T piece of the endotracheal tube.

If the ventilator adds a short inspiratory pause before the expiratory valve is opened, the total thoracic static compliance can be estimated from the volume delivered and the ($P_{plateau}$ – P_{PEEP}) difference; a more accurate measurement requires a longer inspiratory pause and the establishment of zero flow—this is usually only possible in the deeply sedated or paralysed patient.

From Fig. 24.2, it can be seen that the resistance component can be estimated as the difference between peak pressure and plateau pressure and that total respiratory compliance can be calculated using the plateau pressure.

During pressure-controlled ventilation, the same assessment can be made. As long as there is an inspiratory pause with no airflow, the plateau pressure can be used as above to estimate static compliance, however it is not possible to measure the resistance component though because plateau and peak pressure are the same.

Normal Values

- The normal value for total thoracic compliance is 85–100 ml cmH_2O^{-1} but often is less in an anaesthetised, ventilated patient due to atelectasis and changes in the lung gas distribution.

Total Thoracic Static Compliance: Super-Syringe Method

The super-syringe method is the measurement of total thoracic static compliance during stepwise inflation of lung and chest wall compliance in conditions of no

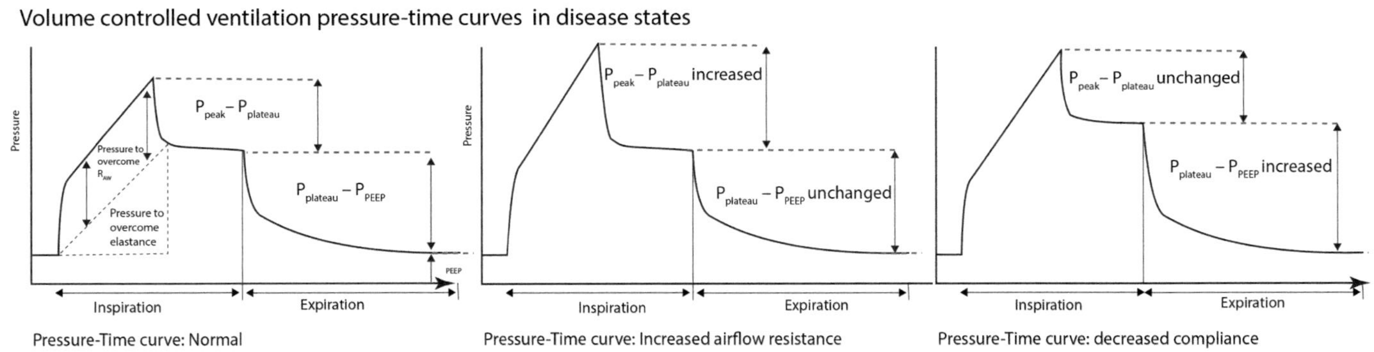

Fig. 24.2 Normal pressure-time curve for volume-controlled ventilation (left), with increased airway resistance; a greater peak pressure is observed (centre), but compliance as determined from plateau pressure remains unchanged. On the right, total respiratory compliance has decreased, but airway resistance is similar to the original

airflow. This is of academic/research interest rather than a clinical tool. The procedure assesses the volume change per transthoracic pressure gradient.

Method

- The procedure is carried out in a sedated, intubated, ventilated patient using the super-syringe method.
- A large syringe is connected to the breathing system, and this is used to increase the volume of the lung incrementally. At each inflation, the airway pressure is recorded and allowed to settle.
- The airway pressure is then equivalent to alveolar pressure.
- Multiple separate manoeuvres are required to construct these compliance curves as the manoeuvre needs to be interrupted to allow for ventilation and oxygenation to occur.

Respiratory: Ventilator Patterns

25

Alan McLintic and Nic Randall

Pressure-Controlled Ventilation (PCV)

Principle

- The desired pressure is set. During inspiration, pressure rises rapidly and then remains constant for the entire inspiratory time. To achieve this, ventilator flow rises rapidly and then decelerates as the lung expands; this is best seen on a flow V time curve (Fig. 25.1). Cessation of flow occurs when the pressure in the ventilator circuit (usually measured within the ventilator itself) is equal to the preset pressure on the ventilator (P_{insp}). Inspiratory pressure approximates alveolar pressure only if flow has stopped, and sufficient time has passed to allow pressure equilbrium between alveoli and the ventilator tubing to occur (at zero flow).
- An inspiratory pause may be added. During an inspiratory pause, the lung is held in inspiration for a set time (usually represented as % of the 'I' time) before the expiratory valve is opened. This allows for a more even distribution of the inspiratory breath.
- Expiration begins with the opening of the expiratory valve, the pressure falls rapidly followed by passive exponential decline in volume, flow and pressure to baseline. Energy for expiration comes from stored potential energy developed during inspiration by the ventilator.

A. McLintic · N. Randall (✉)
Department of Intensive Care Medicine, Counties Manukau Health, Auckland, New Zealand
e-mail: nic.randall@middlemore.co.nz

C. Birch et al. (eds.), *Physics and Measurement for Anesthesia*,
https://doi.org/10.1007/978-3-031-65060-4_25

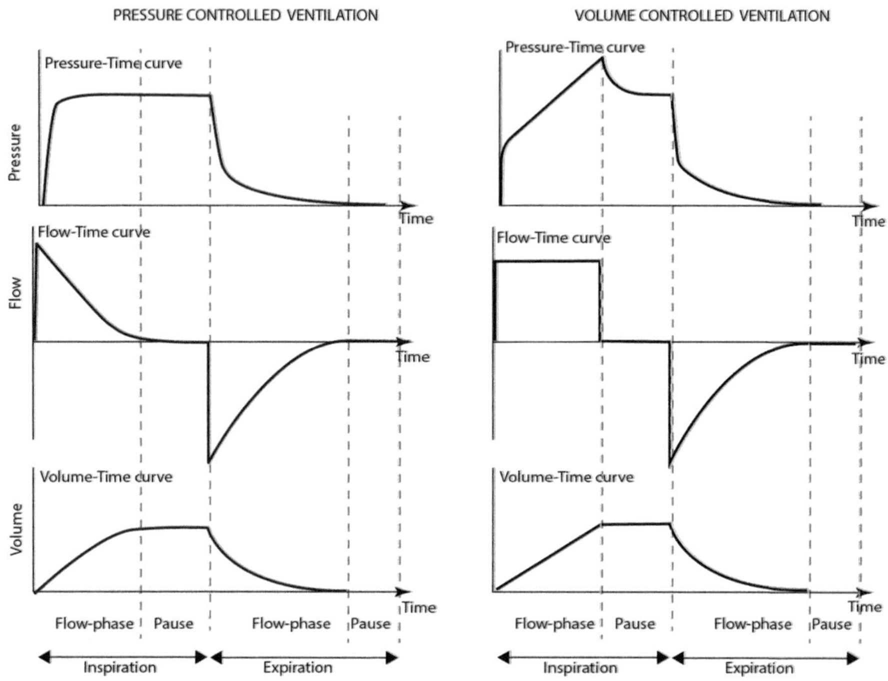

Fig. 25.1 Common ventilator waveform patterns seen in pressure and volume control modes

What Determines the Tidal Volume (V_T)?

- Tidal volume (T_V) is a function of the driving inspiratory pressure and total thoracic (lung, chest wall and equipment) compliance; assuming enough time has been allowed for inspiration in the I:E settings.
- For example, if the inspiratory pressure is set at 10 cmH_2O^{-1} and total thoracic (static) compliance is 50 $mL.cmH_2O^{-1}$, the expected volume delivered would be 500 mL[2].

Lung (Alveolar) Pressure Vs. Ventilator Pressure

The pressure displayed on the monitor is the pressure within the ventilator circuit; alveolar lung pressures can be derived from this only when flow has stopped (equal to zero).

Volume-Controlled Ventilation

Principle

- The tidal volume is set. The ventilator flow rate rises rapidly; in the simplest case, this is followed by constant flow until the set volume is delivered. The T_V can be calculated from the area of the flow-time curve. Modern ventilators may use an inspiratory flow that follows a decelerating pattern (see below).
- The pressures during inflation are a function of the volume set, the airway resistance to flow (equipment and patient) and the total thoracic compliance (lung, chest wall and equipment).
- After the desired volume is delivered, an inspiratory pause is often added; this assists in gas distribution prior to expiration. With cessation of flow, a drop in pressure occurs, due to a loss of inspiratory resistance. The pressure at the end of inspiration (just prior to exhalation) when flow has stopped is called the plateau pressure as is the best representation of alveolar pressure. The difference between peak pressure and plateau pressure gives an indication of inspiratory resistance.
- The plateau pressure during the inspiratory pause is a function of the pressure required to overcome the lung and chest wall elastance.

Auto-Flow Volume-Guaranteed Ventilation

Principle

The aim is to achieve the set volume with the lowest possible pressure. The desired volume is set, but flow rate is decelerating, looking like pressure-controlled ventilation. Flow rises rapidly, then decelerates and adapts to ensure that the volume is delivered. The pressure trace is more or less constant as in PCV. Initial flow is higher than the corresponding square waveform.

Proposed Advantages

- Volume is guaranteed.
- Pressure is minimised.
- If compliance changes, the flow rates are adjusted to maintain preset volume at lowest pressures.

Expiration

Expiration is passive in both PCV and VCV.

Following the opening of the expiratory valve, there is a rapid drop in pressure and an exponential decline to baseline (zero flow).

The rate of decline is determined by the resistance and compliance of the patient and equipment. In a normal anaesthetised patient, the lung volume should decline by 95% in 1.5 s[2]. The greater the airway resistance and lower the compliance, the slower the rate of decline.

The expiratory dynamics can be quantified by a time constant; this is the time taken for equilibrium to occur if the initial flow rate were maintained. Expected values in a paralysed, intubated, anaesthetised patient would be:

- Total airways and equipment resistance: 10 $cmH_2O^{-1}/L.s^{-1}$.
- Total thoracic compliance: 50 mL/cmH_2O^{-1}.
- Time constant = resistance × compliance = 0.5 s.

Ventilator Cycling

Ventilator cycle time is the sum of the inspiratory ('I' time) and the expiratory ('E' time); this is normally presented as the I:E ratio (e.g. 1:2). The ventilator cycle time (s) for a single breath is the respiratory rate divide by 60s e.g. RR of 10 the cycle time is 6s; this is then distributed in the ratio determined by the I:E. The transition from inspiration to expiration is called ventilator cycling. There are a number of different ways in which this can occur.

Time Cycling

Inflation is terminated after a preset time ('I')
T_V is the product of flow and the inspiratory time.
Tidal volume (T_V) delivered depends on the compliance and resistance of the respiratory system.

Volume Cycling

Inflation is terminated after a preset volume has been delivered, and the 'I' time is determined from this.
This guarantees that a certain volume is delivered irrespective of compliance and resistance; however, pressure is a dependent variable.
Pressure alarm limits are required to prevent high pressures being used.

Pressure Cycling

Inflation is terminated when a preset airway pressure is achieved.
This mode is uncommon. Pressure control ventilation uses time cycling with an upper pressure (P_{isp}) that is held.

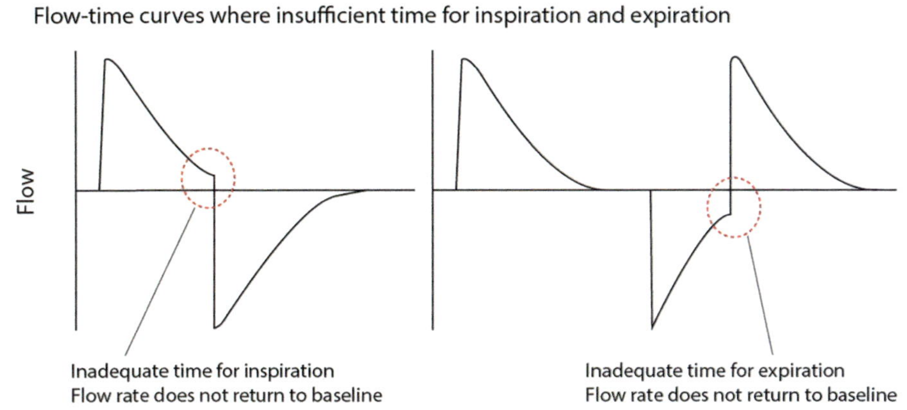

Fig. 25.2 Flow-time curves demonstrating insufficient inspiratory (left) and expiratory (right) time

Consequence of Insufficient Time for Inspiration or Expiration

- The I:E ratio and respiratory rate determine the time for inspiration and expiration (respiratory cycle time). Adjustments of these factors may lead to insufficient time for completion of either inspiration or expiration. Examination of the flow-time trace is a useful way to appreciate if this is occurring. If there is insufficient time for inspiration or expiration, the flow trace will not be seen to return to baseline (Fig. 25.2).

Insufficient Inspiratory Time

Premature inspiratory termination occurs ('clipping') if set volume may not be delivered.

This is seen as a continuous positive flow prior to the onset of the expiratory phase.

Insufficient Expiratory Time

Flow continues throughout the expiratory phase and does not return to baseline (zero) on the flow-time curve.

Gas trapping can occur with increased alveolar pressure and the development of intrinsic PEEP.

There is a risk of tension pneumothorax and barotrauma (especially in patients with acute asthma). It is important to be able to recognise when gas trapping occurring. Management involves increasing the time for expiration through adjustments to the 'E' time. Reducing the RR may also be required to increase the respiratory cycle time to allow sufficient time for expiration. I:E ratio may need to extend out quite considerably eg 1:6 or even further.

Measuring Carbon Monoxide Diffusing Capacity/Transfer Factor

26

Alan McLintic and Michael Webb

Measuring Carbon Monoxide Diffusing Capacity/ Transfer Factor

To exert an effect at tissues, gases must diffuse across the alveolar membrane and into the blood. This process has multiple physiological facets, and a firm grasp of the scientific underpinning of diffusion and diffusion capacity is required to understand the process as it relates to blood gases.

The measurement of diffusing capacity is a laboratory test done to assess the ability of gases to cross the alveolar membrane and is specifically designed to assess the ability of oxygen to diffuse. The test relies upon a measurement of difference in partial pressure of carbon monoxide (CO) in an inspired and expired breath. In this chapter, concepts of the basic science of diffusion of gases, factors germane to the diffusion of oxygen, diffusion capacity vs. transfer factor, use of carbon monoxide as an ideal test gas for diffusion, and a practical laboratory method for the measurement of diffusing are discussed.

Background Principles

Gases must diffuse through the alveolus, and this process follows a consistently observed law. It can be expressed as:

$$\dot{V}\text{gas} = \frac{A}{T} D.\left(P_{\text{alv}} - P_{\text{cap}}\right)$$

A. McLintic · M. Webb (✉)
Department of Anaesthesia and Pain Medicine, Counties Manukau Health, Auckland, New Zealand

C. Birch et al. (eds.), *Physics and Measurement for Anesthesia*,
https://doi.org/10.1007/978-3-031-65060-4_26

where:

- Partial pressure gradient across the membrane ($P_{alv} - P_{cap.}$)
- Area of membrane (A)
- 1/Thickness membrane (T)
- Diffusion coefficient (D)
- 1/Molecular weight of gas
- Solubility in membrane

Oxygen diffusion (not carbon monoxide) is also dependant on perfusion because, at rest and in normal physiological states, oxygen diffusion equilibrium is almost achieved in one pulmonary capillary transit time.

There are rate-limiting steps that govern the speed at which gases move from the alveolus to bind with haemoglobin. These are:

1. Diffusion across the membrane
2. Travel through blood
   - Plasma
   - RBC membrane
   - RBC interior
3. Chemical combination with Hb

The laboratory measurement of "diffusing capacity" is an index of the ability of a gas to diffuse as a result of a pressure gradient. Strictly speaking, it does not account for any other factors than pressure gradients. It is given by the following equation:

$$\text{Diffusing capacity}\left(D_L\right) = \frac{\text{Net transfer}}{\left(P_{\text{alv}} - P_{\text{cap}}\right)}\left(\text{mL.min}^{-1}.\text{mmHg}^{-1}\right)$$

Transfer Factor

To distinguish between simple diffusion along a pressure gradient and the more complex physiological process that involves gas travel through blood and chemical interactions with haemoglobin, the term transfer factor is used. Diffusing capacity is a misleading term because the test measures the rate of uptake from the alveolus, and this is governed not just by diffusion, but by these other two factors.

Carbon Monoxide As a Test Gas for Assessment of Diffusing Capacity

Carbon monoxide (CO) is used to assess diffusing capacity. The unique physiological properties of this substance make it an ideal test gas. Carbon monoxide has 250 times the affinity for haemoglobin as oxygen. This means that the capillary partial pressure of CO remains effectively zero with no back pressure to oppose diffusion. The passage of CO across the membrane is thus governed by the diffusing properties of the blood/gas barrier rather than the amount in the blood. It also simplifies the investigation considerably because there is no need to measure capillary CO partial pressure. Thus, for carbon monoxide, the above equation can be simplified:

$$D_L\text{CO} = \frac{\dot{V}}{P_{\text{alv}}}$$

where $\dot{V}$ is the volume of CO taken up from the alveolar space per minute.

Because of density and water solubility differences, the rate of diffusion of oxygen through the alveolar membrane is faster than that of CO. The rate of reaction with Hb is also faster for oxygen because CO must first displace O_2 from Hb before combining. For this reason, the CO combination rate is altered in the presence of different oxygen concentrations.

Single-Breath-Hold Method of Measuring Diffusing Capacity

- The subject takes a single vital capacity breath of 0.3% CO in 10% helium and holds the breath for 10 s to allow full distribution (Fig. 26.1).
- The subject then breathes out, and the concentrations of CO and helium are measured. The greater the difference between the initial alveolar [CO] and the alveolar [CO] after 10 s, the greater the uptake.
- Although the inspired [CO] is known, the alveolar [CO] is harder to determine because the resident alveolar gases immediately dilute it. Thus, an inert gas such as helium is inspired along with CO.

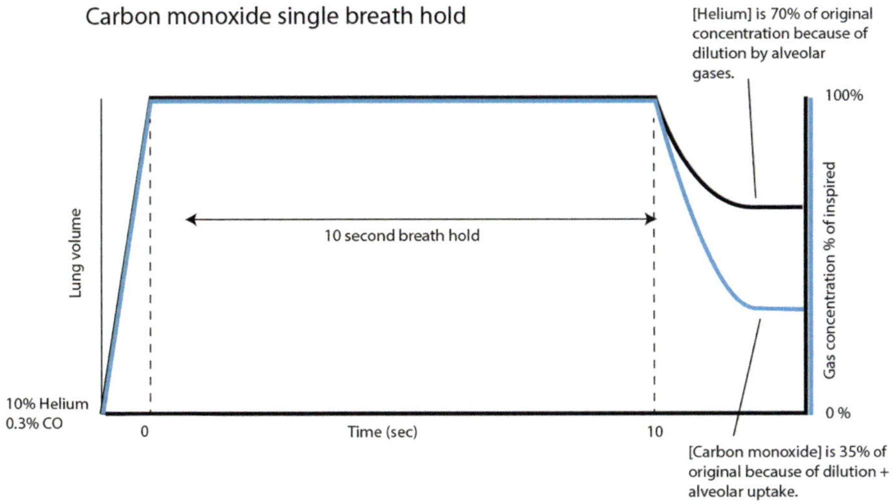

Fig. 26.1 Graphical description of the CO single-breath-hold method

Table 26.1 Factors affecting diffusing capacity

Factors affecting diffusing capacity	
Body size	D_L increases with body size and must be adjusted
Alveolar volume	D_L increases with increasing alveolar volume
Pathological causes of reduced alveolar volume	Multiple pulmonary and extrapulmonary causes of reduced alveolar ventilation will reduce D_LCO
Impaired membrane diffusion	D_L is reduced in collagen diseases, interstitial oedema, alveolitis, fibrosis, etc.
Maldistribution of ventilation	D_L reduced in emphysema
Anaemia	D_L reduced. D_L should be corrected for [Hb]
Polycythaemia	D_L increased
Increased blood volume	D_L increased in exercise and in congestive heart failure

- Helium will not be taken up from the alveoli but will be diluted to the same degree as the CO. Thus, by multiplying the inspired [CO] by the helium dilution factor, we arrive at the initial alveolar [CO]:

$$F_{\text{alv}}\text{CO} = F_{\text{insp}}\text{CO} \times \frac{F_{\text{exp}}\text{He}}{F_{\text{insp}}\text{He}}$$

- The next step is to calculate the rate at which the $F_{\text{alv}}\text{CO}$ changed over 10 s. This is an exponential process because $F_{\text{alv}}\text{CO}$ is declining all the time as CO is being taken up. The rate of change is called K_{CO}.
- The final step is to multiply K_{CO} by the alveolar volume (V_A) at which the measurement was made. The test is usually done at full inflation, and the alveolar volume is usually estimated from the helium dilution used in the test:

$$D_L\text{CO} = K_{\text{CO}} \times V_A \left(\text{mL.min}^{-1}.\text{mmHg}^{-1}\right)$$

- Normal values
- $K_{\text{CO}} \sim$ 6–8 mL.min^{-1}.mmHg^{-1}.L^{-1}
- $D_L\text{CO}$: ~17–25 mL.min^{-1}.mmHg^{-1}

Measurements of diffusing capacity can be altered by a variety of normal physiological and pathological variables. These are summarised in Table 26.1.

Factors Affecting Diffusing Capacity

Further Reading

Gibson GJ. Clinical tests of respiratory function. 3rd ed. London: Hodder Arnold; 2009.

EEG and Depth of Anaesthesia Monitoring

27

Alan McLintic and Nicholas Lightfoot

Introduction

The electroencephalogram or EEG is a cutaneous recording of the voltages (measured in microvolts [μV]) of the post-synaptic electrical potentials generated by groups of cortical neurons. Pyramidal neurons coordinate and communicate with each other to generate large extracellular electrical oscillations, which can be recorded on the scalp. Rather than measuring the electrical activity of a single neuron, the electrical fields that are recorded are the summation of the activity of groups of neurons, analysed using vectoral analysis.

The activity of deeper structures is not easily recorded; however, deeper neurons, such as those in the thalamus or brainstem, can influence cortical activity; the EEG is thought to be a representation of the activity of both cortical and sub-cortical states.

A standard EEG records its potentials using electrodes placed according to the 'International 10–20 system' which standardises their location and connections. Measurements are made of the circumference of the head at the level of the inion (external occipital protuberance) and the nasion (the most anterior point of the frontonasal suture) crossing through the external auditory meatus. Each electrode is placed 10% of this circumferential distance *above* this line and 20% of the circumferential distance *apart*. Readers should refer to standard texts for further information surrounding electrode placement. Overall, there are 20 electrodes which either record potentials or serve as reference electrodes leading to 16 channels being recorded.

A. McLintic · N. Lightfoot (✉)
Department of Anaesthesia and Pain Medicine, Counties Manukau Health, Auckland, New Zealand

C. Birch et al. (eds.), *Physics and Measurement for Anesthesia*,
https://doi.org/10.1007/978-3-031-65060-4_27

Table 27.1 Summary of EEG waveforms and their associations with sleep

Wave	Frequency (Hz)	Amplitude (μV)	
Gamma	25–80		Awake, conscious perception
Beta	13–30	<20	Most common frequency in awake adults. Asynchronous
Alpha	8–12	20–50	Relaxed, eyes closed. Posterior dominance. More synchronous
Theta	4–7	>50	Early sleep
Delta	<4	>75	Deep, non-REM sleep

Normal EEG Rhythms

In the awake state, the EEG appears to be random, with no obvious repetitive patterns. Anaesthesia, sleep and certain pathological states are associated with an increase in cortical synchrony, which is attributed to the influence of neuronal loops between the cortex, thalamus and brainstem.

The awake state is dominated by 'fast' low-amplitude, high-frequency activity in the beta and gamma ranges. Gamma waves are the fastest EEG oscillations and are associated with conscious perception. As the gamma waves are similar in their frequency to the electromyogram or EMG, there is difficulty separating the two, meaning that some researchers have doubted the utility of interpreting this frequency from scalp EEG recordings. As the frequency of the EEG waveform slows or its period increases, the amplitude of the waveforms increases. With sleep, the EEG progresses from beta and gamma dominance to alpha waves when the eyes are closed and the patient is relaxed, then to theta and finally to delta wave activity. Table 27.1 further summarises the waveforms discussed in this section.

Sleep

Neurobiology of Sleep

The control of sleep is centred in the suprachiasmatic nuclei of the anterior hypothalamus. The onset of sleep is associated with the activation of inhibitory neurons, which produce neurotransmitters, particularly GABA that suppresses wakefulness-promoting regions of the brain such as the locus coeruleus. The hypothalamus is where the circadian rhythm is mediated. Signals pass between the retina and the hypothalamus providing cues on the time of the day and day–night cycling. The hypothalamus in turn signals the pineal gland to produce melatonin, which is important in coordinating sleep cycles and regulating the characteristic physiological signs associated with sleep across multiple organ systems.

Rapid eye movement or REM sleep is generated by cholinergic neurons in the mesencephalic and pontine regions. It is here that the cyclical oscillation between REM and non-REM (NREM) sleep arises. This oscillation is called an ultradian rhythm as its recurrent period is less than once per day.

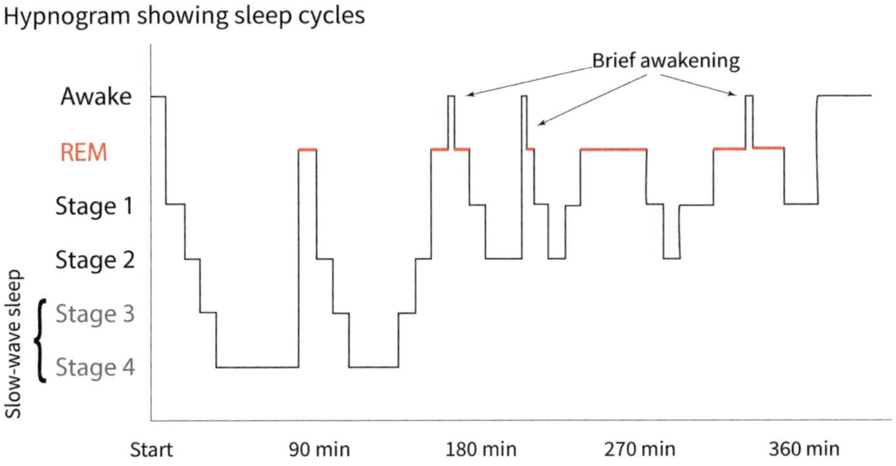

Fig. 27.1 Hypnogram showing sleep cycles over time

Sleep Cycle

Sleep is divided into two phases called NREM and REM sleep. The normal pattern is to cycle between NREM and REM every 90 min meaning that there are between 3 and 6 cycles per night. Initially, NREM comprises around 90% of each cycle, but as the night progresses, the time spent in deep NREM sleep diminishes and the relative proportion of REM sleep decreases; see Fig. 27.1.

As humans age, the production of melatonin decreases meaning the time at which sleep occurs becomes later with a consequent reduction in the amount of deep NREM sleep. During adolescence, the release of melatonin is progressively delayed, which leads to the later sleep times that are characteristic of this age group. The onset of sleep can be altered through a loss of synchrony with external cues, e.g. shift work and jet lag or through sleep disorders which can occur de novo or in conjunction with psychiatric comorbidities.

Stage 1 NREM

This is light sleep with eye rolling at twitching on occasion. Stage 1 NREM accounts for 5–10% of the total sleep cycle in adults with the EEG progressing from alpha when the eyes are closed, and the subject is 'drowsy' to theta waves with deeper sleep.

Stage 2 NREM

During stage 2 NREM, the subject is harder to rouse. This accounts for around 50% of total sleep with the EEG demonstrating theta activity with associated sleep spindles and K complexes. A sleep spindle is a short burst of high-frequency synchronous EEG activity which looks like alpha activity. These complexes originate in the thalamus and may have function in memory consolidation and in moderating disturbances from sleep. K complexes are the largest human EEG wave, which features a brief negative high voltage peak followed by a slower positive complex, and then a final negative peak. These complexes may also play roles in supressing arousal from sleep and in memory consolidation.

Stage 3 NREM/Delta Sleep/Slow-Wave Sleep (SWS)

Slow-wave or stage 3 NREM sleep comprises around 20–25% of the total sleep time. It was previously divided into stage 3 and 4 components, but since 2007, it has been consolidated to one phase. This period is characterised by high-amplitude, low-frequency delta waves which originate in the anterior hypothalamus. During stage 3 sleep, an individual becomes less responsive to external environmental stimuli; as such, this is the most restful and restorative part of the sleep cycle. Stage 3 sleep is associated with reduction in the heart rate and blood pressure, slowing of respiration with a reduction in carbon dioxide sensitivity, muscle relaxation and swallowing at the same rate as when awake.

REM Sleep

In adults, REM sleep accounts for 20–25% of the total sleep time but can be nearer to 50% in infants. REM sleep is generated by mesencephalic and pontine cholinergic neurones and is inhibited by neurones secreting serotonin. Despite the sleeper being at their least responsive to arousal, the EEG exhibits high-frequency, asynchronous waveforms which are like the awake state.

This phase is associated with an increase in the cerebral blood flow and profound muscular relaxation. There may be autonomic dysregulation with increased sympathetic activity and an irregular or increased heart rate and blood pressure. The respiratory rate may also be irregular or increased with periodic airway obstruction which can be manifest as snoring. The ventilatory response to carbon dioxide, like in stage 3 sleep, is again supressed. During REM sleep, there are rapid eye movements, dreaming and bruxism (teeth grinding), and swallowing is markedly reduced. The EEG manifestations of the different phases of sleep are further described in Fig. 27.2.

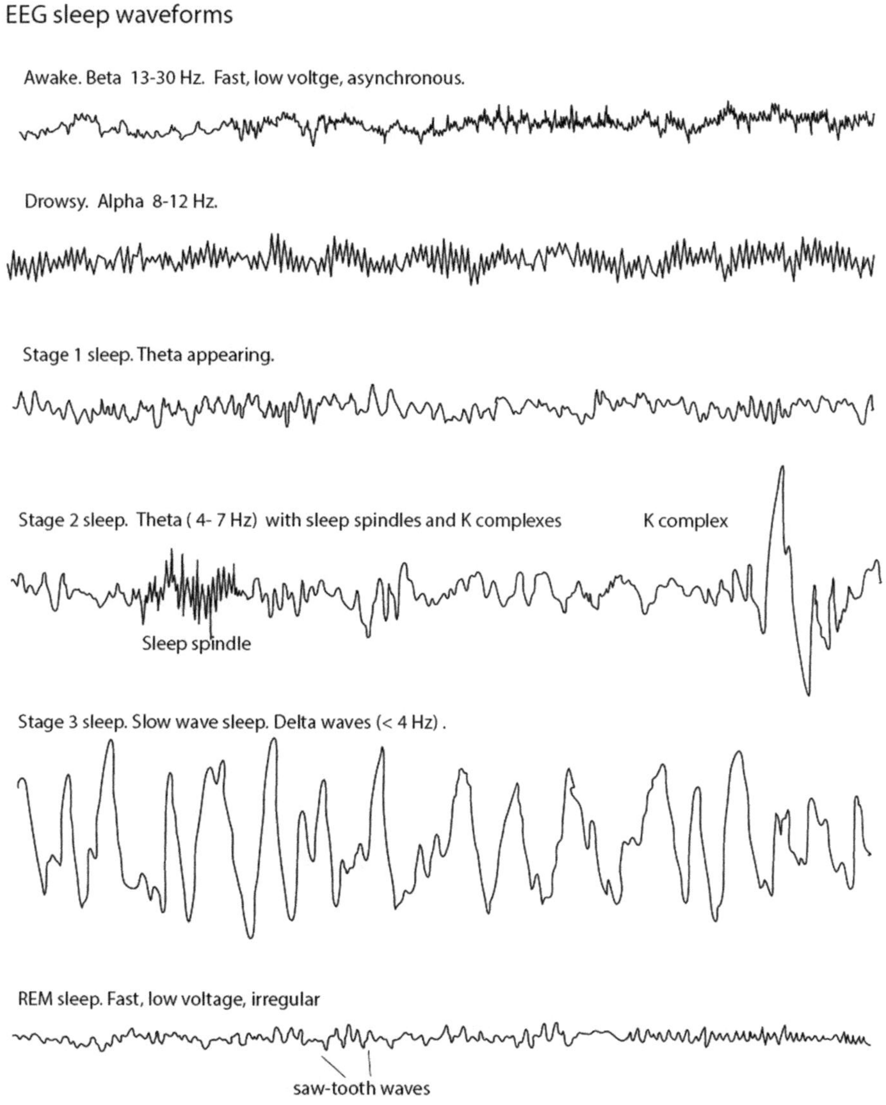

Fig. 27.2 EEG waveforms and their associations with stages of sleep

EEG Under Anaesthesia and Sedation

General Pattern with Propofol and Inhalational Agents

Overall, propofol and the inhalational anaesthetic agents produce suppression of high-frequency activity and activation of low-frequency oscillations. This leads to the waveforms becoming more synchronous. Due to the differential sensitivity of excitatory and inhibitory neuronal circuits to the effects of these drugs, there may be paradoxical excitation with beta wave activity during the early phases of a slow or titrated induction.

As the dose or exposure to the agent increases, there is anteriorisation of cortical activity with frontal alpha waves, and finally at around 1.5 MAC for volatile anaesthetics or an effect site (brain concentration) of propofol of 5–6 μg/mL, burst suppression occurs which is characterised by periods of high-voltage electrical activity ('bursts') alternating with an isoelectric EEG. At approximately 2.0 MAC or a propofol effect site of more than 10 μg/mL, an isoelectric EEG may be induced.

The effects of inhalational and intravenous anaesthetic agents are summarised in Table 27.2. Of note, there are considerable similarities between propofol and the inhalational agents, whereas other drugs, e.g. ketamine or opioid analgesics, produce differing and divergent effects on the EEG. This can have implications when using the processed EEG as a depth of anaesthesia monitor.

Table 27.2 Effects of anaesthetic medications on the EEG

Drug	Anaesthetic level	EEG characteristics
Propofol	Induction bolus	Rapid change from beta to slow delta oscillation
		Burst suppression may occur
	Very slow bolus	Paradoxical excitation and beta activity with very slow bolus
	Maintenance infusion	Slow delta
		Anterior alpha activity ('anteriorisation' of alpha activity)
		Burst suppression and isoelectric EEG at high doses
	Sedation	Anterior alpha plus slow wave (delta)
Inhalational anaesthetics	Guedel stage 1: Sedation	Alpha
	Guedel stage 2: Paradoxical excitation	Beta activity
	Sub-MAC anaesthesia	Alpha, theta and delta with equal power
	Increasing concentration	Delta, burst suppression and eventually isoelectric
Ketamine	Low doses	Increased beta and gamma oscillations
	Hypnotic doses	Increased beta and gamma oscillations
		Theta and slow-wave activity associated with loss of consciousness
		No increase in frontal alpha activity
Dexmedetomidine	Deep sedation	Slow wave with alpha-like anterior spindles. Likened to normal sleep pattern
Nitrous oxide	Anaesthetic adjunct	Prominent beta and gamma oscillation
		No slow-wave or alpha oscillation
		May decrease the power of ether anaesthetics' slow waves
Opioids		Variable but overall, a dose-dependent increase in slow-wave activity

Table 27.3 Methods of assessing the depth of anaesthesia

Methods of assessing depth of anaesthesia		
Category	Example	Notes
Clinical	Clinical acumen	Including knowledge of Guedel stages
	PRST score	Blood pressure, heart rate, sweating, tears
Isolated forearm technique		
EEG processing	BIS	Bispectral index
	Entropy	
	Narcotrend	
	Patient state index	e.g. Masimo SedLine
Auditory evoked responses	Response to active stimulation	

Depth of Anaesthesia Monitors

A depth of anaesthesia monitor is an adjunct which incorporates either clinical signs or monitored parameters to produce an estimate of a patient's cortical activity or level of consciousness in response to a known amount of anaesthetic agent; see Table 27.3.

These monitors can range in complexity from the use of clinical acumen or the monitoring of vital signs to produce a 'depth of anaesthesia score' to monitors which use either the EEG or the auditory evoked potentials in both processed and unprocessed forms to produce an estimate of the depth of anaesthesia.

Special mention is made of the isolated forearm technique, which is used to measure anaesthetic depth in patients receiving neuromuscular blocking agents. Here, an arterial tourniquet is applied to the upper limb to restrict the passage of neuromuscular blocking agents to the forearm. Should the depth of anaesthesia be insufficient, the patient is able to move their arm, indicating to the anaesthetist that the patient may be conscious leading to an increase in the depth of anaesthesia. This is discussed in greater detail later in this chapter.

Clinical acumen and the isolated forearm technique, although simple, do have pitfalls. Especially at sub-MAC concentrations of volatile anaesthetics or in patients receiving intravenous anaesthesia with propofol, movement can occur as the suppression of spinal cord reflex arcs occurs at higher concentrations of anaesthetic agent. Patient movement as such is a less than adequate marker of anaesthetic depth.

Awareness

Accidental anaesthetic awareness describes a state where a patient can form either abstract or concrete memories during anaesthesia. Depending on the clinical circumstance, this may be distressing and in the worst case can be associated with a paralysed patient who has complete recall without analgesia for the surgical procedure. Awareness can lead to psychological and emotional sequelae including

Table 27.4 Incidence of anaesthetic awareness across multiple studies

Incidence of awareness	
• United Kingdom National Audit Project—NAP5	
– Certain and probable awareness	1:25,000
– Certain, probable and possible	1:19,600
– With neuromuscular blockade (NMB)	1:8200
– Without NMB	1:135,900
– Caesarean section	1: 670
• Incidence awareness from other studies	
– 2004 B-aware study of high-risk patients	1:112
– 2014 NAP5 baseline survey	1:15,000
– 2014 Ireland survey	1:23,000

Table 27.5 Risk factors for anaesthetic awareness

Risk factors for awareness from NAP5	
Timing	Induction of anaesthesia
	Towards the end of anaesthesia
Demographics	Female > male
	Younger adults, not children
Type of surgery	Obstetric, cardiac, thoracic, transplant procedures
Others	Use of NMB, particularly with total intravenous anaesthesia (TIVA)
	Out-of-hours emergencies
	Trainee anaesthetists
	Previous awareness
	Converting volatile to TIVA for transport post-op

significant post-traumatic stress, which may affect a patient's long-term functioning following the episode.

The incidence of awareness varies depending on the patient cohort and the group of procedures being studied. The largest study to date was the fifth National Audit (NAP5) from the United Kingdom, which reported its findings in 2014. This cohort studied approximately 2.8 million episodes of general anaesthesia over the course of a 12-month period to produce estimates based on a patient's exposure profile. Overall, the risk factors for accidental awareness can be grouped together as timing of the episode during the procedure, patient demographics, procedural class and others. This is further summarised in Tables 27.4 and 27.5.

Bispectral Index (BIS)

The BIS monitor processes the forehead EEG recordings and compares these to an inbuilt proprietary algorithm to deliver an index of the hypnotic state of the brain scaled between 0—an isoelectric EEG—and 100—the awake state. This algorithm was developed from over 5000 h of raw EEG recordings sourced from 1500 patients receiving commonly used anaesthetic agents. From this, the depth of anaesthesia was graded using a simple clinical score.

Table 27.6 Summary of EEG parameters analysed by the BIS monitor

Summary of EEG parameters analysed by the BIS monitor	
Burst suppression ratio	The fraction of the epoch that is suppressed
QUAZI algorithm	Method to detect burst suppression with baseline wander
Power spectrum analysis	Determines the amount of each frequency in each epoch
Bispectral analysis	The degree of synchronisation between different frequencies
Beta ratio	Ratio of two high-frequency bands

The raw EEG was analysed using both the time and frequency domain methods, which use considerable statistical processing to determine which variables predict differing levels of hypnosis. These variables are then weighted and scored for their predictive value of certain events of anaesthesia, e.g. asleep and unaware versus the awake state. The sum of the weighted variables at any one time produces the dimensionless BIS number from 100 to 0.

When the sensor is applied to a patient, the EEG is processed in 2-s intervals called epochs to determine which patterns are dominant at the current moment in time. As noted above, a value of 100 is a fully awake patient, while 0 indicates an isoelectric EEG. Values between 40 and 60 are regarded as suitable for surgical anaesthesia with minimal risk of anaesthetic awareness. The EEG parameters analysed by the monitor are summarised in Table 27.6.

Time Domain Analyses

Time domain analysis looks at changes in the EEG voltage over time. This is assessed through the burst suppression ratio (BSR) and the QUAZI suppression index ('QUAZI').

Burst suppression (BS) is an alternating pattern of high-voltage activity with interspersed segments of very low or absent voltage. BS occurs in severe head injury and thiopentone coma and with deep anaesthesia. The BSR is the fraction of each epoch where the EEG displays burst suppression. The QUAZI suppression index is similar to the BSR but is tuned to detect burst suppression in cases with a wandering EEG baseline. In some instances, there may be burst suppression superimposed on slow waves, which can 'fool' the usual methods of assessment.

Frequency Domain Analyses

Frequency domain analysis is concerned with the underlying frequencies present in each epoch. The amount of each frequency is quantified by its power, which is the square of the oscillation amplitude. The oscillation amplitude is energy carried by the wave and is proportional to its amplitude squared. Power can be expressed in either μV^2 or decibels. When the amplitude is increased by a factor of two, the power as measured in decibels increases by around 6.02, while doubling the power is an increase of 3.01 decibels.

Power Spectral Analysis

Power spectral analysis determines 'how much' of each frequency is present in each epoch. As noted, with progressive hypnosis, there is the suppression of the high-frequency EEG activity with increasing amounts of low-frequency oscillation. Power analysis occurs through digitisation of the EEG, which is then divided into 2-s epochs. Each epoch then undergoes a fast Fourier transformation (FFT) to determine the dominant frequencies which are present. To convert the amplitude of the waves to a power value, the amplitudes are then squared; this also serves to eradicate negative values. Between algorithms, there may be differences in epoch length and the processing algorithms applied; see Fig. 27.3. Power spectral analysis can be displayed in two main ways.

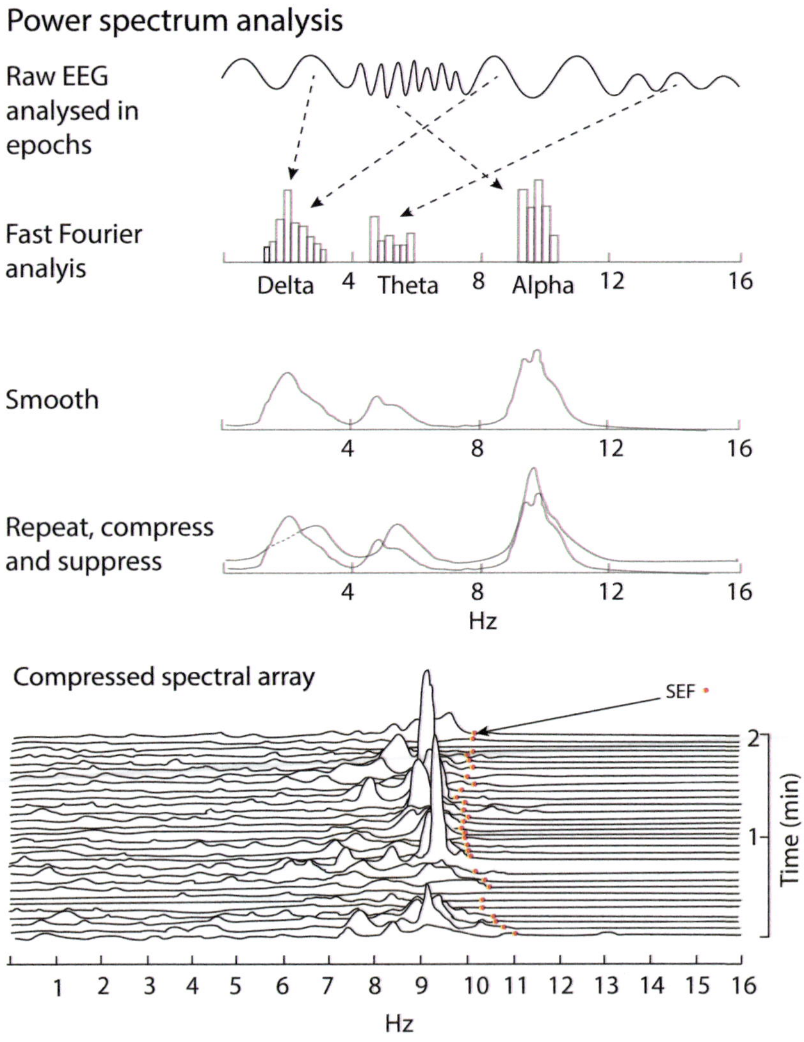

Fig. 27.3 Power spectrum and compressed spectral array analysis of the EEG

Compressed Spectral Array

Some monitors will display not only the dimensionless 'BIS' value but also the frequencies and their power in a compressed spectral array. The frequencies are plotted as a histogram with frequency on the *x*-axis and power on the *y*-axis. This histogram is then smoothed with each subsequent epoch being layered over the previous period to produce a 3D display of frequency, power and time. This layering process is referred to as compressing and supressing.

The spectral edge frequency (SEF) is the frequency below which 95% of all the power lies. This may be marked on the trace by a box, which allows for easy tracking of the depth of anaesthesia. As anaesthesia deepens, the box will move left, towards the lower frequencies.

Density Spectral Array (DSA)

In some monitors such as the Masimo SedLine, a density spectral array (DSA) is used. Here, the *x*-axis reflects time, while the *y*-axis is a range of dots according to the frequencies present in each epoch. The dots are then colour coded according to their power. Blue reflects minimal power, while red is maximal power. As the depth of anaesthesia increases, a wave of red dots passes down through the frequency bands to reflect the increasing dominance of low-frequency, high-amplitude waves with this state.

Bispectral Analysis

Not only do the EEG oscillations become slower with increasing depth of anaesthesia, but they also become more synchronous. This may occur due to a reduction in the number of independent synapses firing with increasing hypnosis. The bispectral analysis compares both the phase and the amplitude alignment of the low-frequency oscillations.

Beta-Ratio

The beta-ratio is the ratio of two frequency bands, one of which is in the beta wave range. This ratio has been shown to give predictive information on light levels of hypnosis and the changes between consciousness and unconsciousness.

Further Parameters

In addition to the parameters already discussed in this chapter, additional information is available from the BIS monitor; this is summarised in Table 27.7.

Table 27.7 Additional information derived from the EEG through the BIS monitor

Additional parameters displayed on the BIS monitor	
Suppression ratio (SR)	Proportion of time over previous 63 secs that the EEG was suppressed
Spectral edge frequency (SEF 95)	Frequency below which 95% of all the power lies
Total power (TP)	The total power of all the component waves
Signal quality index (SQI)	Proportion of all the data that is used in the BIS calculation
Electromyogram (EMG)	Power of the EMG. Range is 30–80 dB. Usual range in awake, unparalysed patient is 40–50 dB. As EMG power increases, the usefulness of BIS declines due to increasing interference

Reliability of BIS

The most recent Cochrane Collaboration systematic review found that when compared with clinical monitoring alone, namely the monitoring of vital signs, BIS reduced awareness and improved early recovery. When compared with protocols which make use of the end-tidal volatile anaesthetic concentration, there was no reduction in awareness. These authors also concluded that beyond the aware versus unaware divide, BIS is an imprecise way to guide anaesthetic depth. Although paediatric sensors have been produced for the BIS monitor, this technique is yet to be prospectively validated for use in children to prevent anaesthetic awareness and titrate the depth of anaesthesia.

Although increasing blood concentrations of both propofol and inhalational anaesthetic agents produce similar depressant effects on the BIS score, this is not the case with all anaesthetic agents:

- Nitrous oxide is associated with decreased delta activity and increased beta and gamma activity. As such, the BIS value is elevated when compared with what is observed for standard anaesthetic agents as measured in minimum alveolar concentration.
- Ketamine, through its unique mechanism of action, produces an active EEG pattern with fast beta oscillations. In patients exposed to significant amounts of ketamine, the BIS is elevated when compared with patients exposed to either propofol or inhalational anaesthetic agent at the same hypnotic level. In the BALANCED study of depth of anaesthesia as measured by BIS monitoring and patient outcomes, the use of ketamine at >25 mg/h was listed as an exclusion criterion.
- Dexmedetomidine produces lower BIS values than propofol for equivalent hypnotic levels.

There is also considerable inter-individual variability between the BIS values observed at seemingly comparable hypnotic levels with a poor correlation between BIS and end-tidal volatile anaesthetic concentrations. The BIS value does not predict an individual's threshold for loss of consciousness or eye opening, and there is no clear-cut transition between the awake and asleep states. Given that the movement in response to a surgical stimulus is a complex interaction between cortical suppression and the activity of spinal cord reflexes, EEG monitors which observe the cerebral cortex are not able to predict the response, e.g. movement to a noxious stimulus. While volatile anaesthetics provide equivalent suppression of both the cerebral cortex and spinal cord reflexes with increasing depth of anaesthesia, propofol has less of a suppressive effect on the spinal cord reflexes meaning that patients may 'move' despite adequate hypnotic effect and lack of awareness. As such, these monitors do not differentiate between differing levels of rousability.

When the electrodes are poorly applied to the patient's forehead or there is perspiration, dirt or makeup, the values produced may be spuriously elevated. Although the signal is filtered prior to analysis to remove ECG, EMG, eye blinking and diathermy effect, these problems are not completely eradicated.

Electromyogram (EMG)

The EMG may produce a high-frequency artefact which can falsely elevate the BIS number. Due to peculiarities of the BIS algorithm, the use of neuromuscular blocking drugs may spuriously reduce the BIS value. Rather than an effect on the cerebral cortex, it is thought that this observation occurs as patients with absent EMG power were by and large deeply anaesthetised in the cohort of patients, which led to the derivation of the algorithm.

Entropy Monitor

The entropy monitor relates the entropy or degree of chaos in the EEG to the behavioural responses of the patient. In the awake state, the EEG appears to be random and without repetitive waveforms. With deepening of anaesthesia, the EEG becomes more synchronous and less chaotic.

The entropy monitor assesses the degree of complexity, irregularity and unpredictability of the EEG. As an example, using a numerical sequence, if the values simply alternate between 1 and 0, the 'system' has zero entropy because it is regular and entirely predictable. A 'system' where the numerical values are produced by a random number generator is unpredictable and has very high entropy. A stylised entropy trace for a case is shown in Fig. 27.4.

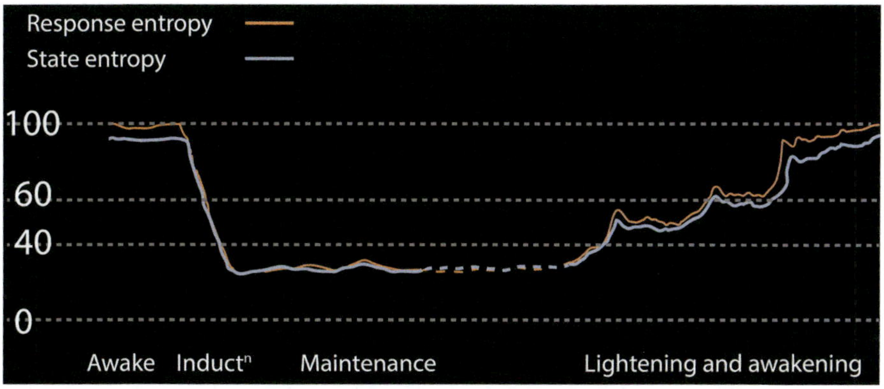

Fig. 27.4 Entropy monitor during various phases of anaesthesia

Basic Principle

The basic premise is the recording of the EEG from three forehead sensors, which then undergoes frequency domain (Fourier transformation) and time domain analysis as well as complex statistical processing. In addition to EEG waveform, the frontalis EMG signal is also processed. The sudden onset of higher frequency and amplitude EMG waveforms can indicate patient arousal to a painful response. As the sampling time for the EMG is shorter than the EEG, the EMG may provide an early warning of arousal.

The entropy monitor follows two distinct entropy states:

- State entropy (SE)—this follows the entropy of the EEG range of frequencies, namely 0.8–32 Hz, and reflects the cortical state of the patient. The sampling window is between 15 and 60 s, and the parameter can take values between 0 and 91 with the scale oriented in the same direction as BIS.
- Response entropy (RE)—this follows the entropy over the 0.8–47 Hz range of frequencies. The higher end of this range includes the EMG-dominant frequencies, which makes this measure more sensitive to patient arousal. The sampling time for the RE is between 2 and 15 s; as such, in a patient who is not deeply paralysed, a peak in the RE value may indicate pain or arousal through surgical stimulation. The RE scale is between 0 and 100 with the scale again oriented in the same direction as BIS.

The interpretation of the SE and RE values is like the BIS monitor with surgical anaesthesia without a high risk of awareness occurring between 40 and 60. At the induction of anaesthesia, both the SE and RE fall rapidly. When neuromuscular blockers have been administered, as there is no EMG signal, the SE and RE will track together and record similar values, and any discrepancy may reflect the differences in sampling rates. On lightening or reversal of neuromuscular blockade, if there is patient arousal, the RE value will spike first, followed by an increase in the SE.

When compared with BIS, the entropy monitor has not been as comprehensively evaluated for the prevention of awareness. There is however evidence that its use is associated with shorter recovery times. As with the BIS monitor, the same provisos exist when a patient is exposed to anaesthetic agents beyond propofol or the inhalational drugs.

Other Depth of Anaesthesia Monitors

There are other monitors which monitor the depth of anaesthesia in addition to BIS and entropy. These are less frequently used and by and large have a lower market penetration when compared with the former.

Patient State Index

This makes use of a proprietary algorithm based on EEG power, frequency and phase information. One such example is the Masimo SedLine monitor. The scale of anaesthetic depth is oriented in the same direction as both BIS and entropy. In addition to the dimensionless depth of anaesthesia variable, the raw EEG is displayed in addition to the density spectral array (DSA, see above).

Narcotrend

The Narcotrend monitor analyses raw cortical EEG using frequency-based and entropic methods. In earlier versions of the monitor, the conscious state was classified on the Loomis scale from stage A = awake to stage F = very deep hypnosis. This has since been refined to include an index scale from 100 to 0. As with both BIS and entropy, the Narcotrend monitor has been associated with a reduction in recovery times. A NICE review from the United Kingdom did not find firm evidence however that the monitor reduces the rate of anaesthetic awareness.

Isolated Forearm Technique (IFT)

The isolated forearm technique has been regarded as the gold standard for preventing conscious awareness under anaesthesia. For practical reasons, this technique is mainly used for research purposes. An upper arm tourniquet is inflated above the maximal anticipated systolic blood pressure prior to the administration of neuromuscular blockade and is kept inflated for around 20 min, or at least long enough to allow the blood level of neuromuscular blocking drugs to fall below paralytic levels. Should the patient move their arm in response to a command during anaesthesia, this may be an indication that the patient is conscious.

Clinical Signs

The use of clinical signs such as heart rate, blood pressure, sweating, lacrimation and pupillary dilation may help to determine the patient's depth of anaesthesia in conjunction with end-tidal anaesthetic gas or estimated blood propofol concentrations. The PRST score makes use of blood pressure, heart rate, sweating and tearing. As noted above, this scale lacks the precision to reliably determine the depth of anaesthesia.

Auditory Evoked Potentials (AEPs)

Auditory evoked potential monitors the response of the brainstem and, to a lesser degree, the cortex to auditory stimuli. These monitors have been superseded by the processed EEG monitors, which have been described above.

A series of clicks are played into one ear, and the brainstem auditory evoked potentials are recorded from forehead and inion electrodes. As the depth of anaesthesia increases, the potentials are delayed and blunted. Surgical stimulation with inadequate depth of anaesthesia could increase the amplitude of auditory potentials.

Fourier Analysis

Fourier Transformation

Mathematically, any complex sine wave can be resolved into its slowest component = fundamental frequency and a series of whole-number multiples or harmonics; see Figs. 27.5 and 27.6. When put together, the complex wave can then be recreated. This technique is used to break down the complex waves of the EEG to the contributing fundamental and harmonic frequencies to allow for a power analysis to take place.

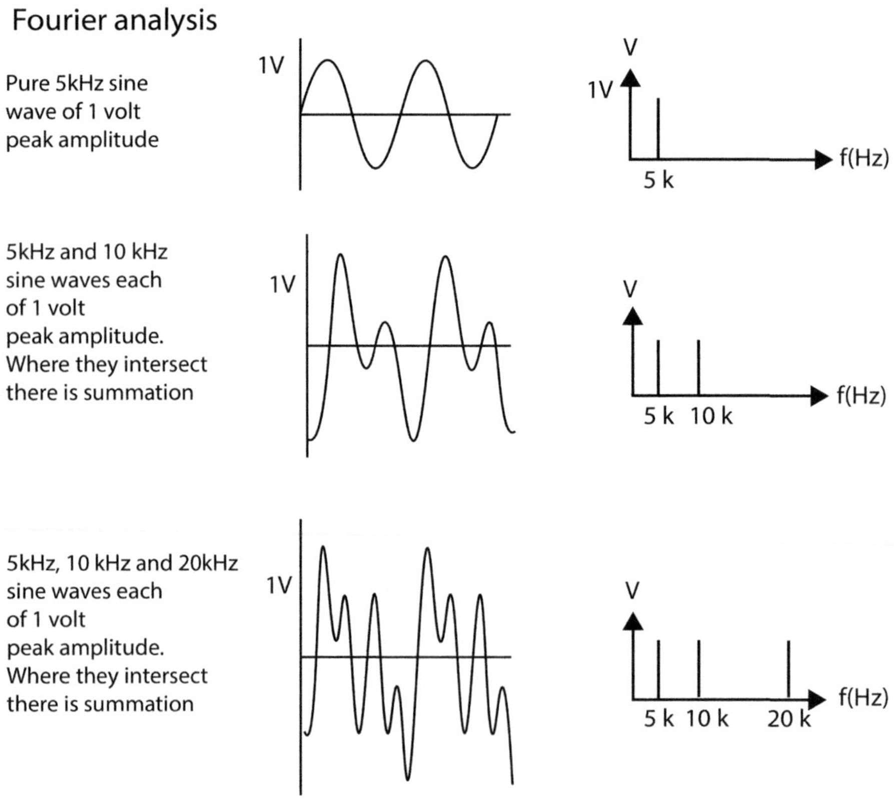

Fig. 27.5 Basic principles of Fourier analysis

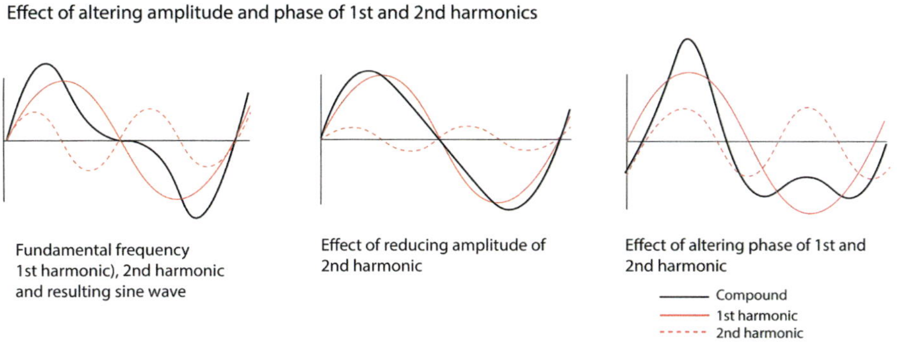

Fig. 27.6 Effects of altering the wave amplitude of harmonics on the composite waveform

Further Reading

Chattopadhyay U, Mallik S, Ghosh S, Bhattacharya S, Bisai S, Biswas H. Comparison between propofol and dexmedetomidine on depth of anesthesia: a prospective randomized trial. J Anaesthesiol Clin Pharmacol. 2014;30(4):550–4.

Jonker WR, Hanumanthiah D, O'Sullivan EP, et al. A national survey (NAP5-Ireland baseline) to estimate an annual incidence of accidental awareness during general anaesthesia in Ireland. Anaesthesia. 2014;69(9):969–76.

Kasuya Y, Govinda R, Rauch S, Mascha EJ, Sessler DI, Turan A. The correlation between bispectral index and observational sedation scale in volunteers sedated with dexmedetomidine and propofol. Anesth Analg. 2009;109(6):1811–5.

Kreuzer M. EEG based monitoring of general anesthesia: taking the next steps. Front Comput Neurosci. 2017;11:56.

Lewis SR, Pritchard MW, Fawcett LJ, Punjasawadwong Y. Bispectral index for improving intraoperative awareness and early postoperative recovery in adults. Cochrane Database Syst Rev. 2019;9:CD003843.

Linassi F, Zanatta P, Tellaroli P, Ori C, Carron M. Isolated forearm technique: a meta-analysis of connected consciousness during different general anaesthesia regimens. Br J Anaesth. 2018;121(1):198–209.

Malver LP, Brokjaer A, Staahl C, Graversen C, Andresen T, Drewes AM. Electroencephalography and analgesics. Br J Clin Pharmacol. 2014;77(1):72–95.

Myles PS, Leslie K, McNeil J, Forbes A, Chan MT. Bispectral index monitoring to prevent awareness during anaesthesia: the B-aware randomised controlled trial. Lancet. 2004;363(9423):1757–63.

Pandit JJ, Andrade J, Bogod DG, et al. The fifth National Audit Project (NAP5) on accidental awareness during general anaesthesia: summary of main findings and risk factors. Anaesthesia. 2014;69(10):1089–101.

Purdon PL, Sampson A, Pavone KJ, Brown EN. Clinical electroencephalography for anesthesiologists: part I: background and basic signatures. Anesthesiology. 2015;123(4):937–60.

Rampil IJ. A primer for EEG signal processing in anesthesia. Anesthesiology. 1998;89(4):980–1002.

Russell IF. Fourteen fallacies about the isolated forearm technique, and its place in modern anaesthesia. Anaesthesia. 2013;68(7):677–81.

Schuller PJ, Newell S, Strickland PA, Barry JJ. Response of bispectral index to neuromuscular block in awake volunteers. Br J Anaesth. 2015;115(Suppl 1):i95–i103.

Shepherd J, Jones J, Frampton G. Depth of anaesthesia monitors—Bispectral index (BIS, E-Entropy and Narcotrend-Compact M'. United Kingdom: National Institute for Health and Care Excellence (NICE), 21 November 2012.

Sleigh J, Pullon RM, Vlisides PE, Warnaby CE. Electroencephalographic slow wave dynamics and loss of behavioural responsiveness induced by ketamine in human volunteers. Br J Anaesth. 2019;123(5):592–600.

Viertio-Oja H, Maja V, Sarkela M, et al. Description of the entropy algorithm as applied in the Datex-Ohmeda S/5 entropy module. Acta Anaesthesiol Scand. 2004;48(2):154–61.

Electromagnetic Principles

28

Alan McLintic and Matthew Taylor

Brief Definitions and Explanations

Electricity

Is a general term for a variety of phenomena resulting from the presence and flow of charged particles (electrons or ions). This includes many well-known physical phenomena such as lightning, electromagnetic fields and electric currents.

Electromagnetic Force

Electromagnetism is one of the four fundamental forces and acts between electrically charged subatomic particles. We say that static charge is surrounded by an electric field but, when current flows in a wire, we say instead that a magnetic field is produced. While the terms are different, they are the same phenomenon. A moving charge creates a magnetic field, and likewise, a moving or time-varying magnetic field can produce an electrical field. Differences in the force fields are simply in the shape, motion and direction of force.

Static Electricity

It is an imbalance of electric charges within or on the surface of a material. A static charge occurs when two surfaces contact and then separate, assuming that at least one of the surfaces is insulated. This results in one surface with a relative surfeit of

A. McLintic · M. Taylor (✉)
Department of Anaesthesia and Pain Medicine, Counties Manukau Health,
Auckland, New Zealand
e-mail: Matthew.Taylor@middlemore.com

C. Birch et al. (eds.), *Physics and Measurement for Anesthesia*,
https://doi.org/10.1007/978-3-031-65060-4_28

electrons and the other a deficit. Certain combinations of materials work better than others in creating a static charge. The triboelectric series lists materials according to how likely they release or accept electrons.

Electric Field

Any object with charge has an electric field around it, the region where it can attract or repel other charges. If a charged object is placed in the field, it will experience a force:

- Opposite charges attract each other.
- Like charges repel each other.

Electric Charge

Charge is the property of matter that causes it to experience a force when it is placed in an electric field. This is a fundamental property of electrons and protons. By convention, an electron is negatively charged, and a proton is positively charged. Charge is quantified in multiples of the elementary unit of charge which is the charge of an electron.

- **The SI unit of charge is the coulomb**. 1 Coulomb is defined as the amount of charge that passes in 1 s when the current is 1 ampere, which corresponds to the charge of 6.24×10^{18} electrons.

Electric Potential

It is an indication of the potential energy of a charge in an electric field. A negative charge in a negatively charged electric field has potential energy to be repelled. This is what moves charge around a circuit.

- **SI unit of electric potential is the volt**. 1 Volt is 1 joule/coulomb.

Electric Current

Current is the rate of flow of charge.

- **SI unit of current is the ampere**. 1 Ampere flows when one coulomb of charge passes a point every second.

The old SI definition of the ampere was 'the current flowing in two parallel wires, 1 metre apart, that would produce a force of 2×10^{-7} newtons between the wires.'

The new SI definition is 'the flow of $1/1.602176634 \times 10^{-19}$ times the elementary charge *e* per second'.

DC Current

Flow of current is in one direction only. The positive pole is, by historical convention, the one from which positive charge carriers would flow to the negative pole. In most cases, however, the positive charges are stationary, and it is the negatively charged electrons that move. Therefore, in most cases, current flows from the negative terminal to the positive terminal.

AC Current

Alternating current (AC) is continuously reversing direction with a sinusoidal waveform. AC current is driven by an electromotive force that also has a sinusoidal wave oscillation.

Voltage

The volt is the unit of electric potential, electromotive force (EMF) and potential difference (PD).

- The EMF is the net difference in electric potential between two terminals of the battery and is the energy available per coulomb to drive charge around a circuit.
- The PD is the energy used or lost per coulomb driving charge through a resistor in a circuit. The volt is therefore the amount of energy available, lost or used per coulomb.
- **The SI unit of electric potential energy is the volt.** 1 Volt is 1 joule per coulomb.

Power

Electrical power is the rate of transfer of energy. The power of an appliance is therefore the product of the potential difference across it and the current passing through. If 10 coulombs are passing through per second (10 amps) and 1 joule of energy is used in the appliance per coulomb, the appliance has a power of 10 watts.

- Power (P) = Current (I) × Potential difference (V).
- As ($V = I.R$), we can also express power as $P = I^2.R$.
- **SI unit of power: Watt. 1 Watt is equivalent to 1 joule per second.**

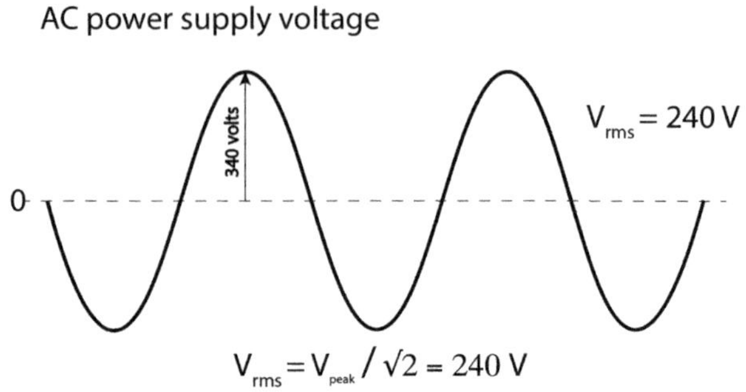

Fig. 28.1 Sinusoidal profile of AC current and how peak voltage relates to RMS voltage

Power Transmission

Domestic power in New Zealand is alternating current at 50 Hz and 230 V_{rms}. Note that this is 230 V_{rms}, not 230 V_{peak}. The average voltage of an AC supply is calculated by taking the root mean square (rms) of the voltage. For a sine wave, this is equivalent to dividing the peak voltage or peak current by $\sqrt{2}$. Thus, a 230 V_{rms} household power supply has a peak voltage of 325 V (Fig. 28.1).

Why Is Electrical Power Transmitted in AC Form?

Domestic power is supplied as AC for a few reasons. Due to the oscillatory nature of AC, production by rotary generators is simplified. Similarly, it also simplifies stepping voltage up and down using transformers (see later). This means that the power can be transmitted at very high voltage, which reduces the transmission current ($P = V.I$). This, in turn, reduces energy loss from resistive heating, which is proportional to the current or, more correctly, the square of the current ($P_{loss} = I^2.R$). Raising the voltage by a factor of 10 reduces the current by a factor of 10 and power loss by a factor of 100. Conversely, over very long distances and underwater, the benefit balance can tip back in favour of high-voltage DC transmission.

Different parts of the system operate at different voltages, optimising trade-offs for the efficiency of distribution and power transfer. Generation is typically around 11 kV AC (2.3–30 kV) utilising generators powered by energy sources transduced to rotary motion. Solar power is generated as DC and converted to AC for distribution. To this end, these voltages are stepped up through a transformer.

For power transmission, three broad voltage categories exist:

- High voltage for national distribution.
- Medium voltage for local distribution.
- Low voltage for domestic supply.

Worldwide, low-voltage domestic supply is most commonly at 110 or 220–240 V. Medium voltage is often quoted at around 11 kV, but considerable range exists depending on the network. The UK system distributes at 6.6–132 kV depending on distances and demands on each section of the local network. High-voltage transmission is generalised to around 220 kV but, again, varies. NZ mostly distributes at 110 or 220 kV AC although some smaller links are as low as 50 kV AC. The "Cook Strait cable" is an HVDC feed at 350 V. UK distributes at 275–400 kV AC.

Note: Resistive losses are also proportional to frequency, so domestic power is transmitted at 50 Hz which is about as low as you can go without perceptible flicker of lighting and other problems.

Resistance

When a potential difference is applied across an electrical component, a current will flow. The magnitude of the current depends on the resistance of the component according to Ohms law:

$$\text{Current}(I) = \text{Voltage}(V) / \text{Resistance}(R).$$

The resistance of a component is determined by the inherent resistivity of the material, its length inversely to the cross-sectional area as well as environmental factors such as humidity, temperature and light.

- **SI unit of resistance is the ohm (Ω).** A component with resistance of 1 ohm and with a potential difference of 1 volt across it has a current flowing through it of 1 amp.

Resistance and Temperature

Metal Conductors

At a constant temperature, the current is proportional to the voltage, so the resistance is constant. Charge is free to move in the form of electrons in a lattice of positive ions. As the metal heats up, the vibration of ions increases causing electrons to collide with them and lose energy. Resistance therefore increases linearly with temperature (Fig. 28.2).

Semiconductors

Semiconductors have far fewer charge carriers than conductors, but, when heated, more charge carriers are released and resistance falls. Thermistors are semiconductors that are used in measuring temperature. There are different types of thermistors, but the type you need to know for the exam is the negative temperature coefficient thermistor (NTC thermistor). The resistance of a typical NTC falls exponentially as temperature increases (Fig. 28.2).

Fig. 28.2 Variation of resistance with temperature

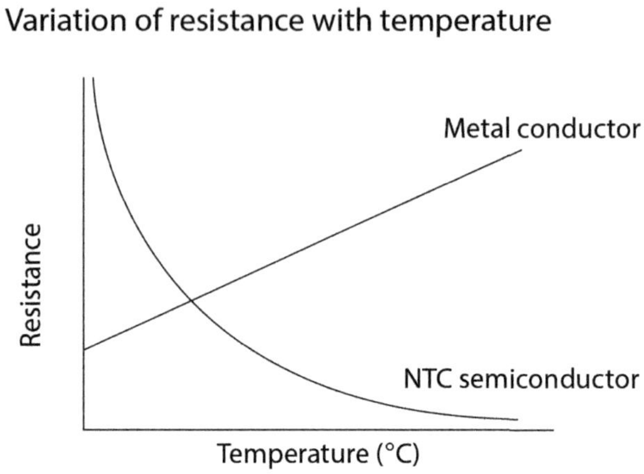

Insulators

Insulators have negligible numbers of charge carriers.

Resistance, Reactance and Impedance

Impedance is a collective concept for the dual concepts opposing charge flow through a circuit, combining the concepts of resistance and reactance. These refer to differing qualities opposing charge flow through a circuit. Resistance refers to the inherent qualities of the component that resist current flow, whereas reactance refers to the properties opposing changes in current.

Resistance

At constant temperature and stable environmental factors, the resistance of many materials is constant and voltage and current have linear relationship with each other ($R = V/I$). These are called ohmic resistors. Their opposition to current flow is simply a factor of the material structure and is termed *resistance*. Resistance does not change with frequency in AC systems.

Reactance

For certain electric components, the opposition to current flow has an additional dimension by varying with the frequency of AC current. This component is called *reactance*.

- Inductor:
  - Reactance increases as frequency increases because of the effect of back EMF (see below), which resists the flow being generated.
- Capacitor:
  - Reactance decreases with increasing frequency because the capacitor is making less and less impact on current flow in the circuit (see later).

Impedance (*Z*)

Impedance is the measure of the total opposition to flow. For an ohmic resistor, impedance = resistance. For capacitors and inductors, the impedance = reactance + resistance.

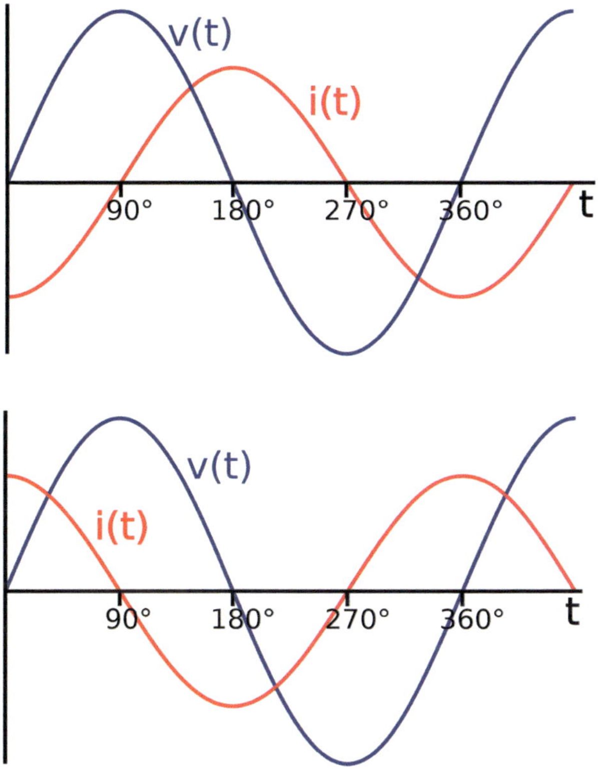

Fig. 28.3 Phase relationship between current and voltage when comparing capacitive (top) and inductance (bottom) systems

Inductors and capacitors are considered separately because their reactance results in current changes that are time dependent but opposite to each other as a function of their properties. Impedance therefore has a phase difference to the AC voltage placed across the system, depending on the various components within the circuit. The value of impedance correspondingly is not a simple additive function and must be considered as a time-dependent variable that changes current in a variable phase to the AC voltage (Fig. 28.3).

Wheatstone Bridge

The output of many sensors is based on changing electric resistance, and this is invariably measured by the highly sensitive Wheatstone bridge. This is a fundamental way of transducing physico-chemical changes in sensors (physiological change generating a resistance change) into an electrical signal that may be manipulated by the monitoring device. Some examples of sensors employing Wheatstone bridges are:

- Hot-wire anemometer flow meters.
- Pressure transducers.

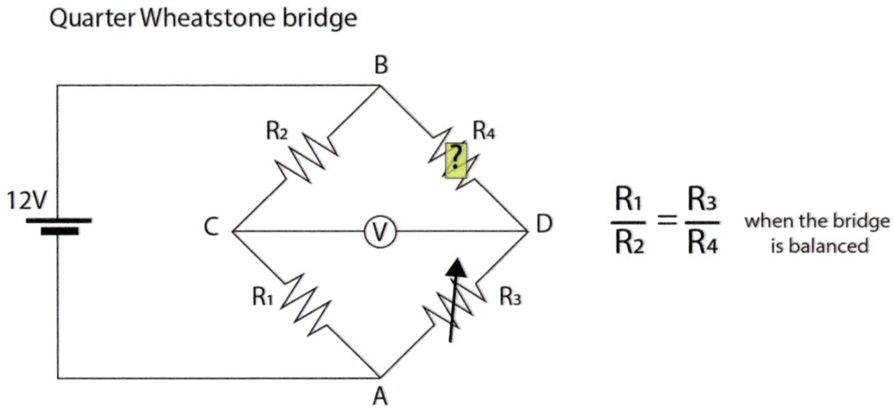

Fig. 28.4 Quarter wheatstone bridge

- Thermal conductivity gas sensors.
- Electronic humidity transducers.
- Thermistors and resistance thermometers.

Quarter Wheatstone Bridge

The simplest Wheatstone bridge is called a 'quarter bridge' because only one of its four resistors is used in the sensor. These are the principal components:

- Battery or other DC power supply (my illustration is 12 V, but will vary according to circumstance).
- Four resistors are arranged in two parallel limbs:
  - Limb 1: R_1 and R_2 are known resistances in series.
  - Limb 2: R_3 is a variable resistor, and R_4 is the unknown resistance, also in series.
- A voltmeter is wired between the two limbs at C–D.

The basic operation is that R_3 is varied until there is no voltage between C and D. As the variation is aiming for minimal/no voltage, it maximises the sensitivity of the system. The bridge is now said to be balanced. When this occurs, R_1, R_2 and R_3 are known, and R_4 can be deduced from $R_1/R_2 = R_3/R_4$ (Fig. 28.4).

Key Points About Drawing the Bridge

The bridge can be drawn in several ways with different labelling of the resistors, with different places for the variable and unknown resistors and in a diamond or rectangular shape. The crucial things are as follows:

- The resistors on the left of the equation must come from one limb, and the resistors on the right of the equation must come from the other limb.

- The numerator and denominator correspond to the same order of resistances. If R_1 comes before R_2 on one limb, R_3 must come before R_4 on the other.
- The voltmeter must be wired between the two limbs from points after the first resistor (i.e. between the resistors).
- Remember to draw a power supply. It will not work otherwise.

The positions of the variable resistor and the unknown resistor are not important. They could be any of the resistors R_1–R_4 in the above equation and drawn in any of the four positions. That is why they appear in different positions in different texts. If we know three of the resistances, we can derive the fourth no matter where its position is in the bridge.

I would suggest drawing the above diagram because it has familiarity with examiners.

How It Works

I believe that this is beyond exam requirement, but I am frequently asked about it.

Key question in understanding: *Why is there no voltage difference between C and D when R1/R2 = R3/R4?*

Work through the following steps:

1. The Wheatstone bridge consists of two parallel circuits, each limb having two resistors in series.
2. The voltage drop across each limb is the same as the battery, 12 V. In each limb, that voltage is divided up between the two resistors in proportion to their resistance. Thus, the sum of the PD across the resistors in each limb must be 12 V.
3. For points C and D to be at the same electrical potential, there must have been the same drop in voltage from A to C as from A to D.
4. Thus, when the bridge is balanced, V_{AC} must equal V_{AD} and, consequently, V_{CB} must equal V_{DB}. Therefore, V_{AC}/V_{CB} must equal V_{AD}/V_{DB} when the bridge is balanced.
5. What is the current going through each resistor? There are two points to remember:
   - The current entering at point A splits in inverse relationship to the total resistance in each limb, which is the sum of the resistors in series ($R_1 + R_2$ and $R_3 + R_4$).
   - At balance, there is no current between C and D, so the current entering points C and D is the same as that exiting C and D. In other words, $I_1 = I_2$ and $I_3 = I_4$.
6. We can now express the resistor voltages in terms of $V = IR$

$$\frac{V_{AC}}{V_{CB}} = \frac{V_{AD}}{V_{DB}} \text{ therefore } \frac{I_1 R_1}{I_2 R_2} = \frac{I_3 R_3}{I_4 R_4}$$

7. Therefore, as the current through the resistors in each pair is the same, ($I_1 = I_2$ and $I_3 = I_4$)

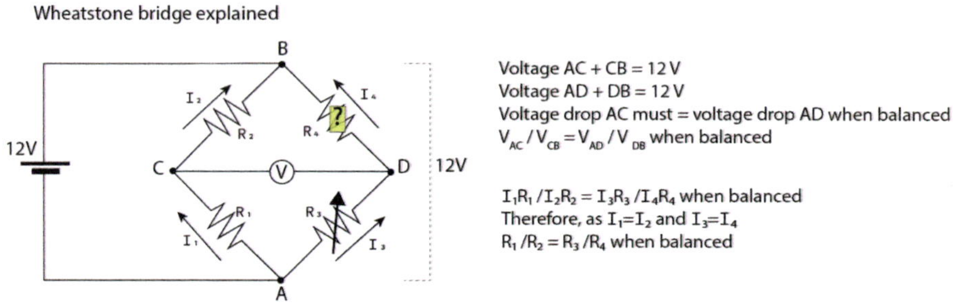

Fig. 28.5 Quarter Wheatstone bridge balancing of current

$$\frac{I_1R_1}{I_2R_2} = \frac{I_3R_3}{I_4R_4} \text{ is simplified to } \frac{R_1}{R_2} = \frac{R_3}{R_4} \text{ when the bridge is balanced}$$

Wheatstone Bridges in Practical Use

Quarter-Bridge Transducers

The unknown resistor (R_4) may be a length of wire or foil on a diaphragm pressure transducer. As the diaphragm bulges, the wire is stretched, its diameter decreases and its resistance increases. Instead of actively balancing the bridge using a variable resistor, the bridge starts balanced and is calibrated by zeroing. From then on, pressure distortions of the diaphragm unbalance the bridge, thereby creating a voltage which is proportional to the pressure change (Fig. 28.5).

Full-Bridge Transducers

Sensitivity can be increased by having all four resistors incorporated on the diaphragm. They are fixed to the diaphragm in such a way to cause maximum unbalancing and voltage production, for a given distortion. Thus, a pressure distortion in one direction might decrease resistance in R_1 and R_4 while increase resistance in R_2 and R_3. This would maximise the difference between R_1/R_2 and R_3/R_4, thereby increasing the voltage and sensitivity (Fig. 28.6).

Test Yourself

Test yourself and reinforce your knowledge with questions about these two bridges (Fig. 28.7). This is an alternative way of drawing them, but I recommend the diamond method because it is familiar. Also note that I have not labelled the variable and unknown resistor because they could be any of the four. Read the electrical 'rules' first.

Full Wheatstone bridge.

Resistor positioning can make R1/R2 vary in the opposite direction from R3/R4, thus maximising the imbalance and the voltage produced.

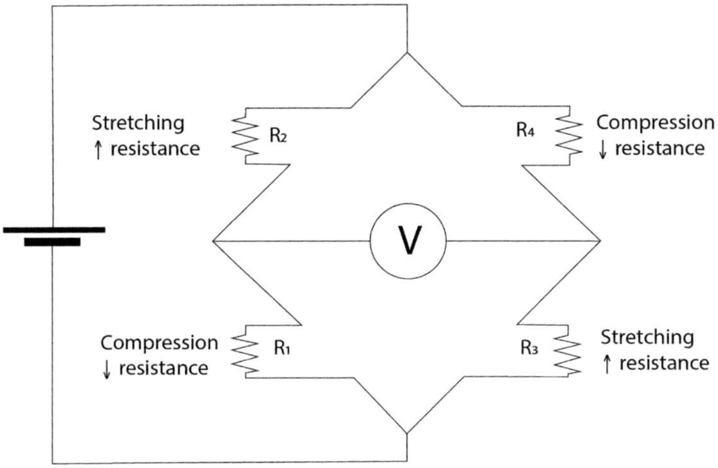

Fig. 28.6 Full Wheatstone bridge indicating increased sensitivity

Reinforce your knowledge

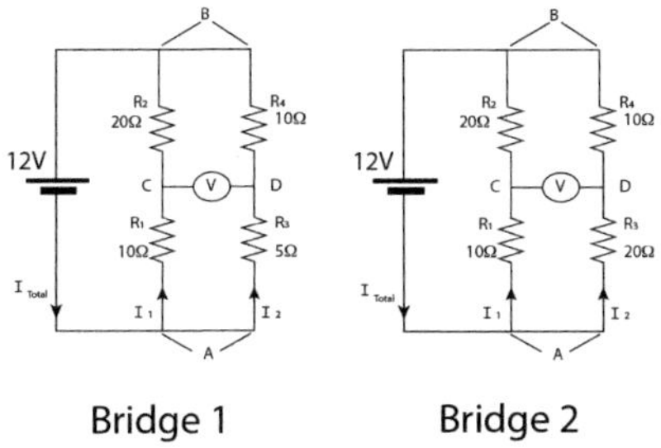

Adding resistance in series: $R_{Total} = R_1 + R_2 + R_3 ...$

Adding resistance in parallel: $1/R_{Total} = 1/R_1 + 1/R_2 + 1/R_3 ...$

Total current in circuit = Voltage / Total resistance

Current divides in parallel circuit in proportion to resistance in each limb.

Current is the same throughout each limb.

Potential difference across each limb is the same as the battery

Potential difference across each resistor is proportional to its resistance

Fig. 28.7 Wheatstone bridge examples

Bridge 1

1. What is the voltmeter reading?
2. What is the total resistance of the circuit?
3. What is the total current in the circuit and current of I_1 and I_2?
4. What are the voltage drops from A to C and from A to D?

Bridge 2

1. What is the total resistance of the circuit?
2. What is the total current in the circuit and current of I_1 and I_2?
3. What are the voltage drops from A to C and from A to D?
4. What is the voltmeter reading?

Bridge 1

1. 0 V. The bridge is balanced.
2. 10 Ω: 1/10 = 1/30 + 1/15.
3. I_{total} = 12 v/10 Ω = 1.2A.
   (a) I_1 = 12 V/30 Ω = 0.4 A.
   (b) I_2 = 12 V/15 Ω = 0.8 A.
   Note: Parallel circuits are 'current dividers'. The current in each limb must add up to the total current.
4. 0.4A × 10 Ω = 4 V and 0.8A × 5 Ω = 4 V. The bridge is balanced, so these voltage drops must be the same if C and D are to be at the same potential.

Bridge 2

1. 15 Ω. 1/15 = 1/30 + 1/30.
2. I_{total} = 12 v/15 Ω = 0.8A.
   (a) I_1 = 12 V/30 Ω = 0.4 A.
   (b) I_2 = 12 V/30 Ω = 0.4 A.
3. 0.4A × 10 Ω = 4 V and 0.4A × 20 Ω = 8 V.
4. 4 V: There is a 4 V difference in potential between C and D. The bridge is not balanced.

Electromagnets

When current flows in a wire, a magnetic field is produced that wraps around the current as described by the right-hand grip rule.

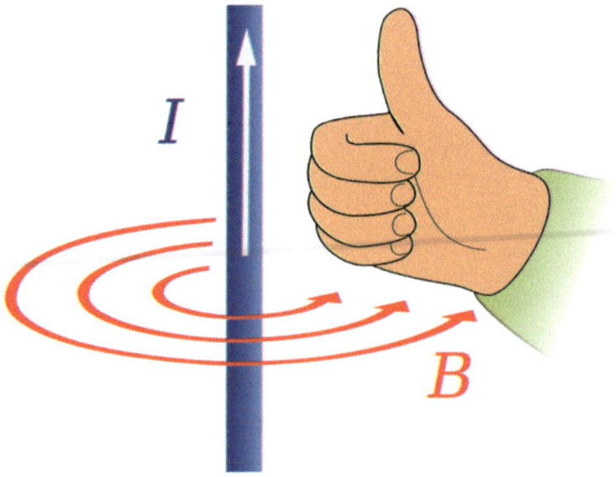

When repeatedly coiled, these summate generating a field with the direction described by the right-hand screw rule. The same hand shape is observed, but signifying different field directions.

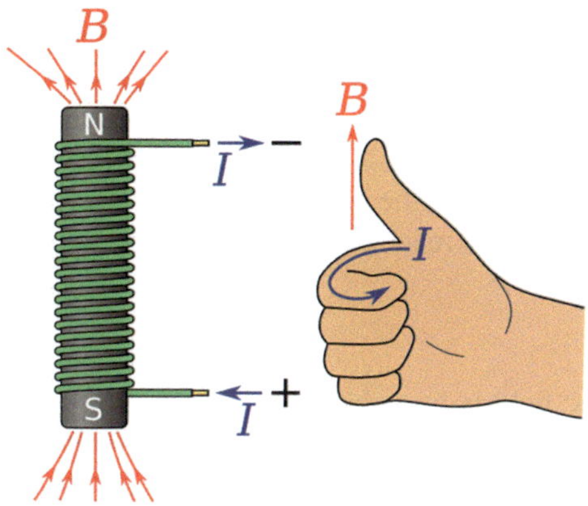

An electromagnet can be made by winding the wire of an electric circuit around an iron core. The strength of the magnet is increased if:

- The number of turns of the coil increases.
- The current is increased.
- The poles are brought together.
- There is an iron core. The iron core concentrates the magnetic flux. The magnetic flux is a measure of the strength of the magnetic field per unit area.

The magnetic field will act on other magnetic fields, ferromagnetic materials and charged particles. The latter is intrinsic to the function of the mass spectrometer.

A simple electromagnet

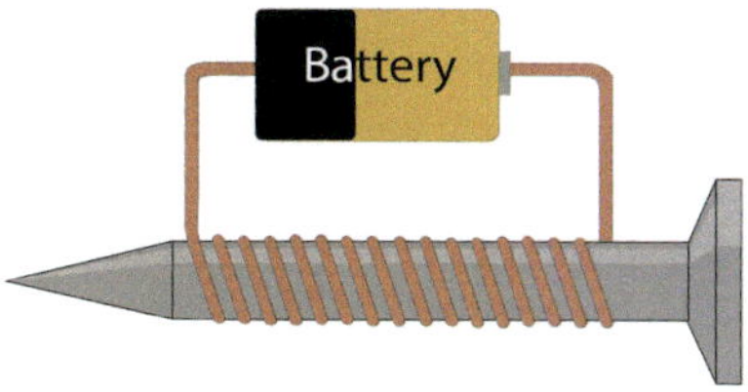

Permanent Magnets

Certain materials exert, or can be made to exert, magnetic fields without the need for an electric current. This is, again, because of electron movement. The electron orbitals of atoms of the material are aligned such that there is communal order in the electron spin, and this produces force-field lines capable of interacting with other magnetic fields.

Inductors

An inductor is a component within an electric circuit with the same basic design as an electromagnet in that it is a coil of wire around an iron core.

The purpose of the inductor in an electric circuit is not so much producing the magnetic field itself, but what that magnetic field is doing to the current flow in the coil that produced it as described above in impedance.

The magnetic field interacts with its own coil to produce an EMF that opposes the current flowing in the coil. This is called a back EMF. The effect occurs with AC and DC circuits. In AC circuits, the greater the frequency of current, the greater the back EMF and the greater the reactance. The purpose in a circuit is to block, reshape or filter AC current.

Electric Motor

If an electromagnetic field is brought close to a permanent magnetic field, a force results that can move things. This is the principle behind electrical motors. The direction of the force is described by Fleming's left hand rule.

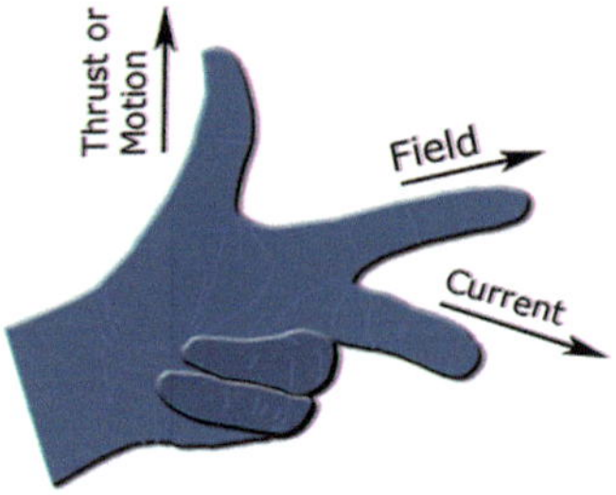

The galvanometer also works on this principle.

Electromagnetic Induction

Electromagnetic induction is the production of electricity from magnetism.

When a conductor is moved back and forwards through a magnetic field, the electrons in the conductor experience a force causing them to move back and forth. This force is in the opposite direction from that seen in the electric motor as they are two sides of the same coin. Electromagnetism is generating force to turn a motor when moving charge (current) in a magnetic field or generating charge flow (current) when moving that wire using force through a magnetic field. Whether the wire or the magnetic field moves does not matter. Thus, an alternating EMF and current have been induced in the conductor. The key point is that the magnetic field lines must be moving in relation to the conductor or there will be no electron movement.

The same phenomenon will occur if:

(a) The magnet is moved and the conductor is stationary,
(b) The conductor is placed in a magnetic field that varies with time (e.g. induced by an AC current),

The rule that governs this directionality for generators is Fleming's right-hand rule (reverse of left hand above).

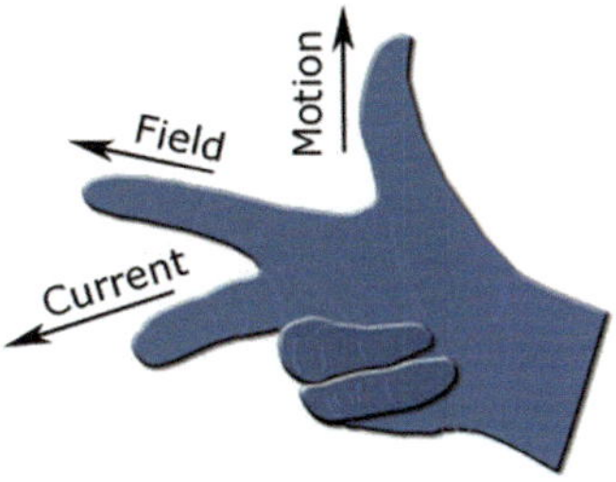

The images below illustrate how this interaction can be generated using wires being moved through a magnetic field or a magnet being moved causing the moving magnetic field to intersect the wires.

Electromagnetic induction

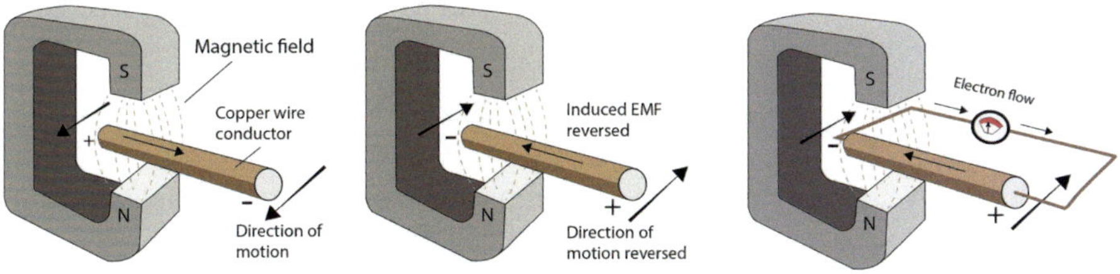

Conducting rod moving through a magnetic field. Electrons experience a force causing them to move and creating an alternating EMF and current.

Electromagnetic induction

Fixed magnet moving in and out of stationary coil produces AC current

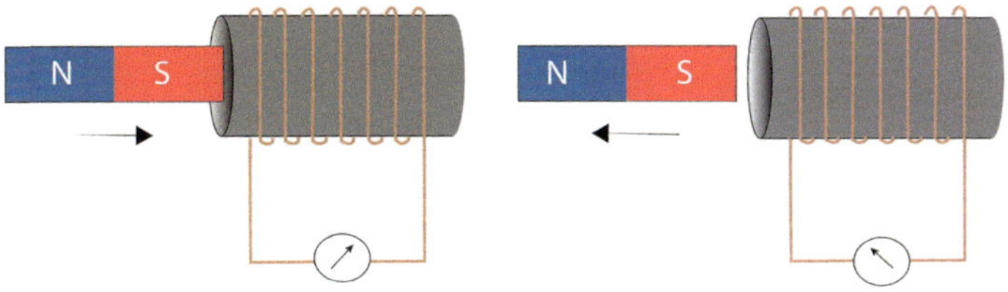

What Determines the Voltage Produced?

- Strength of the magnetic field.
- Flux linkage, which is the linking of the magnetic field with the conductors of the coil:
  - Rate at which the conductor cuts the magnetic field lines (Faraday's law).
  - The number of turns on the coil and the area of the coil exposed to the magnet.

AC Power Generation

A rectangular coil is rotated in a magnetic field. Flux linkage is maximum when plane of coil is at right angles to flux, minimum when they are in same plane and maximum (but reverse direction) after 180° rotation. This produces a sinusoidally varying EMF.

Transformers

A transformer makes use of electromagnetic induction to change the size of the voltage of an alternating current. An AC current flowing through a primary coil induces a magnetic field with moving (time-varying) field lines in the same frequency (but out of phase). These magnetic field lines interact with a secondary coil, creating an alternating EMF and current in the secondary circuit.

- Transformers usually have an iron core to concentrate the magnetic flux and improve efficiency.
- If the secondary coil has more windings than the primary coil, the voltage is stepped up. If the secondary coil has fewer windings, the voltage is stepped down. In an ideal transformer, the voltage ratio between primary and secondary coils is equal to the coil ratio:

$$V_{\text{Primary}} / V_{\text{Secondary}} = N_{\text{Primary}} / N_{\text{Secondary}}$$

N_{Primary} and $N_{\text{Secondary}}$ are the number of primary and secondary windings.
V_{Primary} and $V_{\text{Secondary}}$ are the primary and secondary voltages.

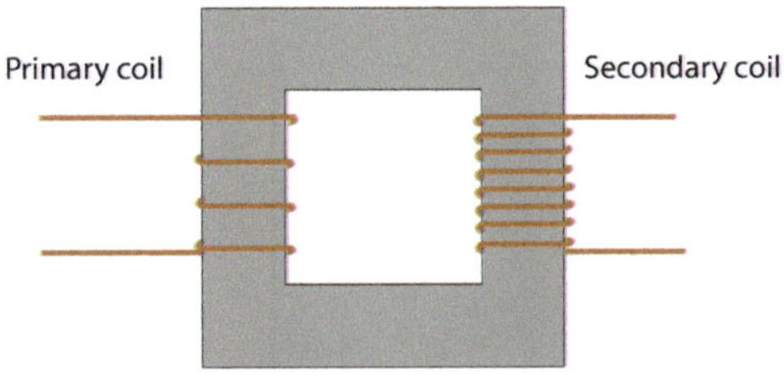

Step-up transformer

Electromagnetic Induction in the Clinical Arena

Induction is utilised in many medical devices. There is an inductor in the patient circuit of a defibrillator to shape and prolong discharge in order to maximise the defibrillation potential, while minimising energy requirement and potential for conductive injuries. Transformers allow AC power supply to be stepped up and down in the national grid and therefore enable power to be transmitted at very high voltages, thus reducing resistive losses (see Power Transmission). Transformers are used to produce isolated power supplies (see Electrical Safety) and to isolate applied parts of medical devices enabling signals to be passed from patient to ECG machine without a direct connection. The patient thus remains isolated from the earthed circuitry (see Electrical Safety).

Coiled wires within equipment may induce magnetic fields and electrical interference in ECG and other monitors. Leakage currents on casings may also be induced this way. This principle is also relevant in the MRI environment where currents may be induced in coiled leads by the strong magnetic environment.

Capacitors

Capacitors are electrical components that store charge. They consist of two plates separated by a dielectric material. Dielectrics are insulators, so electrons cannot cross between the plates. However, the dielectric material itself also becomes polarized, and this reduces the electric field building up on the plates. This, in turn, increases the plate capacitance. The ability of the dielectric to reduce the electric field is called its permittivity.

Capacitor in a DC Circuit

- When the battery circuit is switched on, electrons are pushed around the circuit onto one plate of the capacitor. The negative charge on that plate repels electrons from the other plate, which becomes positively charged.
- As electrons accumulate, it becomes harder to push more on to the plate against the repelling force of the growing negative charge. This causes an exponential decline in current and rate of charge.
- Eventually, current and charging cease when the electrical potential across the plates equals that of the battery. The capacitor is now fully charged.
- When the two plates are then connected together in a secondary circuit, a current will flow momentarily as the negative plate discharges. The electrons are propelled by the electric potential that has developed on the capacitor but, as the potential is declining during discharge, the current falls exponentially during discharge as well.

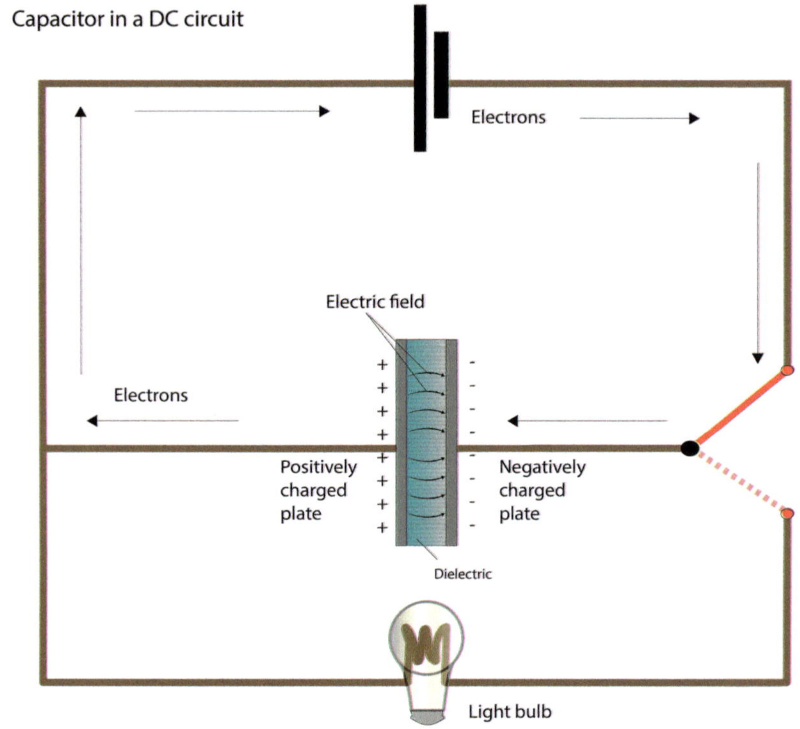

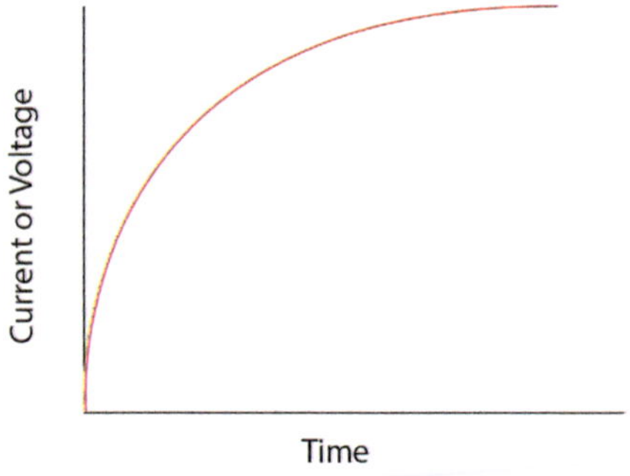

Circuit current and capacitor potential difference during charging

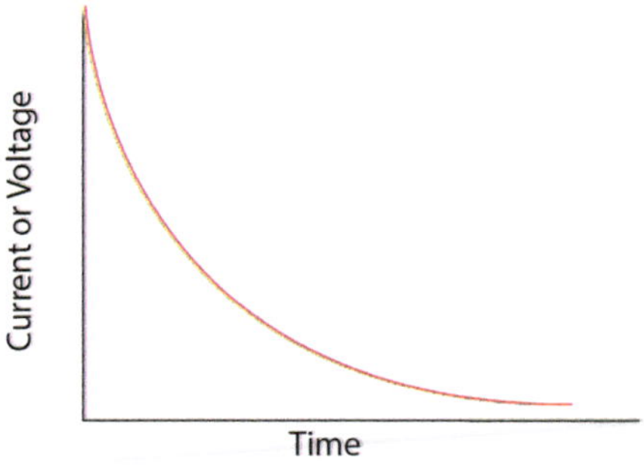

Current and capacitor potential difference during discharge.

Capacitors in an AC Circuit

Capacitors stop DC current from flowing, but they do not stop AC current flow. In an AC circuit, the voltage is constantly changing direction, and the plates are continuously charging and discharging, so the system never reaches a steady state. The faster the current switches direction, the less impact the capacitor has in the circuit.

Thus, the reactance of a capacitor in an AC circuit diminishes as the current frequency increases.

Capacitance

Capacitance is the amount of charge (coulombs) that is stored per volt.

- Capacitance (C) = Charge (Q)/Potential difference (V).
- SI unit of capacitance is the farad. 1 Farad capacitor holds 1 coulomb of charge and has a potential difference of 1 volt across the plates. This would be a very large capacitor. Most capacitors are in μF, nF or pF.

Factors which Increase Capacitance

- Increased surface area of capacitor plates.
- Decreased distance between the plates.
- Dielectric material.

Capacitors in the Clinical Arena

- Defibrillator (see below).
- Electrical filters. Because the function and impedance of capacitors and inductors are closely related to the frequency of AC current, the combination is used in electrical filters and in the production of radiofrequency current.
- An isolating capacitor is a capacitor that allows high-frequency AC current to flow but which inhibits low-frequency current. It is used in electrosurgical units to allow the high-frequency current to flow through the patient but protects the patient against accidental mains (50 Hz) electrocution.
- Capacitance and electrical interference. AC mains current in appliances can produce alternating charge across other surfaces of other equipment such as ECG electrodes. An overhead light with 50 Hz current flowing may then lead to 50 Hz interference in the ECG.

Defibrillator

Defibrillation

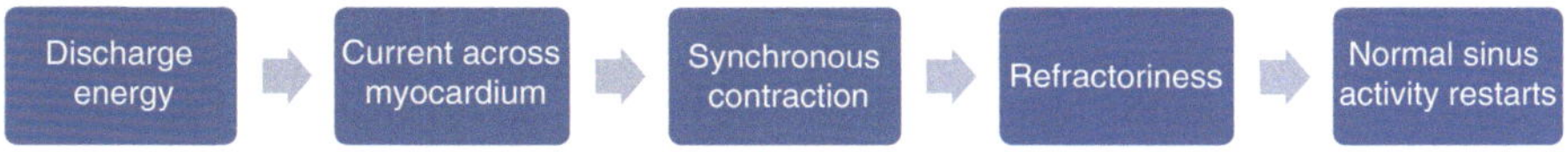

Basic Aim

Drive a current of ~30 A across the heart in a controlled fashion from external surface paddles. This requires two things:

- The capacitor must be charged up with lots of electrons, usually about 100–150 mC.
- Large electric potential across the capacitor to drive the electrons into the thorax (2500–5000 V).

Energy Stored on Capacitor

The energy (*E*) released by the capacitor is determined by the voltage (*V*) across the plates and the number of stored coulombs (*Q*). As the potential difference is falling during discharge, the energy available is ½ *QV* rather than simply *QV*:

$$E = \frac{1}{2}.QV$$

The energy may also be expressed in terms of capacitance (*C*). Remember that capacitance is (*Q*/*V*):

$$E = \frac{1}{2}.CV^2.$$

Illustrative figures for older, monophasic defibrillators:

$$\text{Energy} = \frac{1}{2} \times 160\,mC \times 5000V = 400J$$

Patient Impedance

Defibrillators are generally calibrated for a typical patient impedance of 50–100 Ω. The greater the impedance, the lower the myocardial current and the less chance of success. Some contemporary defibrillators can estimate patient impedance prior to shock and reshape current discharge. Factors affecting impedance:

- Impedance is increased in obesity.
- Impedance is decreased with larger pads and ensuring good contact of pads.
- Increased paddle pressure decreases impedance.

Why Do We Dial Up Energy Rather Than Current?

The myocardial current is the important determinant of successful defibrillation, but the uncertainty of thoracic and skin impedance makes the current uncertain. The energy released from the plates is a surrogate that can be calculated and predicted.

Monophasic Discharge

It is delivered from one paddle to the other. It typically requires 250–400 J energy to achieve adequate myocardial current. The shape of the discharge current is peaked with an exponential decline.

Biphasic Discharge

Current is discharged through the patient and then reversed. This pattern lowers the threshold and energy required for successful defibrillation:

- Better or equal efficiency with lower current and energy.
- Less myocardial injury because of lower peak current.
- Some BFDs sense the electrical impedance of the patient and can extend discharge if there is high impedance.
- Some devices are able to deliver a constant (square-wave), rather than exponential current.

Monophasic and Biphasic Discharge Currents

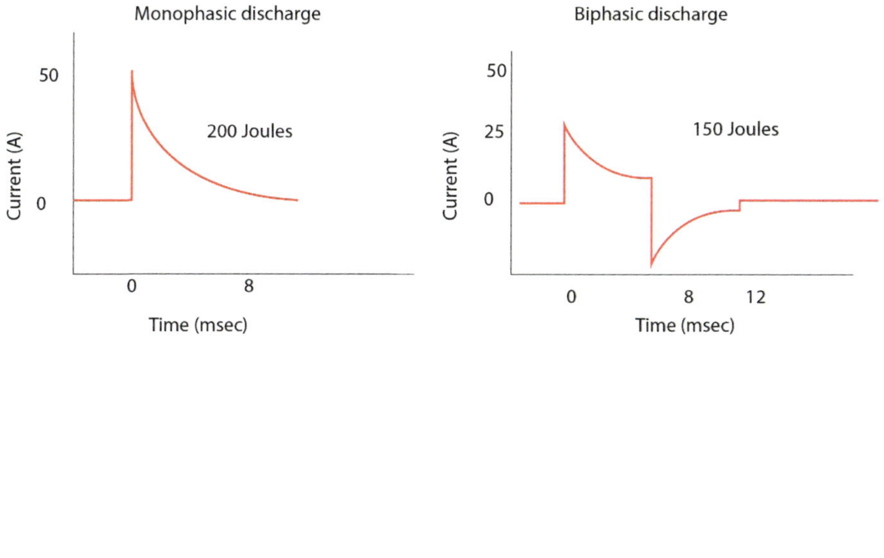

Monophasic Defibrillator Circuit Diagrams

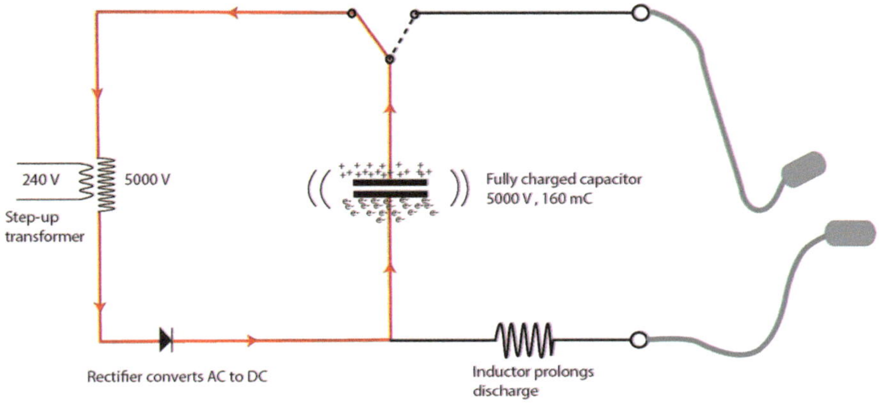

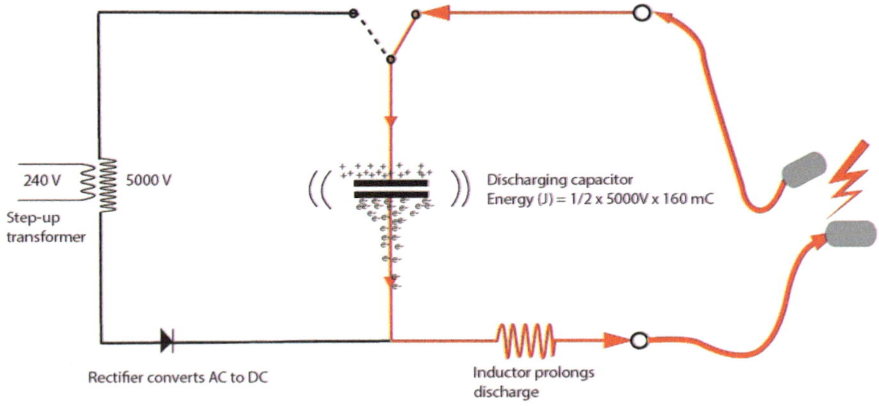

Electrical Safety

29

Alan McLintic and Matthew Taylor

There are many different classifications that apply and can be easily confused:

- **Electrical area classification** refers to the wiring design in the building designed to reduce the risk of macroshock and microshock. This is the "body-safe" and "cardiac-safe" electrical environments (see below).
- **Classification of electrical devices** refers to equipment design to minimise the risk of macroshock. These are termed Class 0, I, II or III.
- **"Applied part" classification** refers to the parts of medical equipment which are in contact with patients and are designed to minimise the risk of transmitting unwanted current into the body. These are types B, BF and CF. They can often be confused with the Electrical area classifications.

Macroshock

Macroshock is electrocution by large amounts of current and occurs when a person accidently becomes part of an electric circuit. The severity of injury depends on the magnitude and duration of the current as well as the direction through the body the current takes. These in turn are impacted by several other factors.

In keeping with Ohm's law, larger voltages generate higher currents for a given resistance, which is reflected in the different effects seen with high-tension power supplies. Lowering skin resistance through wet skin, electrically conductive gels or a medically induced break in the skin's continuity will allow the conduction of larger currents for a given voltage. As a result, skin resistance can vary from a

A. McLintic · M. Taylor (✉)
Department of Anaesthesia and Pain Medicine, Counties Manukau Health, Auckland, New Zealand
e-mail: Matthew.Taylor@middlemore.com

C. Birch et al. (eds.), *Physics and Measurement for Anesthesia*,
https://doi.org/10.1007/978-3-031-65060-4_29

thousand to several hundred thousand ohms. This has considerable influence on the current experienced from 230 V mains supply.

- Current experienced at **1000Ω** skin resistance = 230/1000 = 230 mA. (potentially lethal).
- Current experienced at **100,000Ω** skin resistance = 230/100,000 = 2.3 mA (barely perceptible).

Wet skin reduces resistance and increases the current experienced. The current itself, in its thermal actions on the skin, will further reduce skin resistance worsening the effect. In the event of a shock causing muscle tetany (if the threshold current for "let-go" is exceeded), the skin can break down (burn) during the prolonged contact and conduction causing a fall in skin resistance. The current can rise tenfold or more during prolonged shock.

Current type is also significant in potential risk as it takes three times as much direct current (DC) to produce VF compared with alternating current (AC). Maximum adverse effects are in the low frequencies at which cells produce action potentials (~50 Hz) rather than very-high-frequency currents which do not excite contractile tissue. This forms the basis of electrosurgery.

The risks to patients are not just those of burns (which may be of profound significance) but also in the muscle and nerve depolarisation generated and as an ignition source. Even small currents, when generated in high-risk locations close to the myocardium and at the correct time in the cardiac cycle (R on T), can initiate VF.

Effect of 50 Hz current applied between the hands	
0.1–1 mA	Tingling sensation
5 mA	Pain. Maximum "harmless" intensity
15–20 mA	Muscular contraction. Above this threshold, you cannot let go of the live wire
50 mA	Respiratory arrest
100 mA	VF
>1000 mA	Burns
6 A	Sustained ventricular contraction

Mechanism of Electrocution in Typical "Domestic" Power Supplies and Protective Design

For domestic, low-voltage AC systems, the actual current carried to/from the power supply is in two wires: "active" (sometimes called "live" or "phase") and neutral. The active wire is at 230 V in relation to the neutral wire allowing current flow to/from the device. The neutral circuit is also grounded/earthed through a deep earth stake or via attachment to conductive water pipe. This also occurs at the power generation end at various points (generator, transformer, power lines) in order to provide an alternative return pathway for the current back to the neutral circuit. There are various designs of this each with advantages and disadvantages. Earthing serves firstly to dissipate static charges built up in the network and also to protect against fault currents.

Effectively, the active wire is also at 230 V in relation to the earth. This is termed a neutral grounded power system. The safety aim of this design is in the event of insulation failure of the active connection, either in the power cable or internally. If a device loses its integrity internally through corrosion or deteriorated insulation and the active power pathway forms a link to the chassis, it can allow conducting components of the exterior to become "active" or "live". Equipment design means that same exterior components/chassis is also connected to ground, which allows a low-resistance pathway to conduct the current when compared with a person of intact skin resistance. This is a "class I" design and current will flow through the grounding in a magnitude that burns the fuse protected circuit and cuts the power supply. In practice for modern electrical designs, this will trip residual current devices (RCDs) that disengage the circuit when a differential flow through the active and neutral wires is detected (because of the escape through earth). This is why faulty devices "trip" the power supply when they are connected, and they must be withdrawn from service immediately.

In the theatre environment, people are "isolated from ground." The aim here is to increase the potential for shock by adding another impediment to where the patient could be "grounded" increasing protection over what is seen in domestic supplies. In normal environments, one has a higher skin resistance as the skin is not breached as is can be in the medical area. Without the ground connecting to the chassis and allowing this preferential current flow, a person standing on the ground and touching the active wire or components erroneously connected to the active wire can becomes part of an electric circuit from active wire to earth with a potential difference of 230 V across them and a current dependent on their resistance. They in effect become an earthing path back to the neutral circuit. The electrocution circuit is often described as being from active/phase wire, through victim, through ground and theoretically back up through neutral wire (back at the grounding at the power generator). Of course, the electrons flowing through the victim do not actually return up the neutral wire because the ground is such a massive conductor that they are soaked up in its mass. The important point is that by grounding the neutral wire, the active wire is at 230 V in relation to earth and the current becomes "earth-seeking". If you provide a low-resistance route to earth, the current will pass through you to earth. If, conversely as in "body safe" electrical environments, you are completely isolated from earth, you can touch the live wire without the risk of electrocution via the earth route as there is nowhere for the current to flow back to neutral. This forms the basis of "floating" or "isolated" circuits in the operating room.

The point of the "earth wire" is to provide an alternative pathway at much lower resistance to preferentially conduct the majority of the charge and to also draw off casing leakage currents that arise from capacitance and inductance linkage with other equipment. The point of an RCD is to detect this escape of charge and disengage the circuit rapidly (within milliseconds) to limit any potential current damage to an earthed individual and also to detect faulty equipment, interrupting the circuit before it can place a person at risk. Fuses and circuit breakers protect the circuits from overload and damage by limiting the magnitude of current flowing within the circuit to below that of its design capacity. This is typically still a current magnitude that is capable of electrocution risk so they are

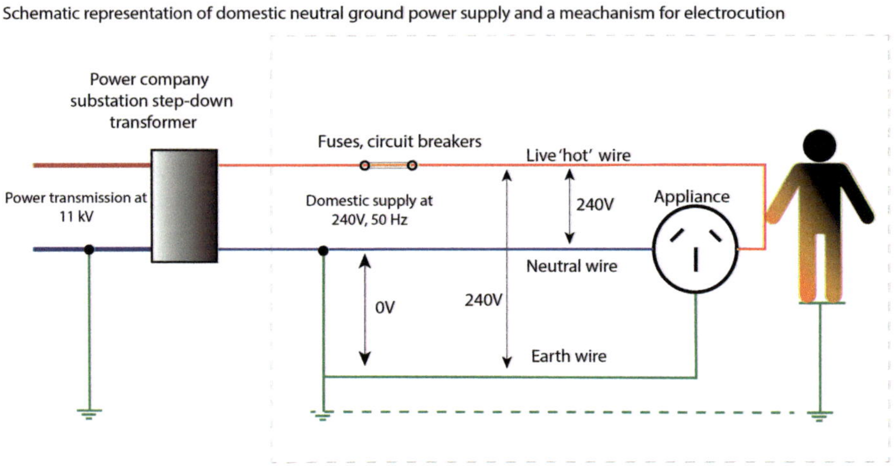

Fig. 29.1 Domestic power supply and earthing

protecting the integrity of the circuit from overload, not people. Bypassing these class I safety designs and touching the live and the neutral wire simultaneously will lead to electrocution with the full 230 V RMS potential (Fig. 29.1).

Classification of Electrical Equipment According to Means of Protection

Class	IEC classification of earthing protection
Class 0	No protective earthing connection, therefore the only protection is insulation between wiring and external components. These have been prohibited in many countries as a single-fault risk for electrocution and additionally RCD/fuse protection would not be protective
Class I	Basic protection in metal casing equipment. Wires insulated from each other and from user, casing earthed. Fuses within equipment and (in the UK) in live terminal plug. If casing becomes live, the current in the circuit is so high that the fuse melts or circuit breaker trips, cutting off the power
Class II	All accessible parts protected by actual or functional double insulation. May have isolating transformer. Casing is not earthed because there are no conductive parts on the exterior to be earthed
Class III	No potentials exceeding 24 V AC or 50 V DC. Separated extra-low-voltage power supply with potentials low enough that are safe to handle without generating dangerous currents. This does not apply in medical environment where the cutaneous barrier is compromised

Residual Current Devices (RCD)/Ground Fault Circuit Interrupters (GFCIs)

As mentioned above, under normal conditions, the current entering an appliance must equal the current leaving the appliance. If there is a fault allowing the current

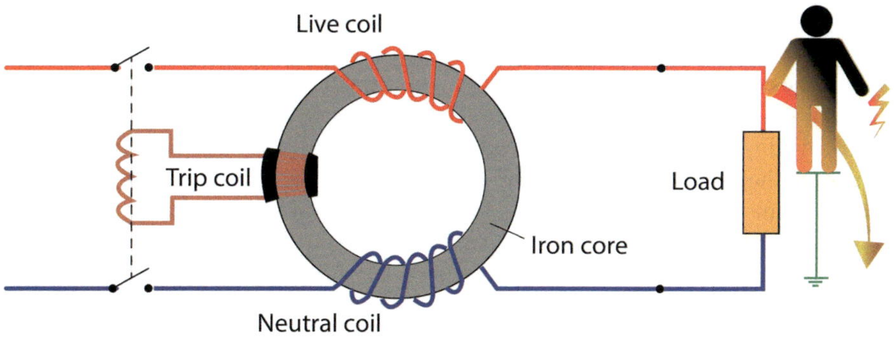

Fig. 29.2 Residual current device

to escape to earth, either through the earthing wire or person, it causes an imbalance in current flow between active and neutral. RCDs are designed to detect this imbalance at a sensitivity of between 5 and 30 mA and cut power within milliseconds. Speed and tripping current differ between devices. In Australian/New Zealand standards, a 10 mA RCD that trips within 40 ms is specified.

The live and neutral wires entering the RCD wrap around an iron core before travelling on to the appliance.

A third "detector" coil connects with a switch in the power supply. Normally, the live and neutral wires produce equal and opposite magnetic fields which cancel each other out. If there is an imbalance between live and neutral currents, a net magnetic field is produced that induces a current in the detector coil that, in turn, snaps the power switch open and cuts off power. RCDs incorporate a test switch that confirms that the unit is capable of cutting off the power supply by inducing a test current. Pressing the switch should shut off power (Fig. 29.2).

Prevention of Macroshock in Operating Rooms (ORs)

Prevention of macroshock
Patient factors
Patient must not be grounded
Equipment factors
Earthing of equipment casing
Fuses and circuit breakers
Isolated power supply and LIMs
Design of equipment

Australian and New Zealand electrical standards require all patient areas to be at least "body safe" in electrical design. This requires circuit design to minimise the risk of macroshock and the use of sensitive RCDs, isolated power supplies (IPSs) and line isolation monitors (LIMs). Cardiac-safe environments add equipotential earthing to this to minimise microshock risk.

Prevention of Patient Connection to Ground

Whilst the earthing wire in Class I equipment is a safety design, many of the electrical issues in medical environments are related to risk when the patient becomes part of a grounding pathway for equipment. When the skin barrier is breached, the magnitude of the current can be amplified and the risk of significant currents at the myocardium is enhanced. Hence, avoidance of conditions leading to patient "grounding" is a concern where the usual domestic protective systems intended for intact skin are inadequate. Patients should be carefully positioned so that they are not touching metal conduits to earth or earthed appliances. In practice, this is frequently the metallic elements of the operating table but may also be faulty electrosurgical cabling, worn ECG cables, etc. that also makes a contact with the grounded circuit. Similarly, a patient should not lie in puddles of moisture both because they may connect the patient to earth and because it reduces the impedance of the skin. For various procedures, especially those with copious fluid irrigation or discharge, this can be difficult to maintain and increased vigilance of these electrical principles must be observed. *This includes staff* interacting with patients as they should avoid the possibility of earthing the patient by touching them. Insulating footwear of 75—100 kΩ should be worn in the theatre environment and staff should not simultaneously touch equipment casing with one hand and patient with the other.

To prevent equipment that does come in contact with the patient (such as ECG electrodes and diathermy) providing a route to earth, floating circuits are employed. Whilst the casing and internal circuitry of the modules of such equipment may be earthed, the patient part of the circuit must "float" free of the rest. The signals may be transferred from patient circuit to processing circuitry optically or via a transformer within the module. The isolating capacitor of a diathermy circuit allows transmission of high-frequency current but is a barrier to low-frequency current.

Isolated Power Supply (IPS)

Isolated power circuits (Fig. 29.3) are used in the operating theatre environment to add further layers of protection by designing a system that requires two faults in order to allow an escape current as well as a monitoring system (line isolation monitor—LIM) that detects the potential for shock due to a failure of one of the levels of protection and alarms. It means that an additional layer of safety arises by an alarm sounding to warn of the increased potential of a fault (due to failure of one of two layers of protection) without tripping RCDs and interrupting the power supply to potentially vital medical equipment. It additionally serves as a barrier to excessive currents being transmitted into the isolated circuit in the event of a lightning strike, solar flare or other overvoltage situations.

In the system design, the mains powered inward circuit is coupled to the isolated circuit through an isolating transformer. Magnetic induction transmits power to the secondary circuit, and the transformer has a load limit preventing conduction of overvoltage. The next protective design is that the secondary circuit is not

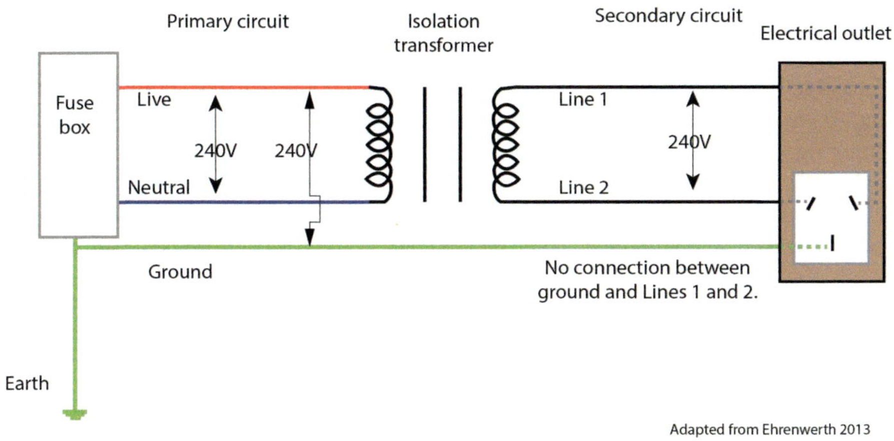

Fig. 29.3 Isolated (floating) power supply

earthed in the way we see in domestic environments. This is because, as mentioned above, standard earthing is an inadequate protection when skin resistance is compromised. The earthing connection seen in the secondary circuit earths the casing/chassis of the equipment to the primary circuit, but the actual secondary circuit remains separated. In theory, one can contact the active wire and, if correctly insulated from ground (appropriate footwear, etc.), no shock will be delivered. Two faults are required to allow current passage, one allowing earthing of the secondary circuit and another allowing contact with the active secondary line. Alternatively coming in contact with both the active and neutral lines simultaneously is a double fault allowing electrocution.

The terminology of earthing/grounding here can get confusing. In domestic supplies, the earth protects by allowing an escape path of lower resistance back to neutral in the event of a fault and then disengaging via a RCD. This minimises shock to a safe level. In OR, this is inadequate, so the isolated system is employed with its two-fault protection. However, earthing points still exist in the OR as all items in the OR environment (beds, patients, staff) can contact ground. This ground is referenced to a common point (unipotential) in order to equalise all the components to the same charge. This is a microshock and electrostatic protective mechanism, not to protect against macroshock and is the basis of "cardiac protected environements".

Line Isolation Monitor (LIM)

A critical part of this system is the LIM. This device continuously measures the integrity of the system isolation, referenced to ground. If a fault develops that allows excessive current leakage, an alarm sounds indicating a failure in the first layer of protection, without interruption of power to the equipment. This means that essential equipment can still function, whilst still warning of a potential (but not yet realised) risk.

Microshock

"Leakage" of a current is charge movement across a boundary that should be insulating. As no insulator can ever be perfect, there will always be an element of leak, and changing electromagnetic fields can induce current in adjacent wiring, generating leakage as well. Part of the function of earthing is providing a route of dissipation of these charges, and electrical equipment can be designed using means to minimise the leakage currents generated. The acceptable levels of leakage currents depend on:

- Equipment classification (I, II, III CF or BF) (see below).
- Differing international standards.
- Where and how you are measuring the current.
- Whether it is under normal conditions or single-fault situations. Max allowable leakage current in single-fault conditions is usually five times that under normal circumstances.

Hence, you will come across several different values attached to CF and BF equipment. I have noted one limit only for each.

"Applied parts" refer to the part of the electrical equipment *that is applied to the patient*. There should not be a direct connection from the power source to the patient, so these items are isolated or "floating" using similar principles to isolated power supplies. The classification of these items is as follows:

Type	Type designation defines suitability for "applied parts" in differing medical environments An applied part is the part of electrical equipment that comes in contact with the patient
Type B	I, II or III equipment: Adequate protection against electric shock with regard to leakage current and reliability. Suitable for external use only. Max patient leakage current in class I equipment under normal conditions of 100 μA
Class BF	No connections between patient and earth. Floating input circuits. Max patient leakage current in class I equipment under normal conditions 100 μA
Class CF	I, II or III equipment. High protection against microshock as very low leakage currents. Considered safe to connect to heart. Max patient leakage currents under normal conditions in class I equipment ≤10 μA

In order to help minimise the flow of leakage currents in cardiac-safe environments, **equipotential earthing** is used.

Equipotential earthing is high-specification earthing whereby all earth points have exactly the same potential. If casings were all earthed separately and with different specifications, it is possible that one casing might still have a little charge on it relative to another. Their relative "earths" would effectively be slightly different. Thus, if you touched both casings at the same time, a current would flow through you. Equipotential earthing should ensure zero potential on all earthed components to prevent these earth variations inducing microcurrents between equipment if bridged through the patient.

Microschock is a potential for harm because small amounts of current delivered at high current density directly into the heart can cause ventricular fibrillation.

Animal studies suggest that microshock can occur at currents of 50–100 μA and AC can provoke VF at lower currents than DC as the myocardium is maximally sensitive at 50 Hz. At higher frequencies (MHz), higher currents can be tolerated allowing safe use for electrosurgical units. Three conditions are required for microshock:

1. A direct conduit for current to pass into, or close to, heart (e.g. central lines, external pacing wires, oesophageal temperature probe, endoscopic equipment). In theory, a saline bridge via IV or arterial access could also do this, depending on the resistance of the entire pathway.
2. Leakage current. This might arise from capacitance or inductance linkage between equipment. Staff might then touch poorly earthed casing and the central line and deliver the current to the myocardium.
3. The patient is accidentally grounded. Again, staff may accidentally ground the patient by touching casing and patient at the same time or being inadequately insulated from ground themselves.

Note: According to AS/NZS 2500 electrical standards, cardiac-safe environments are required for situations where an indwelling electrical conductor is accessible outside the body. These typically refer to pacing wires, intracardiac ECGs and cardiac catheterisation (PA catheters) but not central lines as long as they are in the SVC. Of note: this does not mean that "cardiac-safe is only required for cardiac procedures". In practice, the risk that they could be intra-atrial pending confirmation of placement would suggest that cardiac-safe environments are prudent. Oesophageal probes conducting behind the heart also have the potential for microshock and should be managed thus. Radial artery pressure monitoring is considered, despite the salt bridge through blood vessels, to be a body type applied part and can be monitored in a body-safe environment. The delineation between femoral/brachial arterial lines and cardiac safety is unclear. Many major centres err on the side of cardiac safety when designing operating theatre environments.

Prevention of Microshock

- Equipment that can be positioned close to myocardium must be class CF and must have minimal leakage currents. Max 50 μA (SF) or 10 μA (normal conditions). Some sources define any connection to the bloodstream as requiring CF class applied parts.
- Patient must not be grounded.
- Equipment casing must be efficiently grounded to remove stray currents.
- Staff must avoid providing a route between patient and earth or patient and current.

Electrical Safety Symbols

See Fig. 29.4.

Type B equipment of class I, II or III. Max leakage current under normal conditions is 100 μA. Not safe for direct conduits to heart

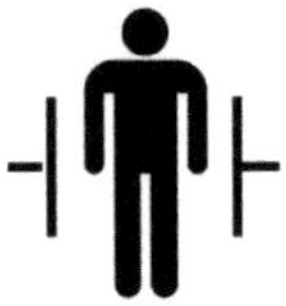

As above but has defibrillator protection.

Type BF equipment of class I, II or III. Similar to B equipment but the patient circuit is isolated (floating) from the rest of the equipment circuitry.

Type CF equipment of class I, II . Designed with very low leakage currents and is safe for direct connection to the heart.
Class 1 limits: Max 50 μA. (SF) or 10 μA. (normal conditions).

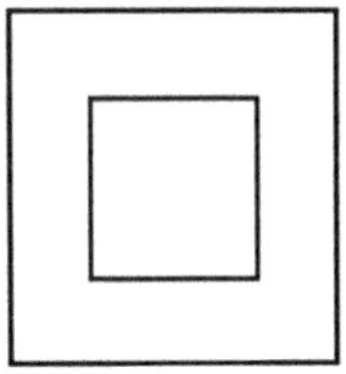

Class II equipment.

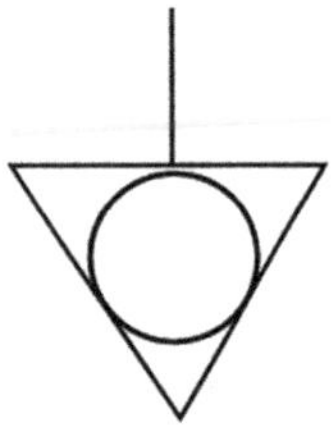

Equipotential earth. All metalwork is earthed to have zero or near zero voltage.

Fig. 29.4 Equipment electrical safety symbols

Laser Surgery

30

Alan McLintic and Craig Birch

What Does LASER Stand For?

Light Amplification by Stimulated Emission Radiation

At the beginning of the last century, Max Planck discovered that light is released, transferred and absorbed in specific amounts of energy called quanta. Electrons are distributed in a number of concentric shells around the nucleus of an atom. If electrons move from one level to another, energy is consumed or liberated in steps called quanta. Quanta of light are called photons. Einstein published a theory shortly afterwards suggesting that most atoms exist in ground energy state Eo. The Eo molecules can be converted to higher energy levels when energy is added to them, and in returning to their ground state, energy is released spontaneously as photons or electromagnetic (EM) waves. If a photon of the same wavelength collides with an excited atom, the two photons are released concurrently and therefore have equal frequencies. This idea of "stimulated emission" was used in the creation of lasers. One of the first lasers was created by using an electrical source to energise a ruby (see the diagram below). The CO_2 laser could emit a concentrated ray of light that was absorbed by water, and thus it was used to vaporise tissue. The neodymium-yttrium-aluminium-garnet (Nd-YAG) laser created coagulation in tissue and so was useful for haemostasis. Thus, several different active media have been used to create new lasers which are used in a variety of subspecialties.

A. McLintic · C. Birch (✉)
Department of Anaesthesia and Pain Medicine, Counties Manukau Health, Auckland, New Zealand

C. Birch et al. (eds.), *Physics and Measurement for Anesthesia*,
https://doi.org/10.1007/978-3-031-65060-4_30

Why Is Laser Light More Powerful Than Ordinary Light?

- Monochromatic: Single specific wavelength.
- Coherent: The photons are in phase, i.e. they have the same wavelength.
- Collimated: The photons move parallel to each other with little beam divergence.
- Negligible loss of energy over distance.

Production of a Laser Beam

The lasing medium can be solid, liquid or gas. The medium determines the wavelength or colour of the laser. It is energised to get the atoms into an excited state; this is usually done with electricity. A large number of atoms are energised, which puts the electrons into an excited state to cause the stimulated emission described. To amplify the energy available, and to allow resonance to occur, the laser device has a pair of mirrors at either end. The photons reflect off the mirrors to move back and forth through the lasing medium, constantly stimulating other electrons. The electrons then release photons of light energy. One of the mirrors is partially transparent, which allows an appropriate density of light to escape through the mirror. This is called the *output coupler*. Figure 30.1 shows a schematic example of a ruby laser.

Key Steps

- Medium put into an excited state by external energy. Often electrical energy:
  - Atoms absorb energy (stimulated absorption) → electrons excited to higher energy level.
- Spontaneous emission of photons in all directions:
  - Electron decays spontaneously and releases a photon.
  - Emitted radiation is of single wavelength but not in phase (e.g. fluorescence, thermal emission).

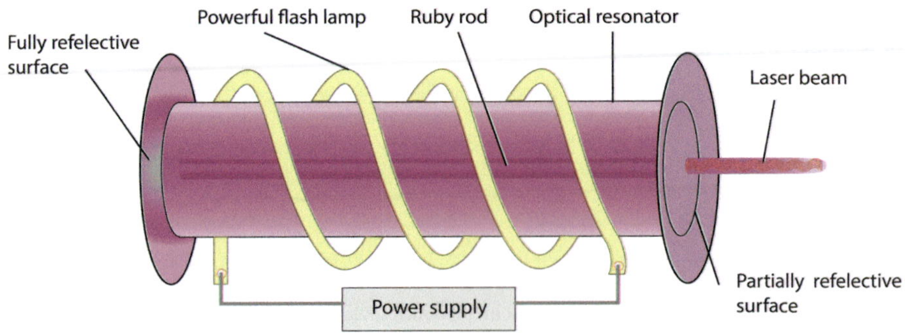

Fig. 30.1 Schematic example of a ruby laser (Dr. AJ McLintic)

- Stimulated emission:
  - A photon interacts with the excited atom to force it back down to lower energy state → stimulated release of identical photon.
  - Stimulated emission therefore produces two identical photons per interaction.
  - For stimulated emission to dominate, more atoms must be in the excited state than in the ground state. This is called population inversion.
  - The emitted light matches the input light in direction, wavelength and polarisation.
- The mirrors reflect these photons, and the process of stimulated emission is amplified: avalanche/cascade process in the mirrored cavity.
- Light impacting the output coupler escapes as a narrow, coherent beam.

Laser Physics Facts and FAQs

Electron Transitions

- An electron transition is the change of an electron from one energy level to another:
  - This causes release or absorption of electromagnetic radiation in the form of a photon.

What Is a Photon?

- Elementary particle; the quantum of electromagnetic radiation such as light:
  - Zero rest mass and always moves at the speed of light within a vacuum.
  - Exhibits properties of both waves and particles.

Are Lasers Really Monochromatic?

- Stimulated emission produces a very narrow bandwidth, but it may not be precisely monochromatic.

What Determines the Interaction with Tissue?

- Energy density.
- Exposure time.
- Wavelength:
  - Infrared: molecular vibration and heating.
  - Visible light: photochemical effects.
  - Ultraviolet: molecular bond dissociation and burning.

Table 30.1 Properties of common LASERs used in medicine (Dr. AJ McLintic)

Laser medium	Type	Colour	Wavelength	Common applications
CO_2	Gas	Far infrared	~10,000 nm	Absorbed by water. Laser 'scalpel'. Skin, ORL
Holmium:YAG	Solid	Mid-infrared	2140 nm	Prostate, lithotripsy including salivary stones and other tissue cutting/ablation requirement
Nd:YAG	Solid	Near infrared	1064 nm	Retina and capsular surgery, skin cancers and tattoo removal, thyroid nodules
Diode	Solid	Red-infrared	800–1000 nm	Hair removal. Laser pointer, barcode scanner
Argon	Gas	Blue-green	350–550 nm	Retinal surgery, AV malformation
Ruby	Solid	Red	694 nm	Hair removal, tattoo removal
Pulsed dye	Liquid	Yellow	390–640 nm	Birthmarks, vascular skin lesions
Excimer (Ar:F)	Gas	UV	193 nm	Skin lesions

Importance of Wavelength

- Different laser mediums produce lasers of different wavelengths.
- Different tissues absorb different wavelengths preferentially:
  - Absorption depends on the rotations, vibrations and transitions of the atoms, which is related to the energy they possess.
- Penetration depth increases with increasing wavelength:
  - Other factors affecting penetration include reflectivity of skin, colour of light and presence of severely absorbing structures such as hair roots (Table 30.1).

Lasers and Theatre Safety

Main Hazards to Patients and Staff

- Eyes.
- Skin burns.
- Ignition.

Maximum Possible Exposure (MPE)

Based on the highest power or energy density that is considered safe. Relates to the probability of causing damage to eye or skin (Table 30.2).

Table 30.2 Risk of LASER injury (Dr. AJ McLintic)

Type	Risk or injury	Risk level
Class 1	Low energy. Not hazardous to skin or eyes. Safe during normal operation	Low
Class 1 M	May cause eye injury if viewed with an optical instrument	Low-medium
Class 2	Visible wavelengths only. Blink response provides safety. Will not burn skin	Low-medium
Class 2 M	As above but hazardous if viewed through optical instrument	Medium
Class 3R	Considered safe if handled carefully. Direct viewing of beam may be hazardous	Medium-high
Class 3B	Direct viewing and specular reflections can cause eye injury	High
Class 4	All medical lasers. Can burn the skin and cause permanent eye damage may ignite combustible materials. Injury possible from reflected beam	Extreme

Patient Safety Issues

ETT Ignition

If the ETT ignites and the patient is being ventilated with oxygen or nitrous oxide, a blow-torch effect can result.

- Laser-resistant tubes.
- Different forms of ventilation, e.g. transglottic or supraglottic jet ventilation cuff rupture.
- Laser-resistant cuffs.
- Double cuffs.
- Cuff filled with saline ± methylene blue as an indicator of cuff rupture.

Gas Mixtures

- Minimise FiO_2.
- Avoid N_2O, which supports combustion.
- Helium carrier gas to reduce FiO_2.
- Avoid pockets of carrier gas under drapes.
- Be aware of high-flow nasal oxygen use with laser.

Others

- Eye protection.
- Aqueous gel on exposed areas including hair.

Staff Safety

- Education and training.
- Good communication in theatre between surgeon and staff regarding laser use.
- Signs on doors and a light warning laser in use.
- Eye protection.
- Matt black instruments to reduce specular reflections.
- Laser safety officer.

Management of an Airway Fire

Primary

- Remove burning ETT.
- Stop flow of all airway gases.
- Disconnect breathing circuit.
- Douse burning area with saline (bowl of saline ready during laser use).
- Re-intubate and ventilate on air.

Secondary

- Bronchoscopy to assess the extent of damage.
- Consider steroids and antibiotics.
- ICU.

Further Reading

Kitching AJ, Edge CJ. Lasers and surgery. Br J Anaesthes CEPD Rev. 2003;8(5):143–6.
Magee P. Physics for anaesthesia magnetic resonance imaging; depth of anaesthesia monitoring; LASER; and light spectroscopy. BJA Educ. 2018;18(4):102e108.

Equipment Considerations When Ambient Pressure Changes

31

Alan McLintic and Craig Birch

Effect of Altitude on Oxygen Partial Pressure

The fractional concentration of oxygen in dry air remains stable at 21% but, as barometric pressure falls with increasing altitude, oxygen partial pressure or PO_2 falls (Figs. 31.1 and 31.2):

- PO_2 in dry air at 100 kPa = 21 kPa.
- PO_2 in dry air at 75 kPa (~8000 ft. altitude) = 0.21 × 75 kPa = 15.75 kPa.

Vaporisers

Variable Bypass with Outlet Splitting Control

In contemporary variable bypass vaporisers with splitting control at the VC outlet, the vaporiser settings to do not need to be adjusted in hypobaric or hyperbaric settings. The simple explanation is that the same mass of molecules is being added to the bypass flow, no matter the atmospheric pressure. Partial pressure is determined by the number of molecules in the vapour phase for a given temperature.

Variable Bypass with Inlet Splitting Control

If the vaporiser splitting control is at the inlet of the VC, the vaporiser will deliver vapour at a slightly different partial pressure when ambient pressure changes. In hypobaric conditions, the partial pressure is a little greater than at sea level, and, in hyperbaric conditions, output partial pressure is lower. This is because the mass of vapour and its carrier volume leaving the VC vary with atmospheric pressure. You

A. McLintic · C. Birch (✉)
Department of Anaesthesia and Pain Medicine, Counties Manukau Health, Auckland, New Zealand

C. Birch et al. (eds.), *Physics and Measurement for Anesthesia*,
https://doi.org/10.1007/978-3-031-65060-4_31

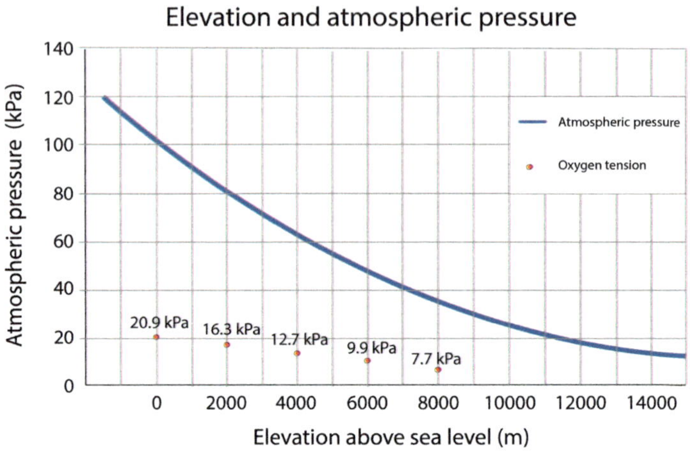

Fig. 31.1 Altitude and atmospheric pressure and the effect on partial pressure of oxygen (pO_2) (Dr. AJ McLintic)

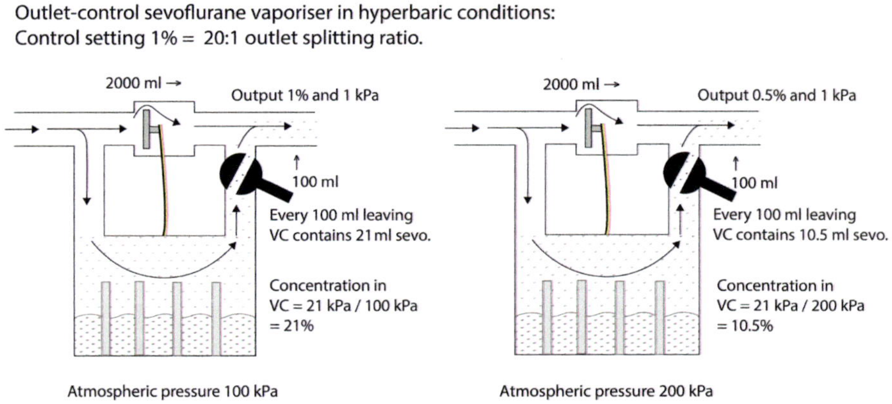

Fig. 31.2 Variable bypass vaporiser with outlet splitting control. Demonstration of an increase in atmospheric temperature to 200 kPa. The same mass of molecules is added to the bypass flow (McLintic)

will see why that is from the examples below and that the differences are clinically trivial (Tables 31.1, 31.2, and 31.3).

Why Emphasise the Difference Between Outlet and Inlet Control Vaporisers?

- Most textbooks and online blogs use schematic diagrams that depict an inlet splitting control, yet describe the function as if it was an outlet control.
- When those texts state that the vaporiser output partial pressure is unchanged in hypo- or hyperbaric conditions, they can *only* be referring to outlet splitting vaporisers, yet the wording and diagrams often imply (incorrectly) inlet splitting.

Table 31.1 Vaporisers at sea level (AJ McLintic)

Sea-level atmospheric pressure 1 bar (100 kPa)		
	Outlet control	Inlet control
Vaporiser setting	1%	1%
Splitting ratio to achieve 1%	20:1	25:1
Volumes if bypass flow is 2000 mL/min	2000 mL/min bypasses and 100 mL/min leaves VC	2000 mL/min bypasses and 79 mL/min enters VC
[Sevoflurane] vaporising chamber	21 kPa/100 kPa = 21%	21 kPa/100 kPa = 21%
Volume control	100 mL/min made to leave VC	79 mL/min made to enter VC
Volume picked up in VC	0.21 × 100 mL/min = 21 mL/min	21 mL/min is picked up to give [VC] of 21% (21/[79 + 21])
Total volume leaving vaporiser	2000 mL + 100 mL = 2100 mL	2000 mL + 100 mL = 2100 mL/min
Concentration leaving vaporiser	21 mL/2100 mL = 1%	21 mL/2100 mL = 1%
Output partial pressure	1% × 100 kPa = 1 kPa	1% of 100 kPa = 1 kPa

Table 31.2 Vaporisers at atmospheric pressure of 75 kPa (AJ McLinitic)

8000 ft altitude ≅ 75 kPa atmospheric pressure (e.g. Addis Ababa, Ethiopia)		
	Outlet control	Inlet control
Vaporiser setting	1%	1%
Splitting ratio to achieve 1%	20:1	25:1
Volumes if bypass flow is 2000 mL/min	2000 mL/min bypasses and 100 mL/min leaves VC	2000 mL/min bypasses and 79 mL/min enters VC
[Sevoflurane] vaporising chamber	21 kPa/75 kPa = 28%	21 kPa/75 kPa = 28%
Volume control	100 mL/min to leave VC	79 mL/min to enter VC
Volume picked up in VC	0.28 × 100 mL/min = 28 mL/min	[a]30.72 mL/min picked up to give [VC] of 28%. (30.72/[79 + 30.72] = 28%
Total volume leaving vaporiser	2000 mL + 100 mL = 2100 mL	2000 mL + 79 mL + 30.72 mL = 2109.72 mL/min
Concentration leaving vaporiser	28/2100 mL = 1.133..%	30.72/2109.72 = 1.46%
Output partial pressure	1.133% × 75 kPa = 1 kPa	1.46% of 75 kPa = 1.1 kPa

[a] If sevoflurane is 28% of the VC flow, the 79 mL of carrier gas must be the other 72% so the total volume in the VC must be 79/0.72 = 109.72 mL The sevo volume picked up must be 109.72-79 = 30.72 mL

Table 31.3 Vaporiser at 2 atm (200 kPa) (AJ McLintic)

Hyperbaric conditions: 2 bar (200 kPa)		
	Outlet control	Inlet control
Vaporiser setting	1%	1%
Splitting ratio to achieve 1%	20:1	25:1
Volumes if bypass flow is 2000 mL/min	2000 mL/min bypasses and 100 mL/min leaves VC	2000 mL/min bypasses and 79 mL/min enters VC
[Sevoflurane] vaporising chamber	21 kPa/200 kPa = 10.5%	21 kPa/200 kPa = 10.5%
Volume control	100 mL/min to leave VC	79 mL/min to enter VC
Volume picked up in VC	0.105 × 100 mL/min = 10.5 mL/min	9.268 mL/min picked up to give [VC] of 10.5%. (9.268/[79 + 9.268] = 10.5%
Total volume leaving vaporiser	2000 mL + 100 mL = 2100 mL	2000 mL + 79 mL + 9.268 mL = 2088.268 mL/min
Concentration leaving vaporiser	10.5/2100 mL = 0.5%	9.268/2088.268 = 0.44%
Output partial pressure	0.5% × 200 kPa = 1 kPa	0.44% of 200 kPa = 0.88 kPa

Tech 6

Measured flow vaporisers deliver the dialled concentration by adding a known mass of vapour into a known flow volume. Thus, the dialled concentration is delivered no matter the ambient pressure:

- 10% desflurane at 100 kPa has partial pressure 10 kPa.
- 10% desflurane at 5000 ft. (~84 kPa) has partial pressure of 8.4 kPa and is therefore less potent:
  - For equivalent potency to 10% at sea level, the dial setting must be increased to 12% at 5000 ft. (12% of 84 kPa is ~10 kPa).

Other Measured Flow Vaporisers

- The Dräger Diva is calibrated for sea-level use and is subject to the same issue.
- The xMAC is, however, altitude corrected.

Gas Analysers

Infrared gas analysers and paramagnetic gas analysers respond to the number of gas molecules (mass) and so are measuring the partial pressure of the gas in question. This is not affected by altitude, but, if the module output converts the pressure to fractional concentration, the output will be incorrect.

Example

- Paramagnetic analyser calibrated at sea level (100 kPa atmospheric pressure):
  - PO_2 in air at sea level is measured at 21 kPa. FiO_2 readout = 0.21.
  - PO_2 in air at 5000 ft. (atmospheric pressure 84 kPa) is correctly measured at 17.64 kPa, but, unless the monitor is recalibrated, the FiO_2 readout will be 17.6 kPa/100 kPa = 17.6%. The correct value remains 0.21. The analyser therefore needs to be recalibrated at altitude.

Flow Sensors

Changes in barometric pressure cause a change in gas density, whereas viscosity changes little or not at all. This can affect flow sensor function.

- A differential pressure flow sensor that ensures laminar flow (e.g. Fleisch pneumotachograph) should be unaltered in function.
- A differential pressure flow sensor where flow is at least partially turbulent will require compensation or recalibration, to account for the change in gas density.
- The Dräger 3000 Oxylog transport ventilator has a differential pressure flow sensor near the patient end, which is intrinsic to accurate flow and volume delivery. Without ambient pressure correction, inspiratory volume delivery can deviate by 44% at 15,000 ft. altitude. There is a further pressure sensor within the machine that registers absolute pressure and automatically compensates flow and volume measurement according to ambient pressure.
- The bobbin of the variable orifice flowmeter (Rotameter) sits in a tapered tube. In hypobaric conditions, there are fewer molecules for a given flow rate impacting and supporting the bobbin. The flowmeter therefore under-reads in hypobaric conditions, and the inaccuracy is greater at higher flows where flow becomes partially turbulent. At 5000 ft. and flows of 8 L/min, the flowmeter under-reads by approximately 8%.

Further Reading

Duncan L. The physics of altitude and anaesthesia. South Afr J Anaesth Analg. 2023;29(5 Suppl 1):S164–6.

Merz TM, Pichler Hefti J. Humans at extreme altitudes. BJA Educ. 2021;21(12):455e461.

Assessing Diagnostic Tests and Screening Tools

32

Alan McLintic and Nicholas Lightfoot

Introduction

In clinical practice, diagnostic or screening tests are often used to detect disease or to determine the risk or chance of an event occurring. These tests serve as surrogates for a 'gold standard' test or procedure, which may not be used as it is either expensive, is difficult to perform or may be associated with unjustified risk when used as a screening test. In other instances, the test is being used to predict the likelihood of an adverse or undesirable event such that a clinician could alter their plan to reduce the likelihood of this occurring.

Examples of diagnostic or screening tests being used against a 'gold standard' include the predictive ability of intraoperative ST depression on a five-lead ECG monitor versus the development of intraoperative regional wall motion abnormalities on either transthoracic or transoesophageal echocardiography to detect myocardial ischaemia or the use of a PSA blood assay versus a prostate biopsy in the diagnosis of prostate cancer. In other instances, clinicians use these tests or scores to predict an outcome—this would include the ability of intraoperative ST depression to predict post-operative cardiac events or the Mallampati score to predict difficult intubation.

The Two-By-Two Contingency Table

To determine a test's predictive ability, data for both the gold standard and the comparator is required and is plotted in a two-by-two contingency table as shown in Table 32.1.

A. McLintic · N. Lightfoot (✉)
Department of Anaesthesia and Pain Medicine, Counties Manukau Health, Auckland, New Zealand

C. Birch et al. (eds.), *Physics and Measurement for Anesthesia*,
https://doi.org/10.1007/978-3-031-65060-4_32

Table 32.1 Two-by-two contingency table

	Disease present	Disease absent	
Positive test	True positives	False positives	Total number of positive tests
Negative test	False negatives	True negatives	Total number of negative tests
	Total number with disease	Total number without disease	Total number of patients

Sensitivity and Specificity

The sensitivity and specificity are parameters which describe the ability of a test to identify or rule out a disease or condition, respectively. These are fixed and do not vary as the disease prevalence changes. Their calculation involves the comparison of the new test or procedure against the current gold standard or standard of practice. The 'gold standard' for the diagnosis of disease is on the horizontal axis of the contingency table, while the predicted or measured results from the new test are on the vertical axis.

The *sensitivity* is the probability of a positive test should the disease of interest be present—as such, it is the number of true-positive tests divided by the total number of patients with the disease. This is the proportion of diseased patients which are picked up by the test. The *specificity* is the probability of a negative test if the patient does not have a disease or condition. This is the number of true negatives divided by the total number without the disease. The specificity is also defined as 1—false-positive rate. A highly specific test will have very few false positives.

For diagnostic tests where there are multiple possible values the result could take, such as the PSA in the example above, the consequences of a positive or negative test, namely invasive investigations or missing a cancer diagnosis, need to be considered when choosing the cut point above or below which a test is defined as abnormal. This has implications for the calculated values of sensitivity and specificity—this trade-off can be further demonstrated through the receiver operating characteristic curve (ROC), which is discussed in greater detail below. The errors associated with these tests can be calculated to determine both the false-positive and the false-negative rates. The *alpha error* or the false-positive rate is 1—specificity, while the *beta error* or the false-negative rate is 1—sensitivity.

The *positive likelihood ratio* or LR+ is used to assess the value of a test in predicting the presence or absence of disease. This is the ratio of true-positive rate divided by the false-positive rate—put another way, this is the sensitivity divided by one minus the specificity. A value of 1.0 means that the test will have little practical significance as the chance of observing a true positive is the same as a false positive, whereas a value of 3.0 indicates that a positive result is three times as likely to occur in a patient with disease compared to one without.

The *negative likelihood* ratio is the ratio of the false-negative rate to the true-negative rate or 1 minus the sensitivity divided by the specificity. Values which are close to or above one indicate that the test will have minimal practical importance

Table 32.2 Formulae to calculate statistical parameters mentioned in this chapter

$\text{Sensitivity} = \frac{\text{True positives}}{\text{Total with disease}}$
$\text{Specificity} = \frac{\text{True negatives}}{\text{Total without disease}}$
Alpha error = 1 − specificity
Beta error = 1 − sensitivity
$\text{Positive likelihood ratio} = \text{LR+} = \frac{\text{Sensitivity}}{1-\text{specificity}}$
$\text{Negative likelihood ratio} = \text{LR−} = \frac{1-\text{sensitivity}}{\text{specificity}}$
$\text{Positve predictive value} = \frac{\text{True positives}}{\text{All positive tests}}$
$\text{Negative predictive value} = \frac{\text{True negatives}}{\text{All negative tests}}$

due to excessive numbers of false-negative results. Values between 0 and 1 increase the utility of a negative test. These formulae are further summarised in Table 32.2.

Positive and Negative Predictive Values

Whereas the sensitivity and specificity are intrinsic properties of a test, the *positive and negative predictive values* (PPV and NPV, respectively) are dependent on the prevalence of disease. These parameters can give considerable insight to the utility of a diagnostic test and whether the test will be useful for screening for disease in a particular population.

The *positive predictive value* is the probability of disease if the test is positive and is defined as the true positives divided by all positive tests. The *negative predictive value* is the probability of absence of disease if the test is negative and is the true negatives divided by all negative test results.

While both the sensitivity and specificity are unaffected by the prevalence of the disease, the positive and negative predictive values are sensitive to changes in the underlying disease rate in a population. The sensitivity and specificity of a test define the false-positive and -negative rate, respectively. When there are large numbers of patients in a population without the disease, application of the test will lead to large numbers of false-positive tests. As the background disease rate is low, there are only relatively few true positives, meaning the false positives grossly outweigh the true positives and reduce the positive predictive value accordingly. If we are aware of the prevalence of the disease in a particular population, the positive predictive value will give insight to determine if the test is appropriate for screening this group.

Table 32.3 Calculation of statistical parameters for two cohorts with differing prevalence of disease

	Disease	No disease		
Cohort A. Prevalence of disease 20%				
Positive test	16	32	48	PPV 16/32 = 33%
Negative test	4	48	52	NPV 48/52 = 92%
	20	80	100	
	Sens^y 16/20 = 80%	Spec^y 48/80 = 60%		
Cohort B. Prevalence of disease 5%				
Positive test	16	152	168	PPV 16/152 = 9.5%
Negative test	4	228	232	NPV 228/232 = 98%
	20	380	400	
	Sens^y 16/20 = 80%	Spec^y 228/380 = 60%		

Example

A diagnostic test has 80% sensitivity and 60% specificity with a 40% false-positive rate (this is calculated as 1 minus the specificity) for identifying a disease. It is then used in two cohorts with differing prevalence of disease:

- Cohort A: 20 out of 100 patients have the disease giving a prevalence of 20%.
- Cohort B: 20 out of 400 patients have the disease giving a prevalence of 5%.

We can draw two contingency tables showing the resultant PPV and NPV; see Table 32.3. This illustrates the effect of changes in the prevalence on the PPV and NPV. In both instances, there is considerable predictive benefit of a negative test, whereas the reduction in prevalence causes a fall in the PPV from 33% to 9.5%, which may lead to considerable numbers of patients undergoing additional investigations depending on the implications of a positive test.

This was seen early in the COVID-19 pandemic with the results of unproven antigen tests in populations with low rates of disease. This led to large numbers of false-positive tests and a resultant reduction in the positive predictive value. As the pandemic developed and the rate of disease in some communities increased in tandem with the accuracy of the tests, the positive predictive value increased accordingly.

Bayesian Methods

Reports of many clinical trials use a frequentist approach where the probability of an event is determined from the current study, and this information is then extrapolated to the general population. The statistics associated with these studies are dominated by dichotomous (YES or NO) based hypothesis testing, which generates p-values. A Bayesian framework calculates the probability of a hypothesis being true by incorporating prior knowledge as new information becomes available.

The prevalence of disease is an example of the prior knowledge that Bayesians seek. This is called the *pretest* or *prior probability*. The probability of disease in

Bayesian terms is called the *post-test* or *posterior* probability; this is equal to the positive predictive value as above, namely the number of positive tests divided by the total number of positive tests. Through Bayes theorem, we can calculate the post-test probability by using both the known baseline prevalence of disease (the pretest probability) and the likelihood ratio.

The incidence of troponin leakage following surgery would be an example of a frequentist probability, whereas through the application of Bayes theorem, we can calculate the probability of troponin leakage following surgery (post-test) in patients with two or more revised cardiac risk index risk factors (pretest). This is one small interaction between frequentist and Bayesian statistics. Bayes theorem has vast applications in science, economics and predictive technologies.

Receiver Operating Characteristic (ROC) Curve

Up to this point, the outcomes have been dichotomous—Does the patient have prostate cancer or is a test 'positive' or 'negative'? Many tests, rather than producing outcomes which are expressed as 'yes' or 'no', are on a continuum. Examples include the CRP for the diagnosis of sepsis or troponin values for the diagnosis of myocardial infarction. For these tests to be clinically useful, we must determine cut points that will be used to codify a test as 'positive' or 'negative'. This can be done with the normal range or by the receiver operating characteristic (ROC) curve.

The normal range can be defined through statistical parameters or based on clinical experience and expert opinion. Using balanced samples of a population, we can take the 95% or 99% confidence interval, defined as the sample mean ± 1.96 standard deviations or the range of values from 2.5 to 97.5 percentile. Both encompass the central 95% of values. For current-generation high-specificity troponin assays, a value of <15 ng/L is termed 'normal' or 'negative'. This range of values encompasses 99% of patients in the sample(s), which was used to define the normal range. In other instances, for example, the diagnosis of anaemia, the reference range has been set by expert opinion using ancillary information such as the amount of haemoglobin which is needed for normal cardiovascular and metabolic functioning. In many populations, the prevalence of anaemia—an abnormal haemoglobin value—is far greater than the 1–5% as outlined above.

Using the continuum of test values, it is possible to compare the sensitivity and specificity of each threshold value when comparing the novel test against the gold standard. For troponin, the gold standard may be the confirmation of myocardial infarction through meeting the diagnostic criteria as prescribed by the Fourth Universal Definition of Myocardial Infarction.

On a receiver operating characteristic (ROC) curve, the calculated sensitivity for each threshold value is plotted on the y-axis, while 1—specificity or the false positive rate is plotted on the x-axis; see Fig. 32.1. In an ideal world, we would have a threshold value with a high sensitivity and a low false-positive rate; however, in reality, there is a trade-off between the two parameters as the threshold is changed. The threshold value which is of the greatest value in clinical use is located towards the top left-hand part of the ROC curve. In addition to maximising sensitivity and

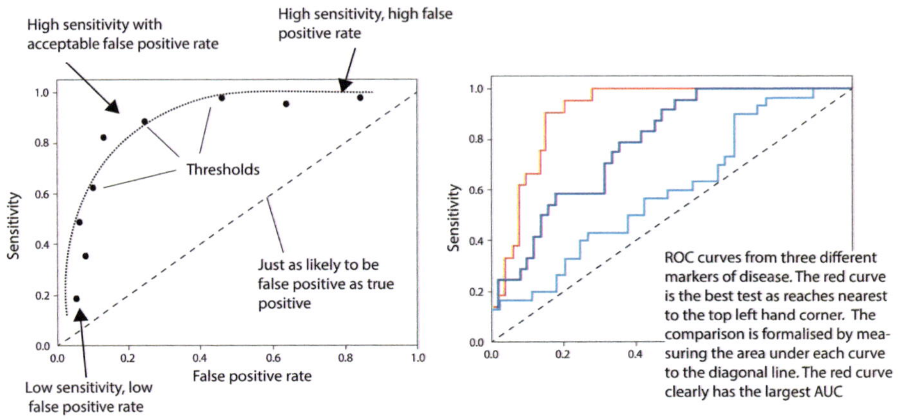

Fig. 32.1 Receiver operating characteristic curve

minimising the false-positive rate, the chosen threshold may also consider the medical, ethical, economic and societal consequences of missing cases versus falsely diagnosing cases.

Depending on the course of action which is mandated after a 'positive' test can also influence the chosen threshold. The use of non-invasive cardiac stress tests to diagnose coronary artery disease prior to non-cardiac surgery is one such example. A positive stress test might lead to coronary angiography with the possibility of coronary stenting. There is some evidence to suggest that preoperative coronary interventions may not reduce the incidence of perioperative myocardial infarction, and coronary angiography by itself can be associated with morbidity and mortality. The decision to order a stress test should include these points in addition to the calculated sensitivity and false-positive values associated with the test.

When there are multiple possible tests which can be used to predict the occurrence of an event, the area under the receiver operating curve (AUC) can be calculated. The testing strategy with the best predictive ability will by and large have the greatest AUC value. This approach can be illustrated by the METS study, which looked at the addition of cardiopulmonary exercise testing (CPET) to standard predictive criteria in determining the risk of death or myocardial infarction/injury following non-cardiac surgery. In comparison to the baseline model, the information produced by a CPET test did not improve the predictive ability of the adverse events as measured by the AUC-ROC.

Further Reading

Petrie A, Sabin C. Medical statistics at a glance. 3rd ed. Chichester: Wiley-Blackwell; 2009.

Wijeysundera DN, Pearse RM, Shulman MA, Abbott TEF, Torres E, Ambosta A, Croal BL, Granton JT, Thorpe KE, Grocott MPW, Farrington C, Myles PS, Cuthbertson BH, On behalf of the METS study investigators. Assessment of functional capacity before major non-cardiac surgery: an international, prospective cohort study. Lancet. 2018;391(10140):2631–40.

Index

C. Birch et al. (eds.), *Physics and Measurement for Anesthesia*,
https://doi.org/10.1007/978-3-031-65060-4

9783031650598